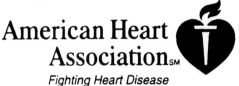

American Heart
Association_{SM}

*Fighting Heart Disease
and Stroke*

Monograph Series

CURRENT AND FUTURE APPLICATIONS OF MAGNETIC RESONANCE IN CARDIOVASCULAR DISEASE

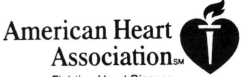

American Heart Associationsm

Fighting Heart Disease and Stroke

Monograph Series

CURRENT AND FUTURE APPLICATIONS OF MAGNETIC RESONANCE IN CARDIOVASCULAR DISEASE

Edited by

Charles B. Higgins, MD

Professor and Vice Chairman
Department of Radiology
University of California at San Francisco
San Francisco, California

Joanne S. Ingwall, PhD

NMR Laboratory
Cardiovascular Division
Brigham and Women's Hospital
Harvard Medical School
Boston, Massachusetts

Gerald M. Pohost, MD

Mary Gertrude Waters Professor of Cardiovascular Medicine
Director, Center for NMR Research and Development
University of Alabama at Birmingham
Birmingham, Alabama

FUTURA

Futura Publishing Company, Inc.
Armonk, NY

Library of Congress Cataloging-in-Publication Data

Current and future applications of magnetic resonance in
    cardiovascular disease / edited by Charles B. Higging, Joanne S.
    Ingwall, Gerald M. Pohost.
        p.   cm. — (American Heart Association monograph series)
        ISBN 0-87993-681-9
        1. Heart—Magnetic resonance imaging.   2. Heart—Diseases–
    –Diagnosis.   3. Nuclear magnetic resonance spectroscopy.
    4. Angiography.   I. Higgins, Charles B.   II. Ingwall, Joanne S.
    III. Pohost, Gerald M.   IV. Series.
        [DNLM: 1.   Heart Diseases—diagnosis.   2.   Magnetic Resonance
    Imaging—methods.   3.   Magnetic Resonance   Angiography—methods.
    4. Nuclear Magnetic Resonance—   methods.   WG 141 C9757   1997]
    616.1'207548—dc21
    DNLM/DLC
    for Library of Congress   97-26138
                                                                    CIP

Copyright © 1998
Futura Publishing Company, Inc.

Published by
Futura Publishing Company, Inc.
135 Bedford Road
Armonk, New York 10504

LC #:
ISBN #:

Every effort has been made to ensure that the information in this book is as up to date
and accurate as possible at the time of publication. However, due to the constant developments in medicine, neither the author, nor the editor, nor the publisher can accept any
legal or any other responsibility for any errors or omissions that may occur.

Printed in the United States of America on acid-free paper.

Preface

This monograph constitutes a timely update of the evolving role of magnetic resonance imaging (MRI) and magnetic resonance spectroscopy (MRS) as clinical diagnostic and scientific investigative tools in cardiovascular disease.

The current volume provides chapters summarizing the application of MRI for the diagnosis of acquired heart disease, congenital heart disease, and vascular disease. Whereas much of the clinical role of MRI at present is directed at depicting morphology, the innate strength of the modality is unparalleled precision in the quantification of cardiac function and blood flow. This potential is amply described in a number of chapters describing the utilization of MR techniques for myocardial tagging, myocardial perfusion, and coronary flow quantification. A series of enlightening chapters describe the continuous pursuit of MRS as a realistic probe for *in vivo* elucidation of myocardial metabolism, myocardial oxidation mechanisms, and myocardial viability.

Magnetic resonance angiography (MRA) has now evolved into an impressive imaging modality for several regions of the circulation. Accordingly, chapters describe the optimal techniques and applications in the thoracic and abdominal aorta, carotid, lower limb, and coronary arteries.

Intensive research continues on two fronts important for the emergence of MR as an important modality in cardiovascular disease. One is the technical developments necessary for the ease of utilization of MR for imaging the heart and vascular system. Second is the continued use of MRI and MRS to gain a fundamental and more quantitative insight into cardiovascular physiology, pharmacology, and metabolism. The information provided in this monograph is a glimpse at a point in time of a rapidly evolving story. This monograph does constitute a compendium of the latest information, but it can be anticipated that future research in the next few years will add considerably to the foundation provided here.

Charles B. Higgins
San Francisco, California

Contributors

Charles M. Anderson, MD, PhD   Associate Professor of Radiology, University of California, San Francisco, CA

Leon Axel, PhD, MD   Professor, Department of Radiology, Hospital of the University of Pennsylvania, Philadelphia, PA

Robert J. Bache, MD   Professor of Medicine, University of Minnesota, Minneapolis, MN

Frank M. Baer, MD   Klinik III fur Innere Medizin, Universitat zu Koln, Koln, Germany

Robert S. Balaban, PhD   Chief, Laboratory of Cardiac Energetics, National Institutes of Health, Bethesda, MD

Georg Bongartz   Assistant Professor, Department of Radiology, University Hospitals, Basel, Switzerland

Paul A. Bottomley, PhD   Professor, Department of Radiology, Johns Hopkins University, Baltimore, MD

Jens Bremerich   Assistant Professor, Department of Radiology, University Hospitals, Basel, Switzerland

Jean Britain, PhD   Department of Electrical Engineering, Stanford University, Stanford, CA

Peter T. Buser, MD   Assistant Professor, Division of Cardiology, University Hospital Basel, Basel, Switzerland

Youngran Chung, MD, PhD   Adjunct Assistant Professor, Biological Chemistry Department, University of California Davis, Davis, CA

Clarence P. Davis, MD   MRI-Center, Department of Diagnostic Radiology, University Hospital, Zurich, Switzerland

Albert de Roos, MD   Associate Professor of Radiology, University Hospital, Leiden, The Netherlands

W. Thomas Dixon, PhD   Assistant Professor, Emory University School of Medicine, Atlanta, GA

Mark A. Fogel, MD   Assistant Professor of Cardiology and Radiology, Children's Hospital of Philadelphia, Philadelphia, PA

Arthur H.L. From, MD   Professor of Medicine, VA Medical Center, Minneapolis, MN

F. N. Gellerich, PhD   Associate Professor, Neurological Clinic, Halle-Saale, Germany

Christoph Gradel, MD   Division of Cardiology, University Hospitals, Basel, Switzerland

Clifford Greyson, MD   Adjunct Assistant Professor of Medicine, University of California, San Francisco, CA

Willem A. Helbing, MD   Division of Pediatric Cardiology, University Hospital Leiden, The Netherlands

Michael Jerosch Herold, PhD   Department of Radiology and Center for Magnetic Resonance Research, University of Minnesota, Minneapolis, MN

Charles B. Higgins, MD   Professor, Department of Radiology, University of California Medical Center, San Francisco, CA

Vincent B. Ho, MD   Clinical Care Center for Congenital Heart Disease, Oregon Health Sciences University, Portland, OR, Department of Radiology and Nuclear Medicine, Uniformed Services, University of the Health Sciences, Bethesda, MD

Bob S. Hu, MD   Assistant Professor, Division of Cardiovascular Medicine, Stanford University, Stanford, CA

Joanne S. Ingwall, PhD   Professor of Medicine, Department of Physiology, Brigham & Women's Hospital and Harvard Medical School, Boston, MA

Pablo Irarrazaval, MSc, PhD   Departamento de Engenieria Electrica, Universidad Catolica, Santiago, Chile

Michael Jerosch-Herold, PhD   Department of Radiology, University of Minnesota, Minneapolis, MN

Thomas Jue, PhD   Assistant Professor, Biological Chemistry Department, University of California, Davis, CA

James B. Kinney, MD   Departments of Pediatrics, Madigan Army Medical Center, Tacoma, WA, University of Washington, Children's Hospital and Medical Center, Seattle, WA

F. D. Laterveer, Msc   Research Associate, Bijvoet Center, Utrecht University, Utrecht, The Netherlands

M. Laudy, Msc   Research Associate, Bijvoet Center, Utrecht University, Utrecht, The Netherlands

Flavian M. Lupinetti, MD   Division of Pediatric Cardiac Surgery, Children's Hospital and Medical Center, Seattle, WA

Albert Macovski, PhD   Professor, Department of Electrical Engineering, Stanford University, Stanford, CA

Warren J. Manning, MD   Assistant Professor, Medicine and Radiology, Harvard Medical School, Boston, MA

Edward T. Martin, MD   Associate in Cardiology, University of Alabama at Birmingham, Birmingham, AL

Barry M. Massie, MD   Professor of Medicine, University of California, San Francisco, Director, Coronary Care Unit & Hypertension Section, San Francisco Veterans Affairs Medical Center, San Francisco, CA

Craig H. Meyer, PhD   Researcher, Department of Electrical Engineering, Stanford University, Stanford, CA

Risto Miettunen, MD   Department of Radiology, University Hospitals, Basel, Switzerland

M. G. H. Nederhoff, Bsc   Technician, Heart Lung Institute, Utrecht University Hospital, Utrecht, The Netherlands

K. Nicolay, PhD   Associate Professor, Department of *in vivo* Spectroscopy, Bijvoet Center, Utrecht University, The Netherlands

Christoph A. Nienaber, MD, FACC, FESC   Division of Cardiology, University Hospital Eppendorf, Hamburg, Germany

R. Andre Niezen, MD   Department of Radiology, University Hospital Leiden, The Netherlands

Dwight Nishimura, PhD   Assistant Professor, Department of Electrical Engineering, Stanford University, Stanford, CA

John N. Oshinski, PhD   Assistant Professor, Emory University School of Medicine, Atlanta, GA

Jaap Ottenkamp, MD   Division of Pediatric Cardiology, University Hospital Leiden, The Netherlands

Roderic I. Pettigrew, PhD, MD   Director, Frederik Philips MR Research Center, Emory University School of Medicine, Atlanta, GA

Gerald M. Pohost, MD   Mary Gertrude Waters Professor of Cardiovascular Medicine, Director, Center for NMR Research and Development, University of Alabama at Birmingham, Birmingham, AL

Martin R. Prince, MD, PhD   Co-Director, Division of MRI, University of Michigan, Ann Arbor, MI

Sidney A. Rebergen, MD   Department of Diagnostic Radiology, University Hospital Leiden, Leiden, The Netherlands

T. Reese, PhD   Research Associate, Bijvoet Center, Utrecht University, Utrecht, The Netherlands

Pierre-Marie Robitaille, PhD   Professor, Departments of Medical Biochemistry and Radiology, Ohio State University, Columbus, OH

Todd Sachs, PhD   Researcher, Department of Electrical Engineering, Stanford University, Stanford, CA

Maythem Saeed, DVM, PhD   Department of Radiology, University of California Medical Center, San Francisco, CA

David J. Sahn, MD   Professor of Pediatrics, Diagnostic Radiology, and Obstetrics & Gynecology, Oregon Health Science Center, University of Oregon, Portland, OR

Hajime Sakuma, MD   Assistant Professor, Department of Radiology, Mie University School of Medicine, Mie, Japan

Heinrich R. Schelbert, MD   Division of Nuclear Medicine, Department of Molecular and Medical Pharmacology, UCLA School of Medicine, Los Angeles, CA

Harald Schicha, MD   Professor of Nuclear Medicine and Chairman, Department of Nuclear Medicine, University of Cologne, Koln, Germany

Gregory G. Schwartz, MD, PhD   Associate Professor of Medicine, Associate Staff, Cardiovascular Research Institute, University of California, San Francisco, CA and San Francisco VA Medical Center

Udo Sechtem, MD   Associate Professor of Medicine and Cardiology, Klinik III fur Innere Medizin, Universitat zu Koln, Koln, Germany

Rolf P. Spielmann, MD   Division of Radiology, University Hospital Eppendorf, Hamburg, Germany

Peter Theissen, MD   Department of Nuclear Medicine, University of Cologne, Koln, Germany

Kamil Ugurbil, PhD   Professor of Medicine, Radiology, Biochemistry, University of Minnesota, Minneapolis, MN

J. Ton, Msc   Research Associate, Bijvoet Center, Utrecht University, Utrecht, The Netherlands

Ernst E. van der Wall, MD   Department of Cardiology, University Hospital Leiden, The Netherlands

F. A. van Dorsten, Msc   Research Associate, Bijvoet Center, Utrecht University, Utrecht, The Netherlands

C. J. A. van Echteld, PhD   Associate Professor, Heart Lung Institute, Utrecht University Hospital, Utrecht, The Netherlands

Yskert von Kodolitsch, MD   Division of Cardiology, University Hospital of Eppendorf, Hamburg, Germany

Gustav K. von Schulthess, MD, PhD   Department of Medical Radiology, University Hospital, MRI Center, Zurich, Switzerland

Eberhard Voth, MD   Department of Nuclear Medicine, University of Cologne, Koln, Germany

Samuel Wang, PhD   Department of Electrical Engineering, Stanford University, Stanford, CA

Michael W. Weiner, MD   Professor of Medicine, Radiology, Psychiatry and Neurology, University of California, San Francisco, Director, Magnetic Resonance Unit, San Francisco Veterans Administration Medical Center, San Francisco, CA

Michael F. Wendland, PhD   Department of Radiology, University of California Medical Center, San Francisco, CA

Richard D. White, MD   Head, Section of Cardiovascular Imaging, Division of Radiology, Cleveland Clinic Foundation, Cleveland, OH

Norbert Wilke, MD   Center for Magnetic Resonance Research, University of Minnesota, Minneapolis, MN

Judith A. Wisneski, MD   Professor of Medicine, University of California, San Francisco; Director, Cardiac Catheterization Laboratory, San Francisco, CA

E. Kent Yucel, MD   Professor of Radiology, Department of Radiology, Boston University School of Medicine, Boston, MA

Elias A. Zerhouni, MD   The Johns Hopkins Medical Institutions, Division of Magnetic Resonance Imaging, The Russell H. Morgan Department of Radiology and Radiological Sciences, The Johns Hopkins Hospital, Baltimore, MD

Jianyi Zhang, MD, PhD   Assistant Professor of Medicine, University of Minnesota, Minneapolis, MN

Contents

Part 3.   Magnetic Resonance Imaging: Function

Part 4. Magnetic Resonance Angiography

Part 5. Magnetic Resonance Spectroscopy

Part 1

Magnetic Resonance Techniques

## Chapter 1

Echoplanar Cardiovascular Imaging

Clarence P. Davis, MD and
Gustav K. von Schulthess, MD, PhD

Introduction

Despite its efficacy, magnetic resonance imaging (MRI) has been hampered by relatively long image acquisition times that limit patient processing and keep costs high. Importantly, long image acquisition times make magnetic resonance (MR) prone to motion artifacts. Therefore, if the advantages of MRI are to be used fully, faster MRI techniques relying on faster data sampling strategies are needed. Two avenues have been pursued in this direction: (1) the improvement of conventional and (2) the development of new imaging techniques that differ fundamentally in the way the raw data is sampled.

Theoretically, the most efficient technique for data acquisition in MR is echoplanar imaging (EPI), as proposed by Mansfield in 1977[1]. In contrast to conventional MRI techniques, EPI allows one to acquire all the data necessary to reconstruct the MR image after a single radio-frequency (RF) excitation. Thus, image acquisition times can be reduced to less than 50 ms, making EPI today's fastest clinically useful imaging technique.

Basic Concepts in Echoplanar Imaging

Using ultrafast MRI, one generally subsumes the strategies that lead to MR images in less than 500 ms. A first step in speeding up

From: Higgins CB, Ingwall JS, Pohost GM, (eds). *Current and Future Applications of Magnetic Resonance in Cardiovascular Disease.* Armonk, NY: Futura Publishing Company, Inc.; © 1998.

image acquisition time was the conception of gradient-recalled echo (GRE) imaging, where the repetition times (TR) have been gradually shortened from 30 ms to 3 to 5 ms on conventional scanners. The problem with GRE techniques and a reduction of TR to just a few milliseconds is a very low signal-to-noise ratio, because the longitudinal magnetization determining the available signal cannot recover to a substantial fraction of the steady-state value.

In order to further reduce imaging time—or for that matter obtain higher resolution images in the same amount of time—hardware improvements have to be made. The most relevant improvement is the combination of higher gradient amplitudes (maximum mT/m) and higher slew rates (mT/m/msec). A second improvement that is only partly a hardware improvement is called "under the ramp sampling." In this mode, data is also collected while the gradient is rising to its final value and continues to be collected while the gradient is falling. With these measures and slew rates the sampling of a single k-line can be reduced roughly by a factor 2 to 3.

EPI goes even a step further by eliminating alpha pulses from the acquisition scheme, collecting all or part of the k-lines after a single RF excitation. This leads to further considerable time savings as every selective alpha pulse is of the order of 1 ms in duration (Figure 1). The major problem with EPI is that the lines are no longer read always at the same point in time during a T2* decay but rather under the decaying T2* curve (Figure 2A). If T2* is relatively fast (ie, = 30 ms), as is the case in heart tissue, the imaging lines read at the end of an EPI sequence have practically no signal left: high-resolution imaging is then not possible. This problem can be remedied by introducing a few (usually 1 to 7) additional alpha pulses into the pulse sequence thereby making it a GRE EPI hybrid, termed segmented or interleaved EPI. As can be seen in Figure 1 in lines 2 and 3, the time penalty for introducing the additional alpha pulses is minimal, but the result is that the signal is spread more evenly among the imaging lines (Figure 2B).

The analysis given above is that of the most simple situation: GRE imaging, in its conventional and echoplanar forms. These sequences are relevant for functinal studies of the brain, heart, kidneys, and for magnetic resonance angiography (MRA). Similarly, spin echo (SE) sequences are shortened by segmentation techniques. Furthermore, a combination of the RARE[2] technique with the EPI technique leads to very short (breathhold) T2 sequences in the form of the so-called GRASE sequence (gradient and spin-echo).[3]

The discussion has also focused on the simplest and most flexible gradient systems, which allow straight ramping. The production of such gradient systems is technically quite challenging and not all manu-

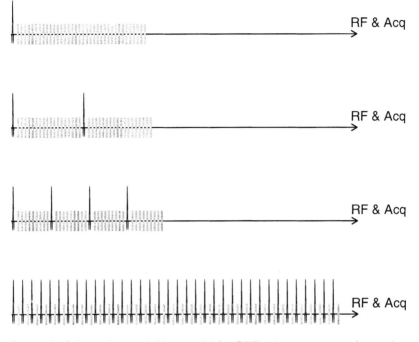

FIGURE 1. Schematic acquisition model for GRE pulse sequences (top to bottom): single-shot EPI, two-shot EPI, four-shot EPI, and conventional GRE sequence with 36 k-space lines. With multiple shot EPI, k-lines are acquired in sets. Data acquisition time increases slightly with increasing number of shots, while overall sampling time savings are maintained compared to conventional techniques. RF & Acq denote RF pulse and data acquisition window, respectively. (Reprinted with permission from Reference 1.)

facturers are currently producing such systems. It is technically simpler to use a sinusoidal gradient rise or a combination of sinusoids; still, the considerations given above remain essentially the same. In fact, the first commercially available ultrafast scanner used such oscillating gradient systems.[4] Finally, the strategy to sample horizontal image lines over the entire image (in k-space) is not mandatory. Other trajectories can be used. The most notable one currently in use is "spiral" scanning recommended by Macovsky et al[5] (Figure 3). In this process, data are collected on a spiral in the (k-space) image. If multiple spirals are used, this acquisition occurs in interleaved or segmented fashion using intertwined spirals.

In the next sections, some of the potential clinical applications of EPI are discussed.

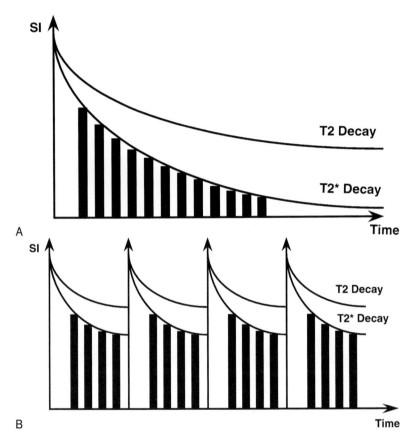

FIGURE 2. Schematic diagram of a single- and four-shot GRE EPI sequence with 16 k-space lines. After the excitation with an α-pulse, all echoes (bars) constituting an image are collected. **Top:** The lines of k-space are sampled during the free induction decay. Since the amplitude of the echo is governed by the T2* decay, lines sampled at the end of the echo train exhibit only little signal. **Bottom:** Increasing the number of shots partly overcomes this problem, because of much shorter read-out period. With each excitation pulse, the signal is recovered, leading to a more homogeneous signal amplitude distribution. (Reproduced with permission from References 49 and 50.)

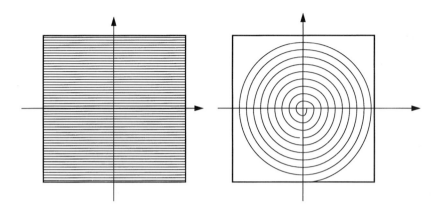

FIGURE 3. Comparison of conventional and spiral data acquisition scheme. In spiral scanning, a magnetic field gradient is oscillating to trace a spiral trajectory in k-space.

Clinical Applications

Cardiac Morphology

Probably the most obvious impact of ultrafast imaging techniques will be on the visualization of rapidly moving structures, such as the heart. In cardiovascular imaging, conventional images are a composite of multiple electrocardiographic (ECG)-triggered acquisitions equal to the desired resolution. Cardiac arrhythmia and respiratory motion can thus substantially degrade image quality limiting the use of MR in the evaluation of cardiac pathologies. Currently, cardiac MRI is routinely performed only for the diagnosis of congenital heart diseases, thoracic aortic diseases, and pericardial masses. This could change with the introduction of ultrafast MR techniques into the diagnostic procedure. Real-time MRI techniques allow imaging of the heart with no need for ECG-gating, virtually eliminating motion artifacts, and significantly reducing scan time. Furthermore, simultaneous morphological and functional studies will become possible. In general, there is considerable data that suggest that ultrafast techniques will permit MR to become the "one-stop shop" examination modality of the heart.

The first real-time images of the heart were published by Rzedzian et al[6] in 1983 and proved that EPI could freeze cardiac motion. Since then a variety of imaging sequences have been tested and technology has been improved. In 1994 our group demonstrated the feasibility of

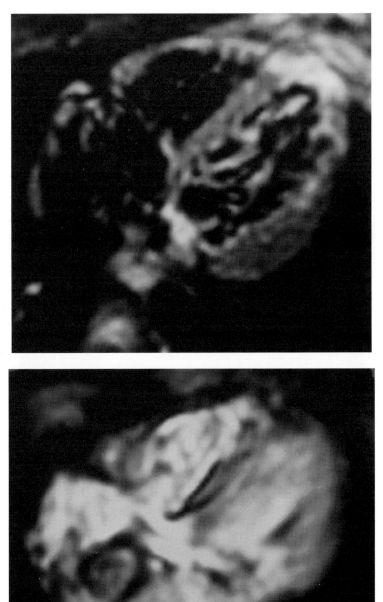

A

B

using single-shot EPI to depict various cardiac structures with diagnostic image quality.[7] SE and GRE echoplanar images were obtained using a TR of 2 cardiac cycles to reduce saturation effects (Figure 4). By progressively advancing the time delay after each R wave consecutive images were acquired at a different time in the cardiac cycle, and thus, a cine loop of the moving heart could be obtained. Both techniques mirrored conventional black-and-white blood heart images. Delineation of cardiac structures was dependent on the intracavitary signal intensity (SI). While the differentiation of myocardial from intraluminal SI was easier on SE images, GRE images, with their high intraluminal SI, allowed visualization of different flow patterns. Small structures like the cardiac valves were not seen with either technique.

Single-shot EPI, however, proved to have serious drawbacks for imaging the heart that primarily result from the rapid $T2^*$ decay, during which the signal has to be sampled, and the resulting limitations in spatial resolution. In the heart, given a $T2^*$ of approximately 20 to 30 ms, the in-plane spatial resolution is limited to a maximum of about 2 mm, which severely compromises the use of single-shot techniques in the heart.

One area in which the limitation in spatial resolution is particularly negative is the visualization of small cardiac structures such as the cardiac valves. In a study undertaken in our laboratory, a sequentially acquired (ie, shots acquired one after the other for each frame) multiple-shot EPI and a single-shot EPI sequence were compared for their ability to delineate the valve leaflets and image their movement over the cardiac cycle.[8] Multiple-shot EPI was found to be clearly superior due to the markedly reduced TE, which rendered intracavitary blood more homogeneous, and therefore facilitated valve leaflet visibility (Figure 5A). Further improvement in image conspicuity could be achieved by acquiring the shots in a nonsequential manner (ie, shots are acquired over several heartbeats), rendering high-resolution EPI images that were, however, no longer real time. Figure 5B highlights the potential of this technique.

FIGURE 4. Transaxial single-shot spin-echo and GRE EPI images of the heart. **A:** On spin-echo EPI images, the left and right ventricular wall is clearly visible. The intracavitary blood is black, due to the wash-out of excited spins. The "wormlike" structures in the left ventricle are probably reflective of various flow patterns. **B:** The cardiac structures are not as well depicted with GRE EPI due to the brighter intracavitary blood signal. Note the substantial susceptibility artifact appearing as signal void along the intraventricular septum. (Reproduced with permission from Reference 50.)

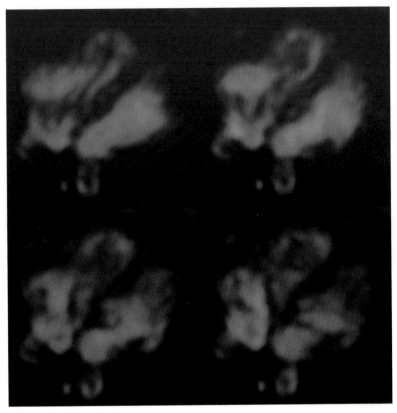

A

FIGURE 5. Four-shot GRE EPI images showing the mitral valves in different positions throughout the cardiac cycle **A:** Sequentially acquired low-resolution images (3.7 × 3.7 mm in-plane resolution). Acquisition time approximately 50 ms per image.

The concept of high-resolution multiple-shot EPI was also studied by Wetter et al[9] who compared a single-shot EPI sequence and four different multiple-shot EPI sequences. All four of multiple-shot techniques evaluated provided better image quality than did the single-shot technique, with little compromise in imaging time. A substantially more homogeneous intracavitary signal allowed better visualization of small cardiac structures and the myocardium. The differences in image quality between the single shot and any of the multiple-shot techniques far outweighted any differences among the various multiple-shot acquisitions.

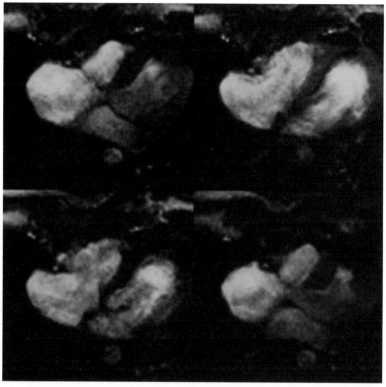

B

FIGURE 5. *(continued)* **B:** High-resolution images (0.75 × 1.5 mm in-plane resolution) acquired over 4 heartbeats (nonsequential acquisition mode). (Figure 5A reprinted with permission from Reference 49, and Figure 5B reprinted with permission from reference 8.)

Cardiac Function

Evaluation of cardiac function is of particular interest in patients with coronary artery disease (CAD) to assess regional myocardial perfusion differences and to establish wall motion irregularities. Futhermore, flow calculation in the big vessels or in the cardiac chambers can help to assess severity of valvular and congenital heart diseases. Ultrafast imaging gives rise to hope that These examinations may eventually become clinical routine because ultrafast imaging speeds up data acquisition and makes breath-held examinations feasible. While the assessment of myocardial wall motion using standard SE and GRE sequences has been performed since the early days of clinical MRI,[10] a new technique referred to as "myocardial tagging" has emerged during the last few years. Tagging uses a virtual grid placed on the myocardial wall, usually of a short-axis cut through the heart.[11,12] The grid is placed during end diastole, when the heart is at rest. With the contraction of the heart during systole, the lines of the grid deform thus allowing instant visualization of the radial and torsional wall motion.[13] This technique can also be performed with EPI, enabling wall motion assessment during apnea.[14] The so-detected wall motion irregularities seem to be a fairly sensitive measure for myocardial dysfunction.

Left ventricular ejection fraction (EF) and cardiac output (CO) measurements are established parameters central to the objective characterization of cardiac performance. Ventricular EF measurements performed by conventional cine MRI have been demonstrated to be accurate.[15,16] However, acquisition and postprocessing is time consuming, therefore, ultrafast imaging strategies are clearly more desirable. Unterweger et al[17] have recently published an ultrafast acquisition strategy based on multiple-shot EPI for the assessment of left ventricular EF and CO. They were able to reduce data acquisition time by a factor of 50 compared with conventional cine MRI, collecting all the data in 40 to 60 heartbeats. Still, they demonstrated multiple-shot EPI to be highly accurate with a correlation coefficient of 0.96 for EF and 0.94 for CO measurements.

Of utmost importance in cardiovascular imaging is the possibility of assessing myocardial perfusion. Conventional techniques are limited by long acquisition times and are of no value in the early assessment of perfusion deficits after myocardial infaction.[18] With the advent of ultrafast techniques, first-pass studies using gadolineium-chelates have become possible and many groups have demonstrated the capability of the latter in detecting regions of ischemia.[19–23]

Any first-pass study monitors the effect of administered contrast media as it passes through the heart. To be applicable in a routine clinical setting an MR approach would therefore have to address the following problems: (1) coverage of the whole heart, (2) sufficient spatial resolution to enable accurate localization of perfusion abnormalities, and (3) adequate temporal resolution to characterize wash-in and wash-out kinetics. Meeting these requirements needs echoplanar capabilities. Preliminary results using EPI have been published.[24–27] Unlike most previously published studies, which use an inversion recovery pulse to increase T1-weighting, Schwitter et al[28] implemented a two-shot SE EPI perfusion sequence with short TRs (Figure 6). This allows coverage of the whole heart in two heartbeats (two shots) with satisfactory T1 contrast and seems to be a reliable protocol for routine clinical patient studies.

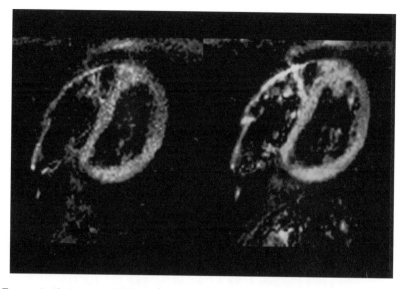

FIGURE 6. Spin-echo EPI images of the heart pre- (left) and post- (right) administration of gadolinium. Note the higher signal intensity of the myocardium after contrast agent application. (Reproduced with permission from Reference 50.)

Cardiac diffusion imaging has also been attempted by Edelman et al[29] who have implemented a stimulated echo EPI sequence for measurement of diffusion in the beating heart. Although results are promising, further studies are needed to evaluate the influence of bulk motion on the myocardial diffusion coefficient and to assess the utility of the method for different heart pathologies.

Phase velocity mapping with ultrafast techniques has been used to assess flow velocity and volume in the great vessels during apnea.[30,31] Eichenberger et al[31] implemented a single-shot phase contrast (PC) technique to perform real time quantification of blood flow in the superior vena cava (SVC) during Valsalva's maneuver. Although limited in spatial resolution, this approach allowed determination of the flow volume with high temporal resolution within 4 to 8 heartbeats. For the first time, they could prove experimentally that venous return to the heart is reduced during Valsava's maneuver due to the collapse of the SVC (Figure 7). Debatin et al,[30] however, compared a segmented k-space PC technique and a multiple-shot EPI PC technique with regard to their measurement accuracy in the thoracic aorta. EPI-PC flow volume measurements correlated well with conventional cine-PC data, taken as the gold standard ($r = 0.98$). Flow volume values obtained with the segmented k-space technique, however, correlated very poorly with Cine-PC data ($r = 0.62$), which was concluded to be a reflection

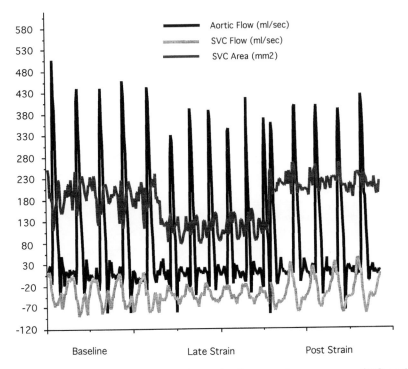

FIGURE 7. Flow and cross-sectional area for the superior vena cava SVC and the simultaneously measured flow curve for the ascending aorta. Curves are plotted for a single subject during normal breathing, late strain, and post strain. The high temporal resolution of the flow profiles allows excellent characterization of the blood flow. (Reproduced with permission from Reference 50.)

of the limited temporal resolution of the segmented k-space technique for vessels with systolic pulsatility.

Although the deficit of temporal resolution precludes segmented k-space techniques from flow quantification in highly pulsatile vessels (ie, aorta), encouraging results have been obtained in vessels with more homogeneous flow profiles, such as the renal arteries[32] and the coronary arteries.[33–37] While most groups concentrate on flow velocity quantification due to limitations in spatial resolution, Clarke et al[38] have demonstrated that breath-hold PC methods can also be applied to measure the absolute flow volume in coronary arteries noninvasively. They compared MR flow measurements with flow data obtained using perivascular ultrasound and found excellent agreement between the two techniques. While they performed the measurements in canine coronary arteries, Grist et al[36] and our group[37] have both been able to obtain reliable results in humans using the same MR technique.

Echoplanar PC strategies for coronary flow quantification are not yet available, but will surely improve measurement accuracy due to their increased temporal resolution. A time-of-flight EPI technique has already been implemented and coronary flow velocity measurements successfully performed.[39]

Ultrafast Magnetic Resonance Angiography

MRA has continuously improved. With the advent of ultrafast gradient systems, breath-hold MRA of various vascular territories now appears practical.

There has been emphasis on coronary artery imaging during the last few years. Inspired by the results of vessel imaging in other body organs, early attempts were made using SE sequences, with very limited success due to respiatory and cardiac motion artifacts.[40–41] In 1991, Edelman et al[42] proposed a new approach using an ultrafast segmented k-space technique, that allowed consistent visualization of the proximal portions of the coronary arteries. Manning et al[43] applied this technique in the assessment of patients with CAD and compared MR and conventional contrast angiography with regard to visualization of substantial (ie, >50%) coronary stenoses. They found MRA to be in high agreement with contrast angiography (specificity = 92%, sensitivity = 90%) and concluded that MR coronary angiography might be most helpful as a screening test for patients with CAD. These promising results have encouraged many groups to follow the same track and segmented k-space MR coronary angiography has become a fairly widespread research application of ultrafast MRI (Figure 8). Nevertheless, it has not had the desired clincial impact, because (1) limitations in spatial resolution persist, which make it impossible to assess the distal segments of the coronary arteries, as well as the septal and diagonal branches with diagnostic accuracy; (2) signal-to-noise ratio is very low, even when using a surface coil; and (3) variation in cardiac position from one heartbeat to the next causes image blurring. Echoplanar strategies, with higher signal-to-noise ratios and shorter image acquisition time may overcome these problems, but systems with whole-body echoplanar capabilities in all three orthogonal axes have only very recently become available and no data has yet been published on this subject. Using an older system, Wetter et al[9] looked at the coronary arteries in a transaxial plane and compared the visibility of four different multiple-shot EPI sequences with a single-shot EPI technique. They found no significant difference between the multiple-shot techniques, but all showed a significantly better depiction of the coronary arteries in comparision to the single-shot approach. This is believed to reflect better temporal

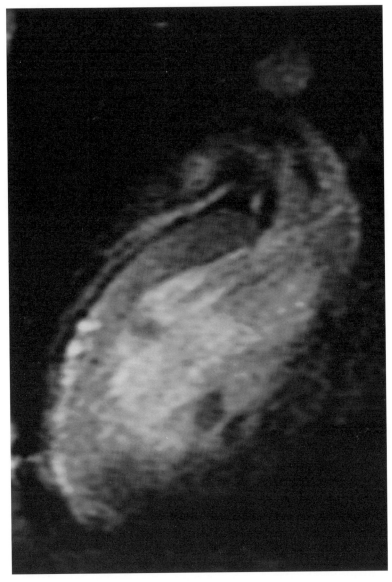

A

FIGURE 8. Five-millimeter thick, breathhold images of the coronary arteries.
A: Left anterior descending artery with a diagonal branch.

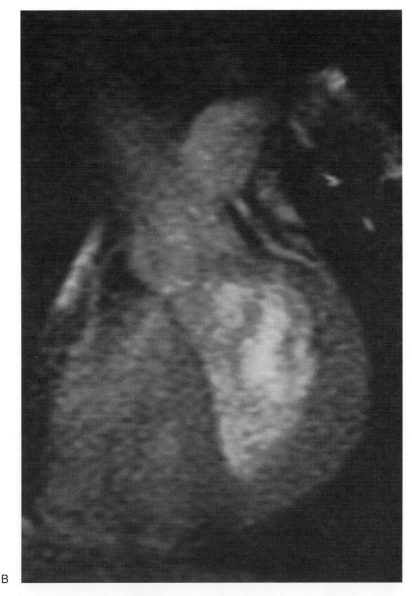

B

FIGURE 8. *(continued)* **B:** Right coronary artery and left main coronary artery with continuation into circumflex coronary artery. (Reproduced with permission from Reference 50.)

resolution achievable using multiple-shot EPI.[44] Yet another approach in ultrafast MR coronary angiography has been chosen by Meyer et al[5] using spiral scanning with promising results.

A shorter data acquisition time also allows better MR angiograms of the trunk because of limited motional artifacts. EPISTAR, an echoplanar technique proposed by Edelman et al[45] is based on alternately acquiring two sets of data that are identical except for the longitudinal magnetization of inflowing arterial spins. By using complex subtraction, vessel images with excellent background suppression can be obtained. A different approach based on three-dimensional (3D) contrast-enhanced GRE data acquisition strategies has recently been proposed.[46,47] By infusing contrast media during the entire acquisition period, the signal in the vessel remains very high (ie, T1 of blood is considerably shortened during the rapid T1-weighted data acquisition), and the background tissue is strongly suppressed due to the 3D acquisition technique. This allows acquisition of aortograms with excellent depiction of branch arteries within a breathhold (Figure 9). Although preliminary data has concentrated on depiction of the renal arteries,[46] the method can basically be applied to every vascular territory including the pulmonary arteries (Figure 10).

Electrocardiographic triggering enables the acquisition of time-resolved ultrafast two-dimensional (2D) data sets of the heart or large vessels in as short as 10 heartbeats. The images can be postprocessed as a 3D data set by means of the maximum intensity projection algorithm. Display of this data set in a movie loop allows visualization of the

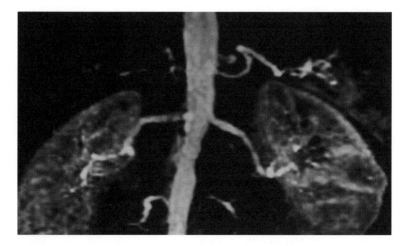

FIGURE 9. Three-dimensional contrast-enhanced breathheld aortogram showing the renal arteries with segmental branches and the splenic artery.

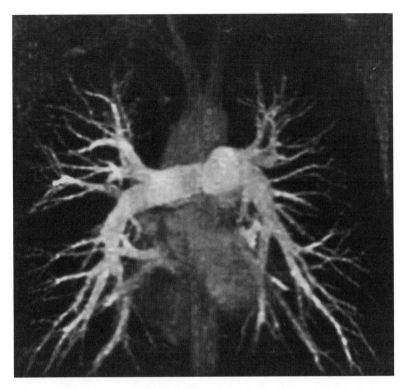

FIGURE 10. Three-dimensional contrast enhanced breathheld acquisition of the pulmonary arteries. Visualization of pulmonary veins can be greatly reduced with adequate timing of the contrast bolus.

flowing blood and thereby differentiation of changing flow patterns from consistent flow voids due to thrombosis or vessel wall narrowing.[48]

Conclusion

EPI has potential as a fast method for the evaluation of the cardiovascular system. At this time it is an evolving method. Technical refinements are clearly necessary before EPI will become a routine clinical tool.

References

1. Mansfield P. Multi-planar image formation using NMR spin-echoes. *J Phys C.* 1977;10:L55–L58.

2. Hennig J, Friedburg H. Clinical applications and methodological developments of the RARE technique. *Magn Reson Imaging*. 1988;6:391–395.
3. Oshio K, Feinberg DA. Single-shot GRASE imaging without fast gradients. *Magn Reson Med*. 1992;26:355–360.
4. Rzedzian RR, Pykett IL. Instant images of the human heart using a new, whole-body MR imaging system. *AJR*. 1987;149:245–250.
5. Meyer CH, Hu BS, Nishimura DG, Macovski A. Fast spiral coronary artery imaging. *Magn Reson Med* 1992;28:202–213.
6. Rzedzian R, Chapman B, Mansfied P, et al. Real-time nuclear magnetic resonance clinical imaging in paediatrics. *Lancet*. 1983;2:1281–1282.
7. Davis CP, McKinnon GC, Debatin JF, et al. Normal heart: evaluation with echo-planar MR imaging. *Radiology*. 1994;691–696.
8. Davis CP, McKinnon GC, Debatin JF, et al. Single-shot versus interleaved echo-planar MR-imaging: Application to visualization of cardiac valve leaflets. *J Magn Reson Imaging*. 1995;5:107–112.
9. Wetter DR, McKinnon GC, Debatin JF, von Schulthess GK. Cardiac echoplanar MR imaging: Comparison of single- and multiple-shot techniques. *Radiology*. 1995;194:765–770.
10. Fisher MR, von Schulthess GK, Higgins CB. Multiphasic cardiac magnetic resonance imaging: Normal regional left ventricular wall thickening. *AJR*. 1985;145:27–30.
11. Zerhouni EA, Parish DM, Rogers WJ, et al. Human heart: Tagging with MR imaging—a method for noninvasive assessment of myocardial motion. *Radiology*. 1988;169:59–63.
12. Axel L, Goncalves RC, Bloomgarden D. Regional heart wall motion: Two-dimensional analysis and functional imaging with MR imaging. *Radiology*. 1992;183:745–750.
13. Buchalter MB, Weiss JL, Rogers WJ, et al. Noninvasive quantification of left ventricular rotational deformation in normal humans using magnetic resonance imaging myocardial tagging. *Circulation*. 1990;81:1236–1244.
14. Tang C, McVeigh ER, Zerhouni EA. Multi-shot EPI for improvement of myocardial tag contrast: comparison with segmented SPGR. *Magn Reson Med*. 1995;33:443–447.
15. Utz JA, Herfkens RJ, Heinsimer JA, et al. Cine MR determination of left ventricular ejection fraction. *AJR*. 1987;148:839–843.
16. Debatin JF, Nadel SN, Paolini JF, et al. Cardiac ejection fraction: phantom study comparing cine MR imaging, radionuclide blood pool imaging, and ventriculography. *J Magn Reson Imaging*. 1992;2:135–142.
17. Unterweger M, Debatin JF, Leung DA, et al. Comparison of echoplanar and conventional cine-magnetic resonance data-acquisition strategies. *Invest Radiol*. 1994;29:994–1000.
18. Krauss XH, van der Wall EE, Doornbos J, et al. Value of magnetic resonance imaging in patients with a recent myocardial infarction: comparison with planar thallium-201 scintigraphy. *Cardiovasc Intervent Radiol*. 1989;12:119–124.
19. Atkinson DJ, Burstein D, Edelman RR. First-pass cardiac perfusion: Evaluation with ultrafast MR imaging. *Radiology*. 1990;174:757–762.
20. van Rugge FP, Boreel JJ, van der Wall EE, et al. Cardiac first-pass and myocardial perfusion in normal subjects assessed by subsecond Gd-DTPA enhanced MR imaging. *J Comput Assist Tomogr*. 1991;15:959–965.
21. Schaefer S, van Tyen R, Saloner D. Evaluation of myocardial perfusion abnormalities with gadolinium-enhanced snapshot MR imaging in humans. Work in progress. *Radiology*. 1992;185:795–801.

22. Wilke N, Simm C, Zhang J, et al. Contrast-enhanced first pass myocardial perfusion imaging: Correlation between myocardial blood flow in dogs at rest and during hyperemia. *Magn Reson Med.* 1993;29:485–497.
23. Eichenberger AC, Schuiki E, Kochli VD, et al. Ischemic heart disease: assessment with gadolinium-enhanced ultrafast MR imaging and dipyridamole stress. *J Magn Reson Imaging.* 1994;4:425–431.
24. Yu KK, Saeed M, Wendland MF, et al. Real-time dynamics of an extravascular magnetic resonance contrast medium in acutely infarcted myocardium using inversion recovery and gradient-recalled echo-planar imaging. *Invest Radiol.* 1992;27:927–934.
25. Wendland MF, Saeed M, Masui T, et al. Echo-planar MR imaging of normal and ischemic myocardium with gadodiamide injection. *Radiology* 1993;186: 535–542.
26. Edelman R, Li W. Contrast-enhanced echo-planar MR imaging of myocardial perfusion: preliminary study in humans. *Radiology.* 1994;190:771–777.
27. Wendland MF, Saeed M, Yu KK, et al. Inversion recovery EPI of bolus transit in rat myocardium using intravascular and extravascular gadolinium-based MR contrast media: dose effects on peak signal enhancement. *Magn Reson Med.* 1994;32:319–329.
28. Schwitter J, Leung DA, Debatin JF, et al. Evaluation of myocardial perfusion: T1-weighted multislice multiphase spin-echo EPI. *Eur Radiol* 1995;5: S37.
29. Edelman RR, Gaa J, Wedeen VJ, et al. In vivo measurement of water diffusion in the human heart. *Magn Reson Med.* 1994;32:423–428.
30. Debatin JF, Davis CP, Felblinger J, McKinnon GC. Evaluation of ultrafast phase-contrast imaging in the thoracic aorta. *MAGMA.* 1995;3:59–66.
31. Eichenberger AC, Schwitter J, McKinnon GC, et al. Phase-contrast echo planar MRI: real-time quantification of flow and velocity patterns in the thoracic vessels induced by Valsalva's maneuver. *J Magn Reson Imaging.* 1995;5:648–655.
32. Debatin JF, Ting RH, Wegmuller H, et al. Renal artery blood flow: Quantitation with phase-contrast MR imaging with and without breath holding. *Radiology.* 1994;190:371–378.
33. Edelman RR, Manning WJ, Gervino E, Li W. Flow velocity quantification in human coronary arteries with fast, breath-hold MR angiography. *J Magn Reson Imaging.* 1993;3:699–703.
34. Keegan J, Firmin D, Gatehouse P, Longmore D. The application of breath hold phase velocity mapping techniques to the measurement of coronary artery blood flow velocity: Phantom data and initial in vivo results. *Magn Reson Med.* 1994;31:526–536.
35. Sakuma H, Globits S, Shimakawa A, et al. Breathhold coronary flow measurement with a cine phase-contrast technique. In: Proceedings of the Society of Magnetic Resonance, 1994; San Francisco, Ca. 1:375.
36. Grist TM, Polzin JA, Bianco JA, et al. Measurement of absolute coronary flow and flow reserve using phase-contrast MRI techniques. In: Proceedings of the Society of Magnetic Resonance and the European Society for Magnetic Resonance in Medicine and Biology. 1995. Nice. 1:19.
37. Davis CP, Hauser M, Gohde SC, et al. Measurement of coronary flow with segmented k-space phase contrast MRI pre and post dipyridamole. In: Proceedings of the Society of Magnetic Resonance and the European Society for Magnetic Resonance in Medicine and Biology. 1995. Nice. 1:319.
38. Clarke GD, Eckels R, Chaney C, et al. Measurement of absolute epicardial

coronary artery flow and flow reserve with breath-hold cine phase-contrast magnetic resonance imaging. *Circulation*. 1995;91:2627–2634.

39. Poncelet BP, Weisskoff RM, Wedeen VJ, et al. Time of flight quantification of coronary flow with echo-planar MRI. *Magn Reson Med*. 1993;30:447–457.

40. Paulin S, von Schulthess GK, Fossel E, Krayenbuehl HP. MR imaging of the aortic root and proximal coronary arteries. *AJR*. 1987;148:665–670.

41. Alfidi RJ, Masaryk TJ, Haacke EM, et al. MR angiography of peripheral, carotid, and coronary arteries. *AJR*. 1987;149:1097–109.

42. Edelman RR, Manning WJ, Burstein D, Paulin S. Coronary arteries: Breathhold MR angiography. *Radiology*. 1991;181:641–643.

43. Manning WJ, Li W, Edelman RR. A preliminary report comparing magnetic resonance coronary angiography with conventional angiography. *N Engl J Med*. 1993;328:828–832.

44. Leung D, Debatin JF, McKinnon GD, et al. Cardiac imaging: Comparison of 2 shot EPI with segmented k-space and conventional cine gradient echo acquisitions. *J Magn Reson Imaging*. 1995;5:684–688.

45. Edelman RR, Siewert B, Adamis M, et al. Signal targeting with alternating radiofrequency (STAR) sequences: application to MR angiography. *Magn Reson Med*. 1994;31:233–238.

46. Prince MR, Bass JRC, Gabriel H, et al. Breath-held 3D gadolinium-enhanced renal artery MRA. In: Proceedings of the Society of Magnetic Resonance and the European Society for Magnetic Resonance in Medicine and Biology. 1995. Nice. 1:539.

47. Holland GA, Dougherty L, Geenman BL, et al. Ultrafast 3D time-of-flight MR angiography with gadolinium of the abdominal aorta and the visceral vessels performed in an breath-hold: preliminary experience. In: Proceedings of the Society of Magnetic Resonance and the European Society for Magnetic Resonance in Medicine and Biology. 1995. Nice. 1:77.

48. Duewell S, Davis CP, McKinnon G, et al. 3 and 4 dimensional MR-angiography with interleaved gradient echo-echo planar sequences. In: Proceedings of the Society of Magnetic Resonance in Medicine. 1993. New York. 1:385.

49. von Schulthess GK, Davis CP. Fast and ultrafast MR-imaging of the heart. *Radiologe*. 1995;35:952–963.

50. Davis CP, McKinnon GC, Debatin JF, von Schulthess GK. Ultra high speed MR imaging. *Eur Radiol*. 1996;6:297–311.

## Chapter 2

Myocardial Tagging
Techniques and Applications

Elias A. Zerhouni, MD

Introduction

A comprehensive understanding of the heart in health and disease requires detailed knowledge of multiple functional parameters such as integrity of the cardiac anatomy, adequacy of vascular supply during both rest and stress conditions, local and global mechanical function and, ideally, underlying metabolism. These parameters are now obtained through a multiplicity of separate methods including echocardiography, radionuclide imaging, coronary angiography, and magnetic resonance imaging (MRI).

Heart Function

Harmonious contraction of myocardial fibers for efficient ejection of blood from the ventricular chambers is the ultimate functional goal of the heart. Accurate study of myocardial contraction is difficult because of the complex motion of the heart during its cycle. Imaging methods that rely either on projectional or on tomographic images cannot display the relative displacement of specific myocardial points during the entire contraction cycle.

Magnetic Resonance Imaging Methods

Given the lack of distinctive anatomic landmarks, it is impossible, for instance, to ensure that end-diastolic (ED) and end-systolic (ES) images of a short-axis plane represent the same myocardial locus be-

From: Higgins CB, Ingwall JS, Pohost GM, (eds). *Current and Future Applications of Magnetic Resonance in Cardiovascular Disease.* Armonk, NY: Futura Publishing Company, Inc.; © 1998.

cause through-plane motion or in-plane shear cannot be detected. Thus, any measure of myocardial mechanical function, such as radial thickening, is inherently flawed. This problem has long been recognized and methods based on the physical implantation of metallic markers into the myocardium have been extensively used in the elucidation of ventricular mechanics. These methods, however, are invasive, disturb to an unknown extent the physiology under study, and are limited to small regions of the myocardium. With the advent of magnetic resonance imaging (MRI), noninvasive, high-resolution and spatially registered images of the entire heart throughout its contractile cycle can be obtained. Nevertheless, conventional MRI has the same limitations as other tomographic imaging methods: the complex cardiac motion patterns and the paucity of natural landmarks prevent "true" analytical description of myocardial function.[1] Methods able to unambiguously encode the intrinsic motion of material points of the myocardial wall would thus be of great value in the characterization of heart function as well as contributing to a comprehensive, integrated cardiac examination.

The intrinsic multiplanar capabilities of magnetic resonance (MR) allow easy evaluation of anatomically complex structures. The intrinsic sensitivity of MR to motion effects can be used advantageously to study flow patterns in vascular structures including the coronary arteries. The high inherent tissue contrast allows sensitive detection of both endogenous and exogenous contrast agents in the intact human. In addition to the standard depiction of myocardial contraction, novel methods using either tissue tagging or multidirectional phase encoding permit unique calculation of three-dimensional deformation within the myocardial tissue during its entire contractile cycle.

Despite its enormous theoretical advantages, MRI has not yet achieved wide clinical acceptance because current scanners cannot perform a comprehensive cardiac study within reasonable examination times. Recent research and development of high-performance hardware and pulse sequences, however, now permit the formulation of more effective study protocols. Faster imaging sequences requiring high-performance gradients have now been implemented successfully and most manufacturers have improved the performance of imaging gradients to the point where routine, clinically effective, high-speed acquisitions can be obtained. This has been greatly enhanced by the use of innovative pulse sequences such as gated single-breathhold segmented k-space techniques and echoplanar imaging (EPI). Although these advances have significantly improved the prospects for successful implementation of an integrated and time efficient cardiac MR examination, current scanners are still hampered by inadequate software design and slow computer systems that are being redesigned to allow near real-time interactive scanning. A consensus is now emerging indicating that dedicated high-speed scanners optimized for cardiovascular applications will be essential to the clinical success of cardiac MR.

Pending successful development of these redesigned specific-use scanners, it is nonetheless currently possible to perform comprehensive cardiac MR examinations. Based on our experience, it is possible to formulate MR examination strategies that, we believe, answer most of the relevant questions in clinical cardiac imaging in a single examination. Although these protocols are likely to evolve in the near future in line with technological developments, they predict the potential of using an integrated approach to clinical cardiac MR. Using standardized imaging protocols that limit the examination to a minimum set of sequences and images while preserving the essential parameters needed for clinical assessment, it is possible to study anatomy, mechanical function, and tissue perfusion in about 1 hour.

Toward this end, MRI offers two distinct approaches to the problem of motion encoding: (1) tissue tagging by localized perturbation of magnetization; and (2) motion detection based on phase-shifts secondary to displacement along magnetic field gradients.

Myocardial Tissue-Tagging Methods

One of the unique properties of MRI is that several intrinsic tissue parameters can be modified by the operator. For example, tissue signal can be modulated by simple implementation of different pulse sequences. One of the main determinants of tissue signal, for instance, is the amount of coherent magnetization of hydrogen atoms within a voxel of tissue at the time of image acquisition. Using a combination of radiofrequency (RF) pulses and gradients, one can selectively modify the local magnetization of tissue, thus generating a difference of signal between regions with modified magnetization versus those with unperturbed magnetization. For as long as differences in magnetization persist within a target tissue after RF perturbation (a time proportional to the longitudinal relaxation time, T1), a difference in signal between the so-tagged regions and the undisturbed regions will be imaged. The myocardial T1 relaxation time (about 600 ms) is long enough to allow visualization of the regions of perturbed magnetization for over 400 ms, thus allowing tracking of tags from ED to ES.

The central concept of modulating the magnetization of specific regions of the myocardium at a given time during the cardiac cycle and tracking the displacement of the tagged regions over a series of subsequent images forms the basis of all current myocardial tagging methods.

The first implementation of myocardial tissue-tagging for the assessment of ventricular function relied on the generation of radial or parallel thin planes of inverted magnetization at ED by using a series of selective RF pulses followed by imaging in planes orthogonal to the tagging planes.[2] Up to 12 radial segments in each short-axis image can thus be generated and tracked at a temporal resolution of 40 to 50 ms. Five or six short- or long-axis images at five or six time points during systole could be acquired during an ECG-gated acquisition of 256 successive heartbeats (Figure 1). A drawback of this method was the need to use a separate RF pulse for each of the radially oriented tagging planes, leading to a separation in time between tags by a few milliseconds and a total tagging time of about 36 ms with a lack of simultaneous tagging. Thus, alternative tagging schemes were subsequently sought and a more efficient method known by the acronym SPAMM (SPAtial Modulation of Magnetization) was developed by Axel and Dougherty.[3,4] The SPAMM method can generate a Cartesian grid pattern in

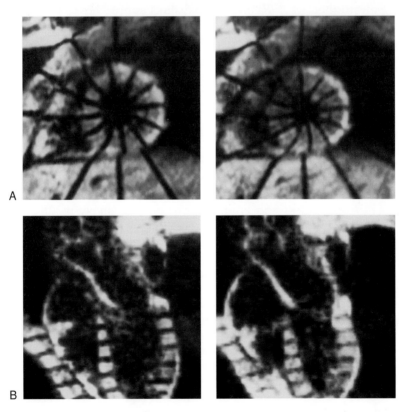

FIGURE 1. **A:** Radial tag pattern in the short axis generated by a series of radiofrequency (RF) pulses at or near end diastole. The image was acquired at 150 ms into systole. Note tag distortion related to in-plane shears. **B:** Example of parallel tags generated with two multispectral RF pulses. Note greater displacement of tag group near base and minimal displacement at apex.

less than 15 ms over the entire image with a series of nonselective RF and gradient pulses. This method, however, suffers from poor edge definition and excessive width of the tags and has subsequently been modified by Mosher et al[5] using a DANTE (Delays Altering with Nutations for Transient Excitation) sequence to overcome some of these drawbacks. Both the radial segmental approach and the Cartesian grid approach offer specific advantages and disadvantages.

The geometry of the heart is better suited to the radial pattern of tagging but no information regarding differential radial thickening between endo and epicardium can be obtained because deformation along the tag plane cannot be recorded. With the SPAMM method, grid points may serve as landmarks to measure endo and epicardial deformation separately. These points, however, do not occur in comparable locations around the myocardium and in most cases only two crossing points are seen across a radial direction. Consequently, differential measurement of epicardial and endocardial deformation is limited. Clearly, a combination of radial tagging, with separately identifiable points rather than lines in the myocardium, or alternatively, very thin grids with a higher tag density than currently achievable, would be desirable.

A combination of the radial tagging and SPAMM method was implemented by Bolster et al[6] to achieve a striped radial tag pattern that allows measurements of both radial and circumferential strains in each layer of the myocardial wall while preserving the advantages of polar coordinates (Figure 2).[6] All of the above methods suffer from the

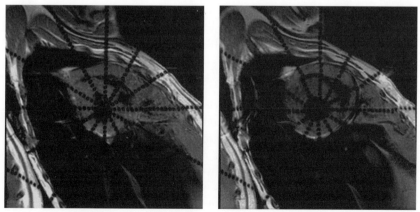

A   B

FIGURE 2. **A** and **B:** Example of striped radial tags allowing study of deformation within the myocardial wall in the radial direction. Three to six loci can be identified and separately tracked for differential studies of endocadial, midcardial and epicardial layers.

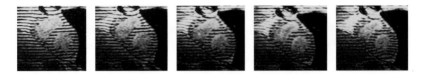

FIGURE 3. Single breathhold tagging technique: Parallel striped SPAMM tagging combined with a fast single breathhold cine-imaging technique allows acquisition of a series of tagged images in 8 to 16 heartbeats thus eliminating respiratory motion artifacts.

long acquisition times required for a cinematic study of ventricular contraction and the attendant dependence on electrocardiographic (ECG) gating during quiet breathing. Diagnostic studies are possible only when cardiac rhythm is regular and the blurring due to breathing motion is limited. Over the past year efforts have been made to develop imaging sequences that can be acquired within a single breathhold[7] and 16 to 32 heartbeats (Figure 3). EPI hardware now becoming available will further reduce these times to 40 to 50 ms per image, thereby increasing the percentage of diagnostic studies and the applicability of the method to the entire patient population.

Phase-Encoding Methods

One of the remaining obstacles to the characterization of contraction in the entire cardiac cycle is the lack of persistence of magnetic tags for sufficiently long periods of time to encompass the entire RR interval.

In the early 1980s, Moran et al[8] demonstrated that the phase of the nuclear magnetic resonance (NMR) signal would be shifted for moving protons relative to stationary ones in the presence of a linear gradient. Thus, if phase detection is performed, any motion of tissue in the direction of an imposed magnetic field gradient could be detected by subtracting images with and without a gradient. This concept was first proposed and preliminarily tested by Van Dijk[9] as a way of studying myocardial wall displacement, but was not further developed because of the extremely long imaging times required. More recently, Pelc et al,[10] using more efficient cine-phase contrast sequences, have generated two-dimensional displacement maps over the entire heart (right and left ventricle) throughout the whole cardiac cycle with temporal resolution on the order of 50 ms. Extension to three-dimensional displace ments should be achievable. Even though the method is very sensitive to other sources of motion artifacts such as respiration and blood motion within the chambers, it is a potentially fruitful approach either alone or in combination with the newer and faster tagging methods. For example, hybrid approaches using in-plane displacement measured via tagging methods and through-plane motion by phase-encoding are being tested and seem promising.

Two-Dimensional and Three-Dimensional Analyses of Tagged Images

The most appealing aspect of myocardial tagging research is its potential for representing, for the first time, the behavior of the ventricle in three dimensions with unambiguous measurement of local regional as well as global myocardial strain at an acceptable temporal resolution. The creation of dynamic displacement and strain maps of the entire ventricle, with separate layer by layer assessment of deformation, may become a unique diagnostic tool in cardiology. No method in existence has yet approached that goal with the degree of accuracy and non-invasiveness of MR tagging. Progress in this regard, however, depends heavily on the development of effective automated image analysis methods in view of the enormous amount of data generated.

Algorithms for automated tag detection and tracking have been developed by research groups active in the field.[11,12] All are heavily dependent on image quality and still require human supervision and editing. Faster sequences now in development, such as EPI, will undoubtedly facilitate this task. The analytical challenge of deriving accurate descriptors and models of myocardial function in health and disease from tagged data sets is now at the center of research efforts. Principles of continuum mechanics and finite element analysis have been adapted successfully for both two-dimensional[13,14] and three-dimensional[15,16] derivations of mechanical strains, deformation, and displacement mapping. The primary approach to three-dimensional reconstruction of the ventricle is currently based on the tracking of material point displacements in two orthogonal sets of cardiac images. These sets of images are congruent at a given time point during the cardiac cycle, with iterative tracking of the subsequent deformation-related displacements, exclusive of rigid body motion. Effective dynamic three-dimensional reconstructions of the ventricle can thus be achieved. Other approaches based on fitting a predefined model to the measured tag points[17] or by dynamic field-fitting methods derived from computer vision methods are being developed. Direct three-dimensional phase-encoding of cardiac wall motion is still under development by Pelc et al[10] and could potentially supplant existing methods.

Applications for MR Tagging Methods

Since its inception, myocardial tagging has been used as a tool for basic physiologic studies of ventricular mechanics in the normal heart to elucidate heretofore unknown patterns of contraction. In the context of ischemia, myocardial tagging has been used in remodeling and in cardiomyopathies to assess its potential clinical value.

MR Tagging and Normal Heart Physiology

In the normal human heart, tagging has demonstrated for the first time the importance of torsion and detorsion (or untwisting) in myocardial performance. Buchalter et al[18] first showed the existence in the normal human heart of marked epicardial-endocardial shears that were heterogeneous from base to apex as well as from posteroseptal to anterolateral locations. Although torsion increased from base to apex, circumferential-longitudinal shear was almost invariant throughout the heart, indicating that our understanding of heart contraction may be enhanced by searching for new defining parameters derived from three-dimensional dynamic data sets. Clark et al[19] showed heterogeneity in segmental shortening with endocardial shortening being greater than epicardial shortening in the normal human heart. Consequently, the definition of new parameters of function, based on more extensive normalized data, is being actively sought. Rademakers et al[20] showed that untwisting of the ventricle in the isovolumic phase of diastole was an important mechanism for efficient diastolic filling and was modulated by catecholamine stimulation. Furthermore, myocardial tagging can be used as a tool for the elucidation of the relationship between myocardial fiber architecture and function. For example, the mechanism by which small amounts of myofiber shortening leads to extensive wall thickening is still unknown given the complex fiber organization of the heart. By correlating data from tagged images and histologic fiber orientation, Rademakers et al[21] have shown that cross-fiber shortening appears more critical in the generation of wall thickening than does shortening in the fiber direction.

Myocardial Pathology and Magnetic Resonance Tagging

The potential impact of MR tagging on the diagnosis and management of ischemic heart disease provides a strong impetus for tagging research. The finding that even normal myocardial contraction is inherently heterogeneous and complex has limited the impact of conventional imaging methods. The sensitive correlation between local perfusion and contractility in the heart, however, make accurate measurements of local deformation a necessity in clinical practice. Furthermore, a more objective and quantifiable assessment of dysfunction could provide the clinician with a guide for appropriate intervention before irreversible decompensation occurs in ischemic heart disease. Are there better indices of function uniquely definable by MR tagging that would allow better discrimination between salvageable and necrotic myocardium? Can one predict the response of the heart to intervention based on a quantified knowledge of its three-dimensional contraction pattern? These are the main research issues now being addressed. Lima et al[22] have validated the accuracy of wall thickening measurements by MR tagging relative to the standard of implanted sonomicrometry in normal and ischemic myocardium. In a series of initial studies in humans with known infarction the topography of segmental shortening was evaluated and showed significant depression of segmental shortening with a persistent transmural gradient in areas of presumed infarction. The noninfarcted regions, however, also exhibited abnormal segmental shortening, suggesting ischemic dysfunction beyond the recognized borders of infarction.[23] The exact significance of these findings is still being investigated. In a sheep model of chronic infarction, similar findings were noted. Increasing ventricular mass and volume with changes from a circumferential to radial direction of maximal elongation from adjacent to remote regions probably reflected post-myocardial infarction remodeling.[24] MR tagging can also be used as an objective tool in the assessment of the effect of drugs on infarct expansion. In left ventricular hypertrophy, MR tagging has shown not only a reduction in rigid body motion and deformation but also a change in the orientation of the principal mechanical strains that may reflect differences in myocardial fiber orientation or cross-fiber shortening.[25] In dog experiments with graded controlled perfusion of the coronary arteries in our laboratory, early results show correlation between the degree of local dysfunction and percent reduction in coronary flow. More studies correlating local perfusion and appropriate mechanical indices derived from MR tagging are necessary to define and match the patterns of mechanical dysfunction with the underlying extent, stage, natural evolution, and reversibility of the ischemic insult. For example, matched contrast-enhanced and tagging studies using iron oxide particles have begun to address such issues.[26] MR tagging can also be used clinically to assess the mechanical impact of myocardial tumors and to differentiate viable muscle from tumor.[27]

Myocardial Tagging and the Integrated Cardiac Examination

The success of an integrated protocol depends in great part on the use of pulse sequences that are flexible enough to allow cine imaging in multiple arbitrary orientations from a single prescription. In addition, these sequences should permit detailed quantitative motion studies using either myocardial tagging or multidirectional phase encoding. The same cine sequence modified in real time at the switch of user-defined control variables can also be used for assessment of perfusion using exogenous contrast agents and coronary imaging. These sequence should allow single breathold acquisitions and be compatible with multicoil array imaging for maximum signal-to-noise ratio (SNR).

Conclusion

The study of ventricular wall motion by motion encoded MRI techniques such as tagging or cine phase-contrast is an unprecedented opportunity to refine our knowledge of myocardial mechanics. Since the inception of the concept of myocardial tagging by MRI, most of the research effort has been directed to the solution of sometimes daunting technological problems. These technological problems include: the ability to acquire artifact free images in a short, clinically realistic time; the ability to generate tag patterns adapted to the application of continuum mechanics for the complete characterization of ventricular contraction in three dimensions with sufficient temporal resolution; and the ability to develop robust image segmentation and tag recognition software, without which realistic and reliable experimental protocols cannot be implemented. More recently, efforts have been directed toward understanding the relationship between fiber arrangement and contraction, the definition of new and more appropriate indices and models of mechanical performance in health and disease, and the correlation of ischemia with tagging-derived three-dimensional strain analysis. In the research laboratory, MR tagging is rapidly replacing or complementing all other existing methods for such purposes. Whether MR tagging will provide useful incremental knowledge for clinical applications is actively being tested. It is likely, however, that even if MR tagging provides significant functional information, its future in the clinical arena will be determined by the successful implementation of other MR methods geared toward direct assessment of the coronary tree and myocardial perfusion, combined in a single, comprehensive and cost-effective MR examination.

Cardiac MR is a very active field of investigation and several new approaches are being proposed for studying myocardial function. It is clear that a period of increased experimentation will lead to rapid changes in the approach to the single step comprehensive cardiac MR examination. The exploitation of novel contrast mechanisms such as blood oxygen dependent contrast (BOLD) may lead to more direct measurements of oxygenation at the tissue level. Perfusion measurements by spin tagging techniques also appear promising and may find a place in the examination protocol of the future. New contrast agents using T2 contrast mechanisms or purely intravascular agents may play a prominent role. Cardiac spectroscopy, which is still a daunting technical challenge, may provide MR with a metabolic dimension of great clinical value. The operator-independent nature of MR examinations and the ability to quantify accurately multiple parameters of flow, perfusion, function and anatomy at spatial and temporal resolutions unmatched by any other existing method is very likely to make MR a cost-effective, high diagnostic value alternative in cardiac imaging.

Acknowledgments

We wish to thank our collaborators, Drs. Elliot McVeigh, Ergin Atalar, Jerry Prince, Michael Guttman, Carlos Lugo-Olivieri, Chris Moore, Anne Bazille, Joao Lima, James Weiss, Walt Rogers and Edward Shapiro for useful discussions, and for supplying of some of the illustrations. We also thank Ms. Mary McAllister for editing and Ms. Nola Miller for manuscript preparation.

References

1. Hunter WC, Zerhouni EA. Imaging distinct points in left ventricular myocardium to study regional wall deformation. In: Anderson, JH, ed: *Innovations in Diagnostic Radiology*. New York: Springer-Verlag; 1989:169–190.
2. Zerhouni EA, Parish DM, Rogers WJ, Yang A, Shapiro EP. Human heart: Tagging with MR imaging: a method for noninvasive assessment of myocardial motion. *Radiology*. 1988;169(1):59–63.

3. Axel L, Dougherty L. MR imaging of motion with spatial modulation of magnetization. *Radiology.* 1989;171(3):841–845.
4. Axel L, Dougherty L. Heart wall motion: Improved method of spatial modulation of magnetization for MR imaging. *Radiology.* 1989;172:349–350.
5. Mosher TJ, Smith MB. A DANTE tagging sequence for the evaluation of translational sample motion. *Magn Reson Med.* 1990;15(2):334–339.
6. Bolster BD Jr, McVeigh ER, Zerhouni EA. Myocardial tagging in polar coordinates with use of striped tags. *Radiology.* 1990;177(3):769–772.
7. McVeigh ER, Atalar E. Cardiac tagging with breath-hold cine MRI. *Magn Reson Med.* 1992;28:318–327.
8. Moran PR. A general Approach to T1, T2, and spin-density discrimination sensitivities in NMR imaging sequences. *Magn Reson Imaging.* 1984;2(1):17–22.
9. Van Dijk P. Direct cardiac NMR imaging of heart wall and blood flow velocity. *J Comput Assist Tomogr.* 1984;8:429–430.
10. Pelc NJ, Herfkens RJ, Shimikawa A, Enzman DR. Phase contrast cine MRI. *Magn Reson Q.* 1991;7(4):229–254.
11. Guttman MA, Prince JL, McVeigh ER. Tag and contour detection in tagged MR images of the left ventricle. *IEEE Trans.* 1994;13:74–88.
12. Prince JL, McVeigh ER. Motion estimation from tagged MR image sequences. *IEEE Trans.* 1992;11(2):238–249.
13. McVeigh ER, Zerhouni EA. Noninvasive measurement of transmural gradients in myocardial strain with MR imaging. *Radiology.* 1991;180:677–683.
14. Axel L, Goncalves RC, Bloomgarden D. Regional heart wall motion: two-dimensional analysis and functional imaging with MR imaging. *Radiology.* 1992;183(3):745.
15. Pipe JG, Boes JL, Chenevert TL. Method for measuring three-dimensional motion with tagged MR imaging. *Radiology.* 1991;181:591–595.
16. Moore CC, O'Dell WG, McVeigh ER, Zerhouni EA. Calculation of three-dimensional left ventricular strains from biplanar tagged MR images. *J Magn Reson Imaging.* 1992;2(2):165–175.
17. Young AA, Axel L. Three-dimensional motion and deformation of the heart wall: estimation with spatial modulation of magnetization—A model based approach. *Radiology.* 1992;185(1):241–7.
18. Buchalter MB, Weiss JL, Rogers WJ, et al. Noninvasive quantification of left ventricular rotational deformation in normal humans using magnetic resonance imaging myocardial tagging. *Circulation.* 1990;81(4):1236–1244.
19. Clark NR, Reichek N, Bergey P, et al. Circumferential myocardial shortening in the normal human left ventricle. Assessment by magnetic resonance imaging using spatial modulation of magnetization. *Circulation.* 1991;84:67–74.
20. Rademakers FE, Buchalter MB, Rogers WJ, et al. Dissociation between left ventricular untwisting and filling. Accentuation by catecholamines. *Circulation.* 1992;85(4):1572–1581.
21. Rademakers, FE, Hutchins GM, Guier WH, et al. LV wall thickening depends on cross-fiber shortening. *Circulation.* (Suppl II)1991;84(4):670.
22. Lima JAC, Jeremy R, Guier W, et al. Accurate systolic wall thickening by nuclear magnetic resonance imaging with tissue tagging: Correlation with sonomicrometers in normal and ischemic myocardium. *J Am Coll Cardiol.* 1993;21:1741–1751.
23. Yeon SB, Reichek N, Palmon LC, et al. Segmental shortening in human myocardial infarction using magnetic resonance tagging. (abstr) AHA 1992.

24. Ferrari VA, Kramer CM, Llaneras M, et al. Mechanical behavior of non-infarcted myocardium adjacent to scarred infarcted tissue during left ventricular remodeling (abstr.) AHA Book of Abstracts 1992.
25. Xie F, Ferrari VA, Palmon LC, et al. Two dimensional analysis of regional systolic rigid body motion and deformation in left ventricular hypertrophy using magnetic resonance tissue tagging (abstr.). AHA Book of Abstracts 1992.
26. Yeon SB, Reichek N, Tallant BA, et al. Imaging function and perfusion defects in myocardial infarction using magnetic resonance tagging and iron oxide contrast (abstract) Proceedings of the Society of Magnetic Resonance in Medicine. 1991:371.
27. Bouton S, Yang A, McCrindle BW, et al. Differentiation of tumor from viable myocardium using cardiac tagging with MR imaging. *J Comput Assist Tomogr.* 1991;15(4):676–678.

## Chapter 3

Magnetic Resonance Imaging
Techniques for Assessing Myocardial Perfusion

Roderic Pettigrew, PhD, MD, John Oshinski, PhD, and W. Thomas Dixon, PhD

Basic Concepts

Ultrafast Magnetic Resonance Imaging to Monitor Perfusion

The development of ultrafast cardiac magnetic resonance imaging (MRI) techniques has made it possible to assess relative perfusion in the heart as well as other organs.[1-4] The ultrafast techniques permit the assessment of perfusion with or without the use of an exogenous contrast agent.[5-7] When a contrast agent is used, image acquisition speed is needed in order to allow imaging at rapid enough intervals to monitor the passage of a contrast agent bolus through the myocardium. For imaging with a contrast agent, temporal resolution of about 1 to 2 seconds is required. When perfusion imaging relies on intrinsic contrast mechanisms, image acquisition speed is needed to avoid artifact from patient respiratory motion. Such artifacts could corrupt the true intrinsic myocardial signal and mask the small intrinsic signal intensity changes caused by myocardial perfusion.

Several ultrafast MRI techniques are currently suitable for assessing myocardial perfusion. These range from turbo-gradient echo-based techniques that can acquire a single, low-resolution (64 × 64 matrix) image in 250 to 500 ms depending on the gradient capabilities, to single-shot echoplanar imaging that can acquire an image in approximately 30

From: Higgins CB, Ingwall JS, Pohost GM, (eds). *Current and Future Applications of Magnetic Resonance in Cardiovascular Disease.* Armonk, NY: Futura Publishing Company, Inc.; © 1998.

ms. It is certainly worth noting that these techniques are continuously evolving as both hardware and software improve. Consequently, the approach that is ultimately used in the routine clinical arena may well have not been developed yet.

Presently, in the most common approach, images are acquired over 250 ms approximately every heartbeat for about 30 seconds after intravenous injection of a T1 or T_2^* agent.[8-10] This temporal resolution permits tracking the contrast bolus into and through the right ventricle cavity, left ventricle cavity, and the left ventricular myocardium. The basic concept is illustrated in Figure 1. An image acquired in 256 ms is obtained after a myocardial signal inverting pulse. The image is acquired at a time during the cardiac cycle when the myocardial magnetization crosses zero, ie, nulled myocardial signal. This allows the signal enhancement from a T_1 shortening agent, eg, gadolinium (Gd), to be easily seen as it enters the myocardium. Acquiring such an image during each heartbeat permits monitoring the change in myocardial contrast agent level.

Method Basics

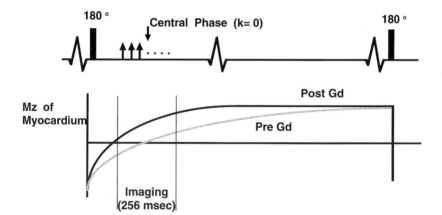

FIGURE 1. Basic methodology of gadolinium (Gd) contrast-enhanced perfusion imaging of the myocardium. Myocardial magnetization (Mz), is nulled precontrast by a 180° radiofrequency (RF) inversion pulse and image data acquired as Mz crosses zero. Note that the central phase-encoding line of image data line acquired at the time that Mz = 0. After the administration of Gd, the previously darkened myocardium becomes bright because of the enhanced growth rate of Mz. Turbo gradient-recalled echo images acquired during sequential heartbeats permits monitoring the transit of Gd through the myocardium. Adapted from Reference 2.

A promising intrinsic contrast-based approach acquires two images within a single 15 to 25 second breathhold, using k-space segmentation to reduce the total acquisition time.[11] The two images are acquired with different echo times (TEs) to allow calculation of T_2^*, which is mediated by the level of myocardial perfusion. This is all accomplished within the breathhold period to avoid respiratory motion artifact and permit an accurate T_2^* calculation. Thus, as indicated above, image acquisition speed is central to the assessment of myocardial perfusion. The details of how this is achieved are given later in this chapter.

Coronary Physiology: Rest vs. Flow

In MRI, as with conventional nuclear single photon emission computed tomography (SPECT) and positron emission tomography (PET) imaging, the assessment of myocardial perfusion for the purpose of identifying coronary artery disease is based on imaging the effects of abnormal coronary flow reserve. This relies on the well-documented observation by Gould et al[12] that abnormal coronary flow reserve, as opposed to simply coronary flow at rest, is a significantly more sensitive indicator of coronary stenosis. As shown in Figure 2, resting coronary flow is maintained at a normal level despite progressive stenosis until the diameter is reduced by 75% to 80%. Under stress, two important changes are observed. First, in normal vessels and those with less than an approximate 50% diameter stenosis, coronary flow is increased

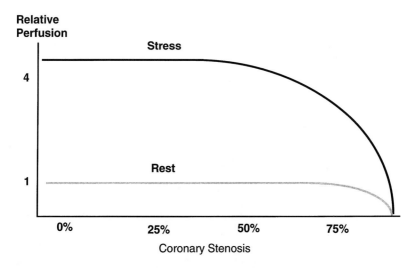

FIGURE 2. The effect of graded coronary stenosis on flow at rest and during stress (see text). Adapted from Reference 12.

by a factor of 3 to 5. Second, for vessels with as little as a 50% diameter stenosis or greater, there is decreased dilatory response to stress with decreased coronary flow relative to normal vessels. Thus assessing flow at stress and relative to resting flow is a more sensitive indicator of stenotic coronary artery disease.[13] This ability to increase flow in response to stress, termed coronary flow reserve, can be indirectly assessed by simple comparison of myocardial perfusion images at rest versus those obtained during stress. In myocardial regions supplied by a 50% or greater stenosed coronary, a perfusion deficit is evident at stress but not at rest unless the degree of stenosis is severe. This is the diagnostic hallmark of ischemic disease.

Pharmacological Stress

To elicit the maximum possible increase in coronary flow during MRI, pharmacological stress must be used. Available agents for which there is a considerable body of human experience are dipyridamole, adenosine, and dobutamine.[14–16] Dipyridamole and adenosine are fundamentally different from dobutamine with regard to both pharmacology and physiologic effects.

Dipyridamole is both a platelet inhibitor and a potent vasodilator. When administered intravenously at a dose of 0.5 mg/kg, it has the desirable hemodynamic effects of decreasing coronary (and systemic) vascular resistance resulting in increased coronary flow. The vasodilatory effects result from an increased level of endogenous adenosine, which is an active vasodilatory agent. Endogenous adenosine is inhibited by dipyridamole from being transported and taken up by red blood cells, thereby producing a higher level of adenosine, as desired.[14–16]

Because adenosine is the actual agent that decreases vascular resistance, it is used rather than dipyridamole in some laboratories. Since it slows conduction time through the atrioventricular (AV) node, it is contraindicated in patients with AV block. Whether dipyridamole or adenosine is used, the effect of interest is the increase in coronary flow, which is blunted in diseased vessels. Adenosine does not increase oxygen demand so that a decrease in regional myocardial function (thickening) is not expected or observed except in cases of severe coronary artery disease.[15,16]

Dobutamine is a synthetic catecholamine that has inotropic (contractility) and mild chronotropic (rate) effects. It decreases vascular resistance, increases heart rate, and increases myocardial oxygen demand. An increase in coronary flow is observed, resulting from the decrease in vascular resistance. When coronary flow cannot be sufficiently increased to meet the increase in oxygen demand, ischemia develops, resulting in decreased myocardial function.[16]

In patients with coronary artery disease, dobutamine stress causes a blunted increase in perfusion (decreased coronary flow reserve) that is insufficient to meet the increase in metabolic demand that is also caused by this agent. Therefore, ischemia develops with an accompanying decrease in myocardial function. In contrast, dipyridamole stress causes only a blunted increased in perfusion without altering metabolic demand. However, with severe stenosis (>80% to 90%) resting perfusion abnormalities, as well as abnormal flow reserve, may also be seen.

Techniques to Monitor Agent First Passage

Turbo Gradient-Echo

There are two central objectives of MRI techniques that are used to monitor the first pass of an agent through the myocardium. First, the image must be completely acquired well within one heartbeat in order to have adequate temporal resolution of 1 to 2 seconds. Second, the image contrast should be optimized so that the arrival and transit of the contrast agent can be definitively observed.[2–4,8–10,17]

The T1 weighted turbo gradient-echo technique designed to meet these objectives has two basic components. The first component is a magnetization preparation period during which the myocardial signal is nulled, followed by the second component that is the image data acquisition period, as illustrated in Figure 3. Electrocardiographic

T1 Turbo GRE

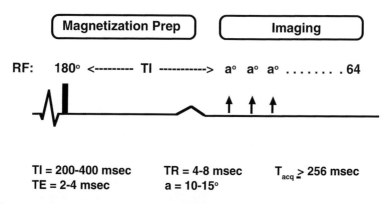

FIGURE 3. Basic method for T1 weighted turbo gradient-recalled echo (GRE) imaging. RF indicates radiofrequency pulse; T1, time of inversion; TE, time of echo; TR, repetition time; a, flip angle of RF pulse; Tacq, image acquisition time.

(ECG) gating is used to minimize motion artifact and to insure that the image is always obtained at the same phase of the cardiac cycle. Nulling of the myocardial signal is achieved by a 180° inversion pulse immediately after the R wave triggers the sequence. After waiting a time T1 to begin, a train a low flip angle radiofrequency (RF) pulses generates gradient echo.[25] The most effective T1 is chosen by trial and error, but typically is in the 200 ms to 400 ms range. The RF flip angle is typically in the 10° to 15° range, with TEs of 2 to 4 ms and TRs of 4 to 8 ms. Thus, to generate an image with 80 lines of resolution the 80 echoes needed can be acquired in 320 ms. The echo that gives the central line in k-space (ie, k = 0) is placed or timed to be acquired during the null point of the myocardial signal (Figure 1).[2–8,9]

When this sequence is used to monitor the first passage of a T1 contrast agent such as gadolinium-based agent, the darkened blood pool and myocardium are progressively seen to enhance or brighten as the agent follows the normal physiologic route. As shown in Figure 4, the brightest enhancement and the earliest is seen in the ventricular lumen or blood pool. The peak normal myocardial signal intensity follows with a maximal enhancement equal to $-\frac{2}{3}$ that of the blood pool. A

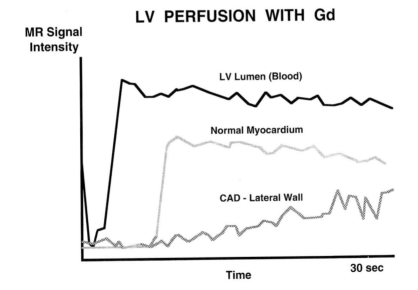

FIGURE 4. Time-signal intensity curves obtained in a patient with high-grade coronary artery disease (CAD). The technique in Figure 3 was used to acquire sequential heart images for 30 seconds after intravenous gadolinium (Gd) administration. Note the prolonged time-to-peak signal, and decreased maximal signal in the lateral wall. Patient had a 90% stenosis of the left circumflex coronary artery.

relative delay in time-to-peak signal, and decreased maximal signal are seen in hypoperfused regions as shown. Indexes of normal versus abnormal perfusion can be extracted from these time-intensity curves generated for the myocardial regions of interest.[3,4,17,18]

If one desires to monitor the first passage of a T_2^* agent (eg, dysprosium), the magnetization preparation component of the sequence must be changed to produced relatively bright precontrast myocardial signal.[3,10,19] This will permit the passage of the susceptibility agent to be seen as it darkens the myocardium. The preparation sequence used to brighten the myocardium should be sensitive to field inhomogeneities and to diffusion-related signal attenuation, in order to be maximally effective.[3] The sequence shown in Figure 5 illustrates an effect T_2^* turbo gradient-echo technique. The magnetization preparation period consist of a 90° RF pulse directed along the x axis, followed by a waiting period T, then a second 90° RF pulse along the -x axis to return the magnetization to the initial upright position (along z). During this waiting period T, the magnetization is allowed to decay by T_2^* mechanisms. In addition, during the imaging component of the sequence there is further signal attenuation produced by diffusion of spins into regions of the susceptibility particles. This occurs during the time between the low flip angle RF pulses and the generation of the echo (ie, TE). Thus the effective TE is a sum of the T period and the TE. For this reason, the

T2* Turbo GRE

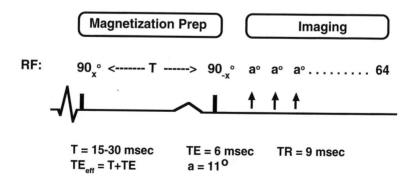

FIGURE 5. Method for T_2^* weighted turbo gradient-recalled echo (GRE) imaging. TE eff indicates effective TE (see text). Adapted from Hu X, Kim SG. A new T_2 weighting technique for magnetic resonance imaging. *Magn Reson Med.* 1993; 30:512–517.

selected TE of 6 ms is longer than the minimum achievable TE. This enhances signal loss from both (1) intravoxel spin dephasing produced by local field inhomogeneities, and from (2) spin diffusion in the inhomogenous regions caused by the T_2^* agent.

Modified Driven Equilibrium

Variations in myocardial signal intensity that are artifactual are a common problem with ECG gated imaging. This largely results from the beat-to-beat variation in the R-R interval producing an inconstant TR. The variation in TR from view-to-view or from the acquisition of one k-space line to the next produces inconsistent image data leading to phase errors in the image data and consequential image artifact. This fundamental problem can be addressed by using a magnetization preparation technique that drives the spins into an equilibrium state that is independent of the residual amount of magnetization from preceding excitations.

This arrhythmia-insensitive approach is diagrammed in Figure 6.[20] Immediately after the R wave trigger, a 90° RF pulse tips any residual magnetization into the X-Y plane. This is then destroyed by a gradient pulse applied along the x axis. After a waiting period T1, there is new magnetization growth along the z axis. The amount of this magnetization growth is determined by the T1 of the tissue and the duration of

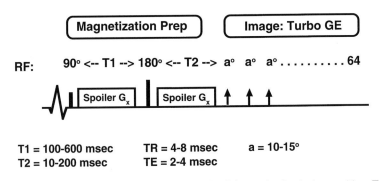

FIGURE 6. Modified driven equilibrium method for arrhythmia insensitive T1 weighted imaging. T1 indicates first interpulse waiting period; T2, second interpulse waiting period; Gx, gradient applied along x axis (see text). Adapted from Reference 20.

the wait period T1. Because of the gradient spoiling, this magnetization is independent of any residual z magnetization from the previous heartbeat or the amount at the beginning of the current heartbeat. After the T1 waiting period, a 180° RF pulse inverts the magnetization in order to null the myocardium. A second waiting period, T2, allows recovery of the inverted magnetization until it reaches the null point at which the central phase encoding gradient echo is acquired as desribed for the T1 turbo gradient-echo sequence. During the waiting period T2, a second gradient pulse is applied along the x axis to spoil or destroy any remaining transverse magnetization. This technique produces T1-sensitive images that are relatively free of artifacts from arrhythmias. Typical parameter values are T1 = 100–600 ms, T2 = 10–200 ms during the magnetization preparation phase, and TE = TE 2–4 ms, TR = 4–8 ms, RF flip angle = 10°–15° during the imaging phase.[3,20]

The contrast behavior with this technique is similar to that observed with a simple T1 turbo gradient-echo technique. The major difference is in eliminating motion artifact from arrhythmias. As such, this currently provides the image quality of choice using conventional systems.[3] For systems that can achieve TE/TR of 2 ms and 4 ms, respectively, 2 to 3 slices can be imaged per 2 seconds, so that the transit of a bolus could be followed through an apex, mid, and basal slice. Covering the entire heart with conventional 1-cm thick short-axis slices would therefore require two scans, each with a bolus injection.

Echoplanar Imaging

Echoplanar imaging (EPI) is now well established as the ultimate high-speed MRI technique, acquiring complete image data in as little as 30 ms to real time.[21] This temporal resolution makes EPI well suited to imaging the transit of a contrast agent bolus through the myocardium. Currently, EPI is the only technique that allows acquisition of enough 1-cm thick slices to cover the entire left ventricle within a single heartbeat.

A T1 weighted echoplanar sequence is illustrated in Figure 7. The magnetization preparation phase consists of a 180° RF inversion pulse followed by a relatively long waiting period T1 of 700 to 900 ms before the imaging phase begins. This allows positive recovery of magnetization (along z axis), which is above zero and can be imaged using a modified spin-echo sequence. During this sequence there is rapid blipping of the phase encoding gradients and switching or oscillation of the read gradient throughout the envelope of the single spin echo. This generates all of the lines of data in the image matrix during the time of a single echo.[3,21] Because all the image data are generated after a single RF pulse, the image is said to be formed in a "single shot."

T1-Echoplanar

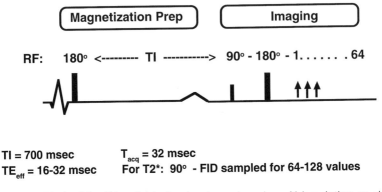

FIGURE 7. Method for T1 weighted echoplanar imaging. Abbreviation as defined in Figures 3 and 5. FID indicates free induction decay (see text).

Because the EPI innovation can be applied after the generation of either a spin-echo or a gradient-echo, the contrast features can be tailored to be either T1 weighted using the spin-echo as above, to T_2^* weighted using a free induction decay (FID) readout.[3,22,23] The effective TE is the time between the 90° RF pulse and the central k-space line acquisition. For T1 weighting this is relatively short, on the order of 16 ms to minimize T_2^* effects. The T1 weighting is provided by the preceding inversion-recovery magnetization preparation period. For T_2^* weighting, the magnetization preparation phase consist of a 90° RF pulse followed by rapid echoplanar sampling of the FID signal with an effective TE of about 30 ms. In either case, the signal-to-noise ratio is decreased compared with the turbo gradient-echo methods. The trade-off is for temporal resolution and spatial coverage within the targeted contrast agent sampling period.

A recent study of Edelman and Li[23] compared these two basic approaches in normal subjects and found the contrast-to-noise ratio to be much better with the T1 weighted approach. In their version, 64 echoes were acquired in 32 ms with an effective TE of 22 ms. To suppress blood pool signal, dephasing gradients were symmetrically placed before and after the 180° RF pulse. The dephasing gradients were of 3-ms duration, placed along the selected slice and frequency-encoding directions. In a report by Grist, diffusion gradients similarly applied to reduce blood pool signal were effective, but also had the effect of compromising the myocardial signal intensity when a stress agent was used, presumably because of the increased motion-related spin dephasing associated with these gradients.[24] Thus, while the temporal resolution and spatial coverage features of single-shot EPI are promising, the approach that balances this concern with that of good contrast-to-noise presently requires continued development.

Techniques to Monitor Intrinsic Contrast

Magnetization Transfer Contrast

The signal intensity of tissues and the resulting image contrast in images obtained with conventional sequences depends predominantly, if not entirely, on the magnetization of tissue water. The magnetization from the protons bound in membrane structures and macromolecules is not believed to contribute to convention clinical images.[25] A contrast mechanism based on the transfer of the magnetization of protons in macromolecules to protons in water, termed magnetization transfer contrast (MTC), was introduced several years ago.[26] Of particular interest in cardiac imaging is the subsequent observation that MTC in cardiac images is also dependent on perfusion.[5]

MTC is a fundamental contrast mechanism wherein the protons in macromolecules are first selectively saturated. This magnetization saturation is then spontaneously transferred to the mobile water protons prior to routine image data acquisition. This transfer likely results from an exchange between the bound and mobile pools involving either chemical exchange or through dipolar interactions. The saturation of the macromolecules is achieved by low-power RF irradiations 5 to 10 kHz off resonance.[24] The reduced magnetization of the macromolecules is then transferred to the water protons, thereby reducing the bulk tissue water magnetization and signal intensity.[28,29] Thus, the effect of MTC on myocardium is to render it darker. When used for magnetization preparation preceding a standard gradient recalled echo acquisition, MTC can enhance the contrast between the blood pool and myocardium.[28–30]

To observe perfusion differences in the myocardium, MTC can be applied as a preparation pulse in a gradient echo sequence as shown in Figure 8. After the R wave trigger, an approximate 1-second pulse is applied, offset by approximately 6 kHz as implemented by Prasad et al.[5] When this preparation pulse is applied before an inversion recovery sequence, the MTC pulse is continued during the inversion period. In the referenced study, there was good correspondence between MTC images and first-pass gadopentetate (Gd-DTPA) turbo gradient-echo images of a rat heart with coronary artery ligation. In these images, the abnormal perfusion was seen as a dark region. Additional rat studies

MTC +T1 Turbo GRE

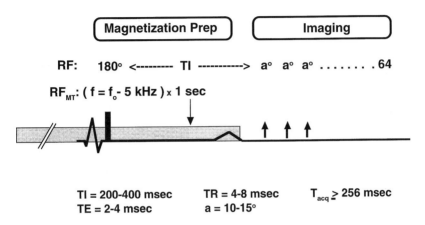

FIGURE 8. Method for magnetization transfer contrast (MTC) prepared T1 weighted turbo gradient-recalled echo (GRE). Produces image with MTC + T1 contrast.[23] f_0 indicates lamour resonant frequency. Abbreviations as above (see text).

from the same group also demonstrated an increase in signal that is linearly related to increasing coronary flow. The authors also noted that this signal increase was greatest with an inversion recovery turbo gradient-echo sequence preceeded by an MTC preparation pulse (Figure 8). Although not yet clinically demonstrated, the authors argue that a 20% change in regional blood flow would produce approximately a 4% change in image signal intensity, which could be detectable in images that are free of artifacts. This methodology has not been applied to studies in humans with coronary artery disease. However, both the theory and preliminary experience with animals indicate that further evaluation is warranted. Advantages include no restriction on the number of slices that could be imaged and the ability to repeat examinations easily, for example with and without dipyridamole.

Blood Oxygen Level Dependent Contrast

Blood oxygen level dependent (BOLD) imaging is, as the name implies, a technique in which the signal intensity is sensitive to the level of blood oxygen. More specifically, the image signal intensity is related to the level of paramagnetic deoxyhemoglobin. The deoxyhemoglobin decreases transverse magnetization consequent to increased magnetic susceptibility. As a magnetic susceptibility agent, deoxyhemoglobin serves as an intrinsic contrast agent. Its concentration decreases as perfusion increases, resulting in increased signal intensity. This effect was initially demonstrated in the brain and is now widely used to observe regional brain activity.[31,32] While this effect is technically more challenging to observe in the heart, it occurs to an even greater degree in the myocardium than in the cerebrum.[11,33] In comparison to the brain, which has a blood volume fraction of approximately 4%, the heart blood volume fraction of approximately 10% is significantly larger. In addition, the cardiac venous blood oxygen saturation of approximately 30% is lower than the 60% typically measured in the brain.[11] Consequently, the theoretical magnitude of the change in signal intensity that can be observed in the heart is greater. Indeed, several investigators have demonstrated the expected changes in myocardial signal intensity on gradient-echo sequences related to the level of deoxyhemoglobin,[6,7,11] or the level increased perfusion induced by dipyridamole,[11,35,36] or decreased perfusion from coronary ligation.[33,34]

Two basic techniques have been preliminarily evaluated in humans. The earliest technique to be explored was a T_2^* weighted EPI method.[34–36] With this approach, ECG gated single-shot EPI gradient-echo images are acquired with a TE = 15 ms and a TE = 29 ms. A trigger delay of 480–600 ms is used to acquire mid-diastolic images. All images are acquired during a breathhold to eliminate respiratory artifact. Comparing signal intensities at the two echo times gives a measure of T_2^*. The signal intensity of the T_2^* weighted images increased significantly with dipyridamole and correlates with magnetic resonance measurements of coronary flow.[36] This group has also shown in patients with coronary artery disease a similar comparison to flow measurements obtained by positron emission tomography.[35]

Recently, a more conventional double-echo gradient-echo technique for assessing the BOLD effect has been demonstrated in humans.[11] This technique is of particular interest because it can be executed on most conventional imagers. This technique is illustrated in Figure 9, and is based on a k-space segmented gradient-echo acquisition. Images at two echo times, TE = 7 ms, and 15 ms, are acquired with interleaved acquisitions as shown. After the initial R wave trigger, a 90° RF pulse is applied followed by a delay TD = 400–700 ms during which dephasing gradients are applied to eliminate any variable residual longitudinal magnetization from the previous excitation. After the TD, the imaging component of the sequence begins in which the appropriate k-space segment data are acquired. As implemented by Li et al,[11] the TR between these RF pulses was a 22.5 ms. Total acquisition time was 15 to 25 heartbeats so that images were obtained with a breathhold to eliminate respiratory artifact and associated data corruption. In addition to eliminating through-plane motion effects, the slice excitation thickness profile during the 90° RF pulse was 4 times wider than that

BOLD for Perfusion

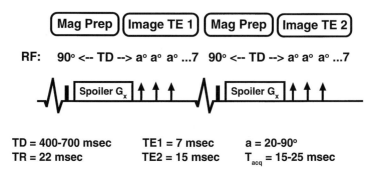

FIGURE 9. Method for generating images sensitive to blood oxygen level (ie, deoxyhomoglobin). Final parameter of interet is T_2^*, calculated from the images acquired at TE1 (echo time for first image) and TE2 (increased echo time for second image of same slice) (see text).

of the slice RF profile for the image data acquisition. The T_2^* image used for analysis of myocardial perfusion was then calculated from the two acquired images by

$$T_2^* = (TE2 - TE1)/\ln (S_1/S_2)$$

where TE2 = 15 ms, TE1 = 7 ms, and S_1, S_2 are the corresponding image signal intensities.

Using this technique, Li et al.[11] have presented promising data from normal subjects that show an approximate 40% change in T_2^* of the myocardium during dipyridamole administration versus an absence of a significant change during dobutamine stress. This observation suggests that this methodology is able to display on images the relation between metabolic oxygen supply and demand; this relation is balanced in normal subjects with dobutamine, (no change in T_2^*) in contrast to an increase in the oxygen supply versus demand with dipyridamole. The greater relative level of oxygen supply results in decreased venous deoxyhemoglobin and increased T_2^*.

In summary, both MTC and BOLD approaches, which are based on intrinsic contrast mechanisms, are relatively new and not yet well explored as techniques for imaging myocardial perfusion. The obvious appeal is that the entire heart can be imaged without the temporal restrictions imposed by efforts to monitor the first passage of a contrast agent. However the concern is the relatively small change in image signal intensity that must be detected. This imposes the need for images uncorrupted by flow or respiratory artifact.

References

1. Pettigrew RI, Avruch L, Dannels W, Bernardino M. Fast field echo MR imaging with Gd-DTPA: Physiologic evaluation of the kidney and liver. *Radiology.* 1986;160:561–563.
2. Atkinson DJ, Burstein D, Edelmann RR. First-pass cardiac perfusion: Evaluation with ultrafast MR imaging. *Radiology.* 1990;174:757–762.
3. Wilke N, Engels A, Weikl A, et al.Dynamic perfusion studies by ultrafast MR imaging: Initial clinical results from cardiology. *Electromedica.* 1990;58: 102.
4. Manning WJ, Atkinson DJ, Grassman W, et al. First pass MR imaging studies using gadolinium DTPA in patients with coronary artery disease. *J Am Coll Cardiol.* 1991;18:959–965.
5. Prasad PV, Burstein D, Edelman RR. MRI evaluation of myocardial perfusion without a contrast agent using magnetization transfer. *Magn Reson Med* 1993;30:267–270.
6. Wendland MF, Saeed M, Lauerma K, et al. Endogenous susceptibility contrast in myocardium during apnea measured using gradient recalled echo planar imaging. *Magn Reson Med.* 1993;29:273–276.
7. Atalay MK, Forder JR, Chacko VCP, et al. Oxygenation in the rabbit myocardium: Assessment with susceptibility-dependent MR imaging. *Radiology.* 1993;189:759–764.
8. Schaefer S, Tyen RV, Saloner O. Evaluation of myocardial perfusion abnormalities with gadolinium-enhanced snapshot MR imaging in humans. *Radiology.* 1992;185:795–801.
9. Wilke N, Simm C, Zhang J, et al. Contrast-enhanced first pass myocardial perfusion imaging: Correlation between myocardial blood flow in dogs at rest and during hyperemia. *Magn Reson Med* 1993;29:485–497.
10. Moonen CTW, Liu G, Gelderen PV, Sobering G. A fast gradient-recalled MRI technique with increased sensitivity to dynamic susceptibility effects. *Magn Reson Med.* 1992;26:184–189.
11. Li D, Dhawale P, Rubin PJ, et al. Myocardial signal response to dipyridamole and dobutamine: Demonstration of the BOLD effect using a double-echo gradient-echo sequence. *Magn Reson Med.* 1996;36:16–20.
12. Gould KL, Lipscomb K, Hamilton GW. Physiologic basis for assessing critical coronary stenosis. *Am J Cardiol.* 1974;33:87–94.
13. Klocke FJ. Measurements of coronary flow reserve: Defining pathophysiology versus making decisions about patient care. *Circulation* 1987;76:1183.
14. Beller G. Dipyridamole cardiac imaging. *JAMA.* 1991;265:633.
15. Crystal GJ, Downey HF, Bashour FA. Small vessel and total coronary blood volume during intracoronary adenosine. *Am J Physiol.* 1981;24:H194–201.
16. McGuinness ME, Talbert RL. Pharmacologic stress testing: Experience with dipyridamole, adenosine, and dobutamine. *Am J Hosp Pharm.* 1994;51: 328–346.
17. Burstein D, Taratutra E, Manning W. Factors in myocardial "perfusion" imaging with ultrafast MRI and Gd-DTPA administration. *Magn Reson Med.* 1991;20:299–305.
18. Wilke N, Kroll K, Merkle H, et al. Regional myocardial blood volume and flow via first pass imaging in concert with polylysine-gadolinium-DTPA. *J Magn Reson Imaging.* 1994;1995;5:227.
19. Rendel P. Snapshot MRI with T_2^*-weighted magnetization preparation. *Magn Reson Med.* 1993;30:399–402.

20. Tsekos NV, Zhang U, Merkle H, et al. Fast anatomical imaging of the heart and assessment of myocardial perfusion with arrhythmia insensitive magnetization preparation. *Magn Reson Med* 1995;34:530–536.
21. Stehling MK, Turner R, Mansfield P. Echo-planar imaging: Magnetic resonance imaging in a fraction of a second. *Science.* 1991;254:43–50.
22. Wendland MF, Saeed M, Masui T, et al. Echo-planar MR imaging of normal and ischemic myocardium with gadodiamide injection. *Radiology.* 1993;186: 535–542.
23. Edelman RR, Li W. Contrast-enhanced echo-planar MR imaging of myocardial perfusion: Preliminary study in humans. *Radiology.* 1994;190:771–777.
24. Grist TM, Korosec FR, Fisher DJ, Mistretta CA. Echo-planar imaging in patients with myocardial perfusion abnormalities. In: *Proceedings of the Society of Magnetic Resonance Annual Meeting,* August 1994, 106.
25. Dixon WT. Use of magnetization transfer contrast in gradient recalled echo images (editorial). *Radiology.* 1991;179:15–16.
26. Wolff SD, Balaban RS. Magnetization transfer contrast (MTC) and tissue water proton relaxation in vivo. *Magn Reson Med.* 1989;10:135–144.
27. Wolff SD, Eng J, Balaban RS. Magnetization transfer contrast: method to improve contrast in gradient-recalled echo images. *Radiology.* 1991;179: 133–137.
28. Balaban RS, Chesnick S, Hedges K, et al. Magnetization transfer contrast in MR imaging of the heart. *Radiology.* 1991;180:671–675.
29. Scholz TD, Ceckler TL, Balaban RS. Magnetization transfer characterization of hypertensive cardiomyopathy: Significance of tissue water content. *Magn Reson Med.* 1993;29:352–357.
30. Balaban RS, Ceckler TL. Magnetization transfer contrast in magnetic resonance imaging. *Magn Reson Q.* 1992;8:116–137.
31. Kwong KK, Belliveau JW, Chesler DA, et al. Dynamic magnetic resonance imaging of the human brain activity during primary sensory stimulation. In: *Proceedings of the National Academy of Science of the United Status of America* 1992;89:5675–5679.
32. Ogawa S, Menon RS, Tank DW, et al. Functional brain mapping by blood oxygenation level-dependent contrast magnetic resonance imaging: A comparison of signal characteristics with a biophysical model. *Biophys J.* 1993; 64:803–812.
33. Balaban RS, Taylor JF, Turner R. Effect of cardiac flow on gradient recalled echo images of the canine heart. *NMR Biomed.* 1994;7:89–95.
34. Stillman AE, Wilke N, Jerosch-Herold M, et al. BOLD contrast of the heart during occlusion and reperfusion. In: *Works in Progress Supplement, SMR, 1st Meeting, Dallas 1994.* p. S24–S25.
35. Poncelet B, Weisskoff RM, Zervos G, et al. FPI detection of changes in coronary flow velocity and myocardial tissue perfusion during hyperemia in patients with coronary artery disease. In: *Proceedings of the Society of Magnetic Resonance. Third Scientific Meeting and Exhibition, Nice, France.* 1995, p 20.
36. Niemi P, Poncelet BP, Kwong KK, et al. Myocardial intensity changes associated with flow stimulation in blood oxygenation sensitive MRI. *Magn Reson Med.* 1996;36:78–82..

## Chapter 4

Magnetic Resonance Angiography
Techniques

Martin R. Prince, MD, PhD

Magnetic resonance angiography (MRA) is used increasingly to evaluate arterial and venous diseases.[1-11]. Although the resolution of magnetic resonance is not as high as conventional arteriography, it is sufficient to evaluate pathological conditions in large vascular structures, including the aorta and its major branches. It is especially useful in patients who cannot tolerate the risks of iodinated contrast or arterial catheterization. This includes patients with a serum creatinine greater than 2 mg/dL or with a history of major allergic reaction to iodinated contrast.[12]

There are numerous MRA techniques, and every year more and more are introduced that take advantage of the tremendous variety of magnetic resonance imaging (MRI) effects and capabilities. This chapter reviews the underlying principles of the five most basic and useful techniques and demonstrates examples of how these techniques are used in clinical practice.

Black Blood Imaging

The most important pulse sequence for imaging large vascular structures is the T1 weighted spin-echo sequence with the parameters optimized to allow intravoxel dephasing within the blood vessels. This intravoxel dephasing destroys the signal within flowing blood, causing

Supported in part by National Institutes of Health grant HL46384.

From: Higgins CB, Ingwall JS, Pohost GM, (eds). *Current and Future Applications of Magnetic Resonance in Cardiovascular Disease*. Armonk, NY: Futura Publishing Company, Inc.; © 1998.

a black-blood effect. To obtain images in which the blood appears black (as a flow void), it is necessary to obtain the standard T1 weighted image with a sufficiently long TE so that the blood flows away and disperses its signal between the 90° pulse and the echo. Generally, a TE of 20 to 30 ms is adequate for arteries and veins with normal flow.

The black blood effect creates image contrast between black vessels and the surrounding tissues that have typical T1 contrast with bright fat and intermediate intensity of the muscles and organs. This contrast allows evaluation not only of the vessel lumens but also of the aortic wall. It is especially useful in patients with vasculitis, which may cause thickening of the aortic wall. The ability to see the relation between the vessels and the surrounding structures also helps to evaluate anatomic variations, whether congenital or acquired.

With extremely slow flow, such as in patients with heart failure or with aneurysmal disease, even very long TE's may not result in complete flow voids. In addition, the poor signal-to-noise of flow voids makes it difficult to resolve smaller vessels with black blood images. For these reasons, a number of bright blood techniques have been developed.

Time of Flight

The most basic of the bright blood MRA techniques is known as time-of-flight imaging. Time-of-flight images are acquired by giving the magnetic resonance pulses rapidly using a very short TR of approximately 10 to 50 ms. These pulses are so rapid that none of the tissues have time to recover their longitudinal magnetization. Thus, all tissues are dark. Only where fresh blood flows into the plane of imaging is there bright signal. This is because the blood flowing into the image plane has not been exposed to any previous pulses and thus has its full longitudinal magnetization available to give off signal.

In time-of-flight imaging, the signal is acquired as quickly as possible after each magnetic resonance pulse (ie, with a TE as short as possible, <10 ms) in order to capture the signal before blood flow causes phase dispersion. In fact, with time-of-flight imaging, there is not enough time for the 180° refocusing pulse; the 180° pulse is eliminated. The pulse sequence used for time-of-flight MRA is known as a gradient-echo pulse sequence. Thus, fresh blood flowing into the imaging plane has bright signal, but the background is dark. This technique works best when the slices are thin and perpendicular to the direction of blood flow in order to maximize the fraction of blood that has been refreshed by inflow into the image plane.

It is important to make the TR as short as possible for time-of-flight imaging, but still long enough to allow blood to flow into the imaging plane. A typical blood velocity is approximately 1 mm per 10 ms (10 cm/sec). At this velocity, for a slice thickness of 3 mm, the TR needs to be about 30 ms in order to have optimal inflow of fresh, unsaturated spins. If the slice thickness becomes much thicker or the vessel is not perpendicular to the image plane, or the patient has particularly slow flow in the artery of interest, then either the TR must be increased, the slice thickness must be decreased, or the flip angle must be decreased in order to have sufficiently bright blood. Some large arteries may have faster flow particularly during systole that may allow using shorter repetition times.

Time-of-flight images come in two varieties, two dimensional and three dimensional. Two-dimensional time-of-flight is very fast but lower in resolution and can be degraded by slice misregistration artifacts. Slice misregistration is the failure of one slice to line up perfectly with the next slice because of variations in patient positioning from coughing, breathing, or moving. Three-dimensional time-of-flight has higher resolution and eliminates misregistration, but is much slower. The two-dimensional time-of-flight imaging is well suited for evaluating for deep venous thrombosis (Figure 1) and for evaluating the runoff from the distal aorta to the ankles where it is necessary to cover a long distance in a reasonable length of time. Three-dimensional time-of-flight imaging, however, is best for renal arteries, the circle of Willis, and the carotid bifurcation, where it is possible to spend 10 to 20 minutes of imaging time on a small region of the body and high resolution is essential.

Time-of-flight images can be confusing when there is bright signal in both the arteries and veins. This can be remedied by using presaturation pulses. Presaturation pulses are pulses that are applied prior to the imaging radiofrequency pulse in order to change the magnetization of the tissues in advance of imaging. Because arteries and veins typically flow in opposite directions, application of a presaturation pulse above or below the plane of imaging will generally selectively saturate either the arteries or the veins. By using a chemically selective preparatory pulse applied within the plane of imaging, it is also possible to selectively saturate fat (the brightest background tissue). This is sometimes referred to as fat saturation.

In order to eliminate respiratory motion, time-of-flight MRA may be performed during breathholding. More sophisticated respiratory gating and navigator echo techniques are being developed to reduce respiratory motion artifacts without requiring breathholding. ECG gating is also possible for minimizing vascular pulsation artifacts. By trig-

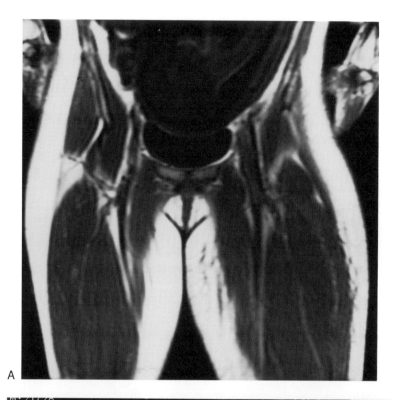

A

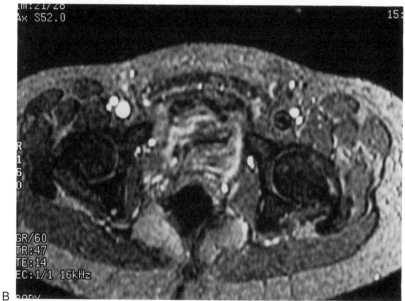

B

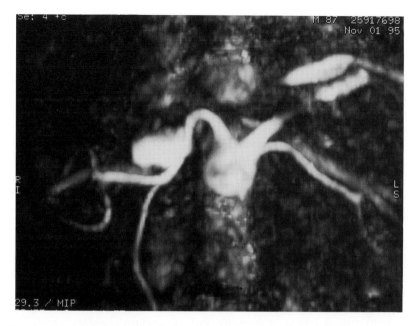

FIGURE 2. Three-dimensional phase contrast magnetic resonance angiography (MRA) in an 87-year-old patient. The data are displayed with brightness corresponding to velocity. Note that the renal arteries (with faster flow) are brighter than the renal veins.

gering off the R wave and using an appropriate delay, data can be acquired during either systole or diastole. Because only a small segment of image data (k-space data) can be acquired during each R-R interval, this approach is sometimes referred to as a segmented k-space acquisition.

Phase Contrast

Magnetic resonance physics allows for encoding additional information in addition to the spatial position of spins. One example used in MR angiography is known as phase contrast imaging (Figure 2). With

FIGURE 1. Nineteen-year-old female of 26 weeks gestation with deep venous thrombosis of left common femoral vein. **A:** T1 spin-echo image shows the left leg is swollen compared with the right leg and the left common femoral vein does not have a black flow void. **B:** Two-dimensional time-of-flight at the level of the femoral heads shows normal in-flow enhancement of the right common femoral vein but no in-flow enhancement of the left common femoral vein.

this technique, flow direction and velocity information are encoded into the image data set. This can be very useful for quantitating blood flow and for determining the flow direction in a particular vessel of interest. Of course, the additional time required for the encoding process can double or triple the amount of time required to collect the image data, depending on how many flow directions need to be encoded.

Phase contrast MRA also requires specifying the range of velocities to be encoded. The image quality is directly related to how accurately the velocity encoding (known as Venc) is selected. The optimal Venc is generally selected by trial and error, which becomes less tedious with increasing experience.

Cine

In arteries that have pulsatile flow, this variation in flow with the cardiac cycle can be evaluated with the cine technique. With cine imaging, data are acquired while monitoring the ECG such that multiple images at the same location are reconstructed to represent multiple phases of the cardiac cycle. This enormously increases image acquisition time by a factor of 5 or 10. But for certain diseases, this extra information is crucial. For example, in aortic dissection, cine allows evaluation of the flow in the true and false lumens and can freeze the motion of the intimal flap so that the presence and extent of aortic dissection can be assessed with greater confidence. It is also extremely useful for evaluating valvular disease. By combining cine and phase contrast imaging, it is possible to quantitate pulsatile flow.

Gadolinium-Enhanced Magnetic Resonance Angiography[7-10]

The preceding MRA techniques all take advantage of the exquisite sensitivity of magnetic resonance for detecting motion to differentiate between moving blood and stationary vessel walls and surrounding tissues. These techniques work well in normal arteries that have normal laminar blood flow. But in patients with vascular disease, where the flow is disturbed, these techniques are not as effective. Patients with aneurysmal disease, poor cardiac output, or with tortuous vessels are particularly problematic for the standard MRA techniques. In these patients, it is useful to image the arteries with a bright blood technique, which does not depend on blood flow. Bright blood images, based on anatomy, are obtained by injecting a sufficient dose of gadolinium to make the blood T1 shorter than the T1 of all surrounding tissue (Figures 3–5). For the gadolinium compounds currently available, a dose of at

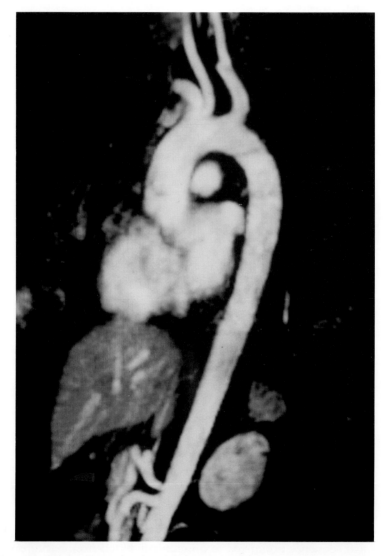

FIGURE 3. Three-dimensional gadolinium-enhanced magnetic resonance angiography (MRA) of a normal thoracic aorta. Reprinted with permission from Reference 8.

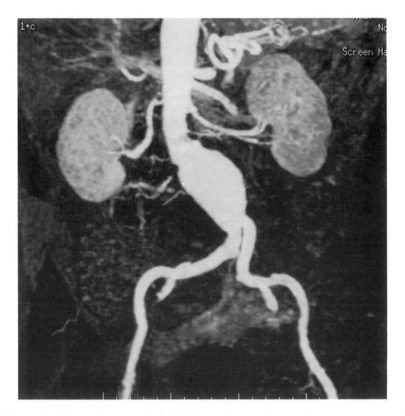

FIGURE 4. Three-dimensional gadolinium-enhanced magnetic resonance angiography (MRA) of abdominal aortic aneurysm.

least 0.2 mmol/kg (double dose) is required to reduce the blood T1 to less than that of fat (T1 = 270 ms), the brightest background tissue. In general, the higher the dose of gadolinium the better the vascular enhancement, up to about 0.5–1.0 mmol/kg where the T_2^* effects can begin to reduce signal on T1 weighted gradient-echo images if the TE is not short enough.

Once the T1 of blood is shortened with a gadolinium infusion, a T1 weighted sequence optimized to differentiate blood from background tissues is required. The three-dimensional spoiled gradient echo pulse sequence is particularly useful. This sequence provides high-resolution images with near isotropic voxels and minimizes pulsatility and misregistration artifacts. The blurring effect of vessel motion occurring during systole results in the images primarily representing the anatomic appearance during diastole. Surprisingly, these images show

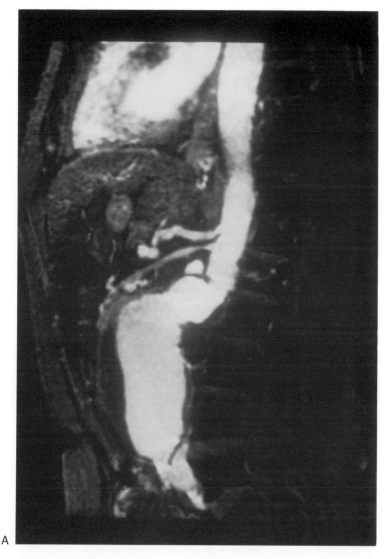

A

FIGURE 5. Sagittal **(A)** gadolinium-enhanced two-dimensional time-of-flight of abdominal aortic aneurysm and **(B)** conventional aortogram.

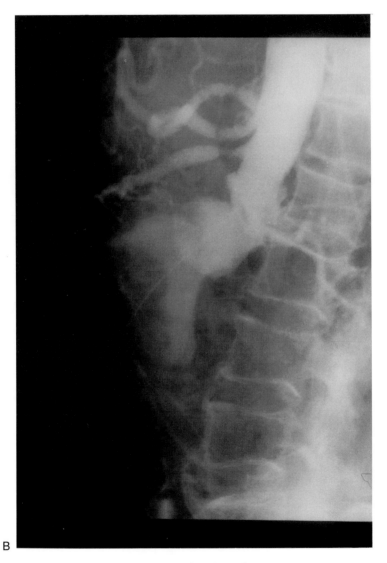

B

FIGURE 5. *(continued)*

minimal cardiac motion artifacts, even in the ascending aorta, without requiring ECG or peripheral gating.

The degree of T1 weighting is modulated by adjusting the flip angle. For a TR of approximately 25 ms with a gadolinium dose of 0.2–0.3 mmol/kg infused over 2 to 3 minutes, a flip angle of 40° is appropriate. If the TR is substantially reduced, the flip angle may have to be reduced such that for a TR of 15 ms a flip angle of 30° is more appropriate. If the dose is increased, better signal-to-noise and contrast-to-noise may be obtained by increasing the flip angle. It is also essential to use a TE where fat and water are out-of-phase. At 1.5 T, echo times of approximately 2.3 or 6.9 ms are appropriate.

By imaging during the infusion of contrast, it is possible to preferentially enhance the arteries. This allows evaluation of the aorta and its branch vessels without the confounding effect of excessive venous enhancement. This preferential arterial enhancement is maximized by timing the gadolinium infusion such that the period of maximum arterial gadolinium concentration corresponds with the acquisition of the center half of k-space. For most gradient-echo pulse sequences, the center of k-space is acquired during the middle of the acquisition, so it is important to maintain the highest infusion rate during the middle of the acquisition.

When using a dynamic infusion, the infusion rate must be sufficient to maintain a high intra-arterial gadolinium level, and it must last for most of the acquisition. Thus, it is crucial to not have a too long an acquisition time. For a gadolinium dose of 0.2–0.3 mmol/kg, an acquisition time of 3 to 4 minutes is acceptable. In the abdomen, it is useful to keep the acquisition under 1 minute so that it can be performed in a single breathhold.[13] It is also useful to standardize one volume of gadolinium contrast to use in every patient in order to get used to the timing of the infusion. Generally two bottles of gadolinium (42 mL) is an appropriate dose for most patients.

Appendix

THORACIC AORTA PROTOCOL

PATIENT PREPARATION

Valium 5-10 mg.

Respiratory Comp.

EKG Gating

IV

	Contrast Type:	Omniscan
	Contrast Amt.	<90 lbs.--21cc
		<200 lbs.--42cc
		>210 lbs.--63cc

PATIENT POSITIONING

ENTRY: Head First

POSITION: Supine

COIL: Body

LANDMARK: Nipple line

If pt. is small, decrease FOV on localizer to 40 cm

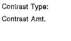

ALIGNMENT OF EACH SERIES

SERIES 2: AXIAL T1 BLACK BLOOD

-From just above the arch down to
diaphragm. Use sufficient skip to cover with
one acquisition.

SERIES 3: AXIAL FASTCARD (OPTIONAL)

-Two slices only

-1 at rt pulmonary artery

-1 through ventricles

SERIES 4: SAG 3D DURING GADO

-Top edge 3 cm. above arch

-Right to include right edge of ascending
aorta

-Left to include left edge of descending aorta

SERIES 5: AXIAL FASTCARD POST GAD (OPTIONAL)

-4 slices through arch

-1 at right pulmonary artery *

-1 at aortic valve

-1 through ventricles *

* at same levels as pre gad fastcard images

SERIES 6: AXIAL 2DTOF POST GAD

-8 skip 10 to cover from arch down to aortic
bifurcation

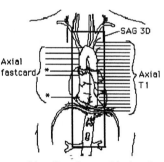

* location of pre gad fastcards

FILMING INSTRUCTIONS

-All series filmed 12 on 1.

-For series 1 and 2, film all images.

-For series 3, film the single best image at each location.

-For series 4, film on Windows workstation; coronal, sag & sag obl. protocols

-For series 5, film the single best image at each location.

-For series 6, film all images.

-Transfer all images to the Windows workstation.

BILLING

-MRA Chest with or without contrast (771555)

-Contrast enhanced exam (799070)

THORACIC AORTA

SEQUENCE	1 COR LOC	2 AXIAL T1 BLACK BLOOD	3 AXIAL FASTCARD (OPTIONAL)	4 SAG 3D DURING GADO	5 AXIAL FASTCARD POST GAD (OPTIONAL)	6 AX 2DTOF
SCAN PLANE	CORONAL	AXIAL	AXIAL	SAGITTAL	AXIAL	AXIAL
MODE	2D	2D	2D	3D	2D	2D
PULSE SEQUENCE	SPIN ECHO	SPIN ECHO	GRE	VASC TOF SPGR	GRE	GRE
IMAGING OPTIONS	RC EKG GATING NP	RC EKG GATING NP	FC GATING SEQ. NP FAST GRAPHIC RX	FAST GRAPHIC RX	FC GATING SEQ. NP FAST GRAPHIC RX	FC NP SEQUENTIAL RC GRAPHIC RX
PROJECTION IMAGES				COLLAPSE / 0		
USER CVS			0		0	
FLIP ANGLE			60	30	60	45
# OF ECHOES	1	1				
TE	20	20	MINIMUM	MINIMUM	MINIMUM	MINIMUM FULL
TR						23
BANDWIDTH			16kHz	16kHz	16kHz	
GATING-TRIGGER TYPE	AUTO LEAD	AUTO LEAD				
EFFECTIVE TR	1RR	1RR				
TRIGGER DELAY	MINIMUM	MINIMUM				
TRIGGER WINDOW	15	15				
INT. SEQUENCE DELAY	MINIMUM	MINIMUM				
CARDIAC PHASES	SINGLE	SINGLE				
TRIGGER TYPE			AUTO LEAD		AUTO LEAD	
TRIGGER WINDOW			15		15	
VIEWS / SEGMENT			8		8	
FOV	40 or 48	32	32	36	32	32
SLICE THICKNESS	8	10	8	2-3 (2.5)	8	8
SLICE SPACING	3	5	0		0	10
SAT PULSES						
SCANNING RANGE	P80-A63		GRAPHIC	GRAPHIC	GRAPHIC	GRAPHIC
# OF SLICES	14		2	28	7	
MATRIX-FREQUENCY	256	256	256	256	256	256
MATRIX-PHASE	256	256	128	256	128	256
FREQUENCY DIR.	SI	RL	RL	SI	RL	RL
PHASE FOV				1		
NEX / SCAN TIME	2 / 8:54	2 / 8:54	4 / 1:06 PER SLICE	2 / 3:52	4 / 1:06 PER SLICE	4 / :22 PER SLICE
REPS BEFORE PAUSE			NONE		NONE	1
CONTRAST	NO	NO	NO	YES	YES	YES

AAA PROTOCOL

PATIENT PREPARATION

Valium 5-10 mg
Respiratory Comp.
IV with custom MR tubing set

Contrast Type: Omniscan
Contrast Amt: < 90 Lbs.--21cc diluted with NaCl to 42cc
                   <210 Lbs.--42cc
                   >200 Lbs.--63cc

PATIENT POSITIONING

ENTRY: Head First

POSITION: Supine

COIL: Body--If pt. is very thin (≤100 lbs.) use torso
             array coil

LANDMARK: Mid-kidney (between xyphoid and iliac crests)

Landmark

ALIGNMENT OF EACH SERIES

SERIES 2: COR 3D DURING GADO

    -top edge at diaphragm

    -ant. edge at bend in SMA, anterior to left renal vein

    -post. edge at mid-kidney

    -you will miss the anterior edge af AAA

SERIES 3: SAG 2DTOF

    -6-8 slices centered on celiac and SMA

SERIES 4: AXIAL 2DTOF

    -contiguous slices through celiac, SMA & renal arteries

    -5 extra slices of abdominal aorta and iliacs below renals

SERIES 5: AXIAL 3DPC POST GADO

    -cover renal arteries

    -include SMA and celiac if possible

    -If creatinine is >2.0, then decrease VENC to 20

Sag 2dtof

Axial 3dpc

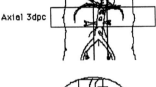

Coronals

Axial 2dtof

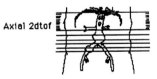

FILMING INSTRUCTIONS

SERIES 1:   12 on 1--2 sheets of film
SERIES 2:   Film on Windows workstation
SERIES 3:   12 on 1 with cross reference
SERIES 4:   12 on 1 with cross reference
SERIES 5:   Film on Windows workstation
      TRANSFER ALL IMAGES TO WINDOWS WORKSTATION

BILLING

-MRA Abdomen with or without contrast (774185)
-Contrast enhanced exam (799070)

AAA

SEQUENCE	1 SAG T1 LOCALIZER	2 COR 3D DURING GADO	3 SAG 2DTOF	4 AX 2DTOF	5 AXIAL 3DPC
SCAN PLANE	SAGITTAL	CORONAL	SAGITTAL	AXIAL	AXIAL
MODE	2D	3D	2D	2D	3D
PULSE SEQUENCE	SPIN ECHO	VASC TOF SPGR	GRE	GRE	VASC PC
IMAGING OPTIONS	RC NP	FC	FC SEQUENTIAL	FC NP SEQUENTIAL	FC
		GRAPHIC RX	FC	RC GRAPHIC RX	GRAPHIC RX
PROJECTION IMAGES		COLLAPSE / 0			COLLAPSE / 0
ACQ. FLOW DIRECTION					ALL
ADDITIONAL IMAGES					R/L FLOW
FLOW RECON TYPE					PHASE DIFFERENCE
VELOCITY ENCODING					30 CM/SEC
FLIP ANGLE		40	45	45	35
# OF ECHOES	1			1	
TE	MINIMUM FULL	6.9	MINIMUM	MINIMUM FULL	
TR	385	26	33	23	24
BANDWIDTH		16kHz			
FOV	40-48 (44)	(36)-40	36	32	30
SLICE THICKNESS	8	2.5-3 (2.7)	6	8	2
SLICE SPACING	INTERLEAVE			0	
SAT PULSES					
SCANNING RANGE	L92-R92	GRAPHIC		GRAPHIC	GRAPHIC
# OF SLICES	24--2 ACQUISITIONS	28	6 TO 8		60
MATRIX-FREQUENCY	256	256	256	256	256
MATRIX-PHASE	256	256	192	256	128
FREQUENCY DIRECTION	SI	SI	SI	RL	RL
PHASE FOV		1	1		
NEX / SCAN TIME	2 / 7:11	1 / 3:36	4	4 / :22 PER SLICE	1 / 13:07
REPS. BEFORE PAUSE				1	
CONTRAST	NO	YES	YES	YES	YES

RENAL ARTERY PROTOCOL

PATIENT PREPARATION

Valium 5-10 mg.

Respiratory Comp.

IV with custom MR tubing set

Oxygen if pt. will have trouble breathholding

Contrast Type: Omniscan

Contrast Amt: < 90 Lbs.--21cc

                    <210 Lbs.--42cc

                    >200 Lbs.--63cc

PATIENT POSITIONING

ENTRY: Head First

POSITION: Supine

COIL: Body--If pt. is very thin (≤100 lbs.) use

             torso array coil

LANDMARK: Mid-kidney (between xyphoid and

             iliac crests)

Landmark

ALIGNMENT OF EACH SERIES

SERIES 2: CORONAL BREATHHOLD TOF (optional)

    -Center at top edge of kidneys

    -Anterior to aorta at level of SMA

    -Posterior edge at mid-kidneys

    -No more than 21 slices--3 slices per breathhold

SERIES 3: AXIAL T2 FAT SAT KIDNEYS

    -Cover kidneys

Axial
T2 fat
sat

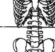

SERIES 4: CORONAL 3D DURING GADO

    -Use foam cushions to elevate arms

    -Top edge at diaphragm (below the heart)

    -Anterior to left renal vein

    -Posterior to mid kidneys

    -Try to keep slice thickness at 2 mm

    -47 second breathhold

      -scan delay=5 seconds

          =15 seconds if CHF

    -If pt. cannot breathhold, use series 2 from AAA protocol

celiac-

sma

left renal
vein

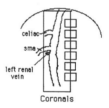

Coronals

SERIES 5: AXIAL PHASE CONTRAST

    -Cover renal arteries with top edge above celiac if possible

    -Do not change slice thickness

    -If pt. older than 70, has heart disease,or creatinine >2,

    use VENC of 30. If creatinine>3, VENC=20

Axial
PC

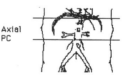

FILMING INSTRUCTIONS

SERIES 1 & 3:   12 on 1--2 sheets of film

SERIES 2:   Do not film

SERIES 4:   1 sheet of 11 coronal MIP images per windows protocol (set batch movie loop).

SERIES 5:   1 sheet of 11 axial MIP images per windows protocol (set batch movie loop).

          TRANSFER ALL IMAGES TO WINDOWS WORKSTATION.

BILLING

      -MRA Abdomen with or without contrast (774185)

      -Contrast enhanced exam (799070)

RENAL ARTERY

SEQUENCE	1 SAG LOC	2 COR 2DTOF BREATHHOLD (opt)	3 AXIAL T2 FAT SAT KIDNEYS	4 CORONAL 3D DURING GADO	5 AXIAL 3D PC
SCAN PLANE	SAGITTAL	CORONAL	AXIAL	CORONAL	AXIAL
MODE	2D	2D	2D	3D	3D
PULSE SEQUENCE	SPIN ECHO	VASC TOF SPGR	SPIN ECHO	VASC TOF SPGR	VASC PC
IMAGING OPTIONS	FC NP	FC NP SEQ ED	FC FAST	FAST	FC
		GRAPHIC RX	GRAPHIC RX	GRAPHIC RX	GRAPHIC RX
USER CVS			1		
PROJECTION IMAGES		COLLAPSE / 0		COLLAPSE / 0	COLLAPSE / 0
ACQ. FLOW DIRECTION					ALL
ADDITIONAL IMAGES					R/L FLOW
FLOW RECON TYPE					PHASE DIFFERENCE
VELOCITY ENCODING					30-50 CM/SEC
ETL			8		
FLIP ANGLE		30		45	35
# OF ECHOES	1		1		
TE	MIN FULL	6.9	102	MINIMUM	
TR	385	20	3000		24
BANDWIDTH				32 kHz	
FOV	40	32	32-36	28-32 (30)	28-32 (30)
SLICE THICKNESS	8	2.9	7	2.2	2
SLICE SPACING	INTERLEAVE		2		
SAT PULSES			SI /FAT		
SCANNING RANGE	L92-R92	GRAPHIC	GRAPHIC	GRAPHIC	GRAPHIC
# OF SLICES	24–2 ACQUISITIONS		17 PER ACQ	28	60
MATRIX-FREQUENCY	256	256	256	256	256
MATRIX-PHASE	256	128	256	128	128
FREQUENCY DIRECTION	SI	SI	R/L	SI	R/L
PHASE FOV			1	1	
NEX / SCAN TIME	2 / 7:11	2 / :11 PER SLICE	3 / 5:00 PER ACQ	1 / 0:47	1 / 12:34
REPS. BEFORE PAUSE		1	NONE		
CONTRAST	NO	NO	NO	YES	YES

References

1. Anderson CM, Edelman RR, Turski P. *Clinical Magnetic Resonance Angiography.* New York: Raven Press; 1993.
2. Edelman RR. Basic principles of magnetic resonance angiography. *Cardiovasc Intervent Radiol.* 1992;15:3–13.
3. Grist TM. Magnetic resonance angiography of renal artery stenosis. *Am J Kidney Dis.* 1994;24:700–712.
4. Higgins C. *Essentials of Cardiac Radiology and Imaging.* Philadelpia: J.B. Lippincott; 1992.
5. Nienaber CA, von Kodolitsch Y, Nicolas V, et al. The diagnosis of thoracic aortic dissection by noninvasive imaging procedures. *N Engl J Med* 1993; 328:1–9.
6. Potchen E, Haacke E, Siebert J, et al. *Magnetic Resonance Angiography: Concepts and Applications.* St. Louis: Mosby-Year Book, 1993.
7. Prince MR. Grist TM, Debatin JF. *3D Contrast MR Angiography.* New York, Springer; 1997.
8. Prince MR. Gadolinium-enhanced MR aortography. *Radiology.* 1994;191: 155–164.
9. Prince MR, Narasimham DL, Stanley JC, et al. Breath-held 3D gadolinium MRA: New developments for imaging the abdominal aorta and its major branches. *Radiology.* 1995;197:785–792.
10. Prince MR, Narasimham DL, Jacoby WT. Three dimensional Gd-enhanced MR angiography of the thoracic aorta. *AJR.* 1996;166:1387–1397.
11. Yucel E. *Magnetic Resonance Angiography: A Practical Approach.* New York: McGraw-Hill; 1995.
12. Prince MR, Arnoldus C, Frisoli JK. Nephrotoxicity of high-dose gadolinium compared with iodinated contrast. *J Magn Reson Imaging.* 1996;1:162–166.
13. Prince MR, Grist TM, Debatin JF. *3-D Contrast MRA.* Heidelberg: Springer-Verlag; 1977.

## Part 2

Magnetic Resonance Imaging: Morphology

## Chapter 5

Magnetic Resonance Imaging in Myocardial and Pericardial Disease

Richard D. White, MD

Introduction

Magnetic resonance imaging (MRI) is well suited for the evaluation of acquired cardiac conditions, including nonischemic myocardial diseases and pericardial diseases. Because of its ability to provide valuable information about the associated structural, histological, and functional (contraction, relaxation/filling, and hemodynamic) manifestations of these two disease groups, MRI has unique capabilities compared with other imaging modalities.

Myocardial Diseases

Nonischemic myocardial diseases are represented by the entities more often referred to as the cardiomyopathies (CMs). The CMs constitute a group of diseases in which the dominant feature is pathology of the heart muscle unrelated to ischemic, hypertensive, congenital, valvular, or pericardial diseases.[1,2]

A variety of schemes have been proposed for classifying the CMs.[3] The following categorization is helpful: (1) dilated CM causing ventricular dilatation, contractile dysfunction, and symptoms of congestive heart failure; (2) hypertrophic CM associated with inappropriate hypertrophy of the left ventricle (LV), often with asymmetric septal involvement, and usually preserved or enhanced overall contractile function,

From: Higgins CB, Ingwall JS, Pohost GM, (eds). *Current and Future Applications of Magnetic Resonance in Cardiovascular Disease.* Armonk, NY: Futura Publishing Company, Inc.; © 1998.

despite frequent regional impairment; (3) restrictive CM characterized by impaired diastolic filling; and (4) right ventricular CM causing dilatation and regionally or globally impaired contractility of the right ventricle (RV) related to dysplasia, with partial to total replacement of the myocardium by variable amounts of adipose and fibrosis tissue.[1,2] The distinctions between these categories are not absolute; there is often overlap.

Dilated Cardiomyopathy

MRI can readily define the abnormally enlarged cavity size (Figure 1) and globally depressed function (Figure 2) of the LV and RV in cases of dilated CM.[4,5] In contrast to normals, patients with dilated CM fail to demonstrate a gradient of progressively increasing systolic wall thickening from base to apex and have significantly decreased ejection

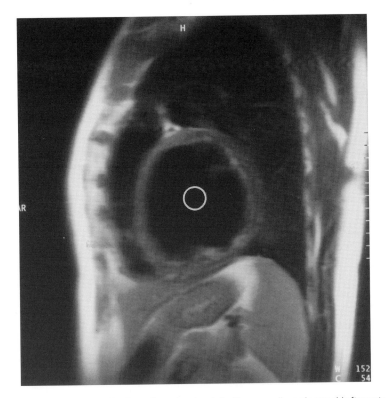

FIGURE 1. Dilated CM (spin-echo; short axis). Abnormally enlarged left ventricular cavity size (open circle).

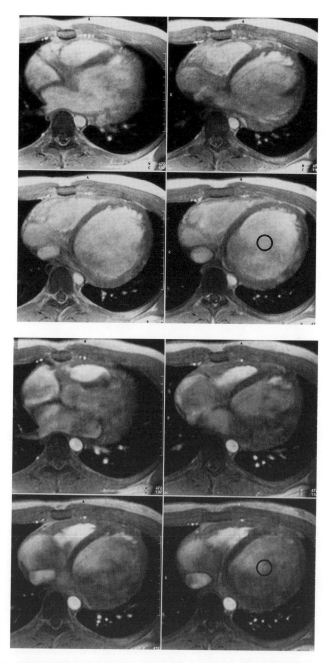

FIGURE 2. Dilated CM (cine gradient-echo; adjacent transaxial). Globally depressed left ventricular systolic function with minimal change in size of cavity (open circles) from end diastole (**A**) to end systole (**B**).

fractions on cine MRI,[6,7] although improvement in left ventricular ejection fractions (LVEF) from afterload reduction by angiotensin-converting-enzyme (ACE) inhibitor therapy has been demonstrated.[8] The effects of therapy with an ACE inhibitor on diastolic dysfunction have also been assessed using cine MRI in patients suffering from dilated CM with and without mitral regurgitation; analysis of LV time-volume curves revealed improvements in both peak-filling rate/end-diastolic volume ratios and ejection fractions in the group without, but not in the group with, mitral regurgitation.[9]

A fundamental limitation of ventricular volumes and ejection fraction as indices of myocardial performance in dilated CM is that they are both dependent on hemodynamic loading conditions.[10] Of the approaches to load-independent evaluation of myocardial performance, those related to systolic cardiac elastance have attracted the greatest attention. However, the systolic chamber elastance method, although valuable in assessing acute alterations in contractile state, is limited in value in both serial studies of chronically diseased hearts and comparative studies of populations of subjects with and without long-standing heart disease.[10] In order to compensate for this restriction related to chronic compensatory changes in the myocardium (eg, chamber remodeling and hypertrophy), MRI estimates of ventricular wall stress may provide an alternative to catheter measurement of intracavity ventricular pressures.[11-13] The calculation of ventricular wall stress is simplest for meridional stress, the force applied along the length of the ventricle to achieve shortening of that length; an analogous calculation can be used for circumferential stress, the force applied in the circumferential direction in the short-axis plane to achieve circumferential shortening.

Cine MRI has been applied for reproducible quantification of left ventricular wall stress at end systole and end diastole, using graphic recordings of the carotid pulse for timing of the cardiac cycle and systemic arterial or ventricular pressure recording.[7,8,11-15] End-systolic left ventricular wall stress determined from cine MRI has been determined to be abnormally elevated in patients with dilated CM, and inversely proportional to regional ejection fraction.[15] In patients with dilated CM, significant increase in peak-systolic wall stress, compared with normal subjects, has also been demonstrated.[7] However, decreased end-systolic wall stress following afterload reduction by ACE inhibitor therapy has been shown using cine MRI.[8]

Hypertrophic CM

Various patterns of left ventricular hypertrophy in hypertrophic CM (Figure 3) have been defined using MRI.[16-19] Unfortunately, spin-

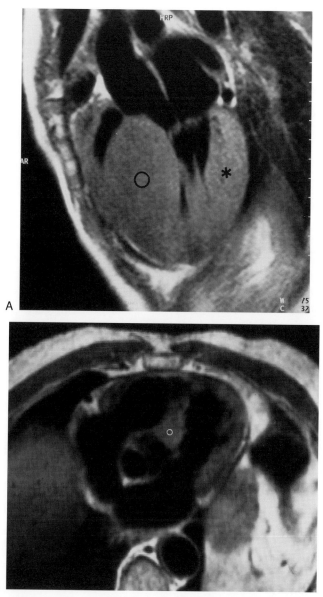

FIGURE 3. Hypertrophic CM (spin-echo). Various patterns of left ventricular hypertrophy, including the following: (1) diffuse asymmetric septal hypertrophy (**A**) horizontal long-axis) with hypertrophy of the interventricular septum (black open circle) exceeding that of the free wall (asterisk); (2) basal-septal hypertrophic bulge (**B**) Transaxial) with a focal muscle prominence of the interventricular septum (white open circle) below the aortic valve; and (3) apical hypertrophy (**C**) vertical long-axis) with obliteration of the cavity at the apex due to pronounced hypertrophy (closed circle).

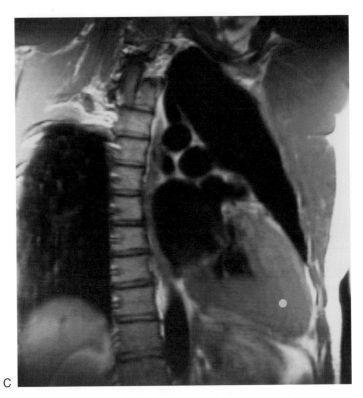

C

FIGURE 3. *(continued)*

echo signal characteristics of the myocardium in hypertrophic CM have not been shown to differ from those found in normals or in patients with physiologic left ventricular hypertrophy.[20] Pathophysiologic characteristics associated with hypertrophic CM have also been demonstrated with MRI; in the setting of this condition, cine MRI has been used to evaluate asymmetric left ventricular systolic wall thickening, subaortic post-stenotic flow related to systolic anterior motion of the anterior mitral leaflet and related mitral regurgitation (Figure 4).[21-23]

FIGURE 4. Hypertrophic CM (cine gradient-echo; adjacent horizontal long-axis). Fixed narrowing of the LV outflow tract at end-diastole (**A**) with decreased distance between the interventricular septum and the anterior mitral leaflet (arrowheads). Associated pathophysiologic characteristics in early-systole (**B**) and mid-systole (**C**) include the following: (1). subaortic post-stenotic flow (open circles) related to systolic anterior motion of the anterior mitral leaflet; and (2) mitral regurgitation (arrowheads).

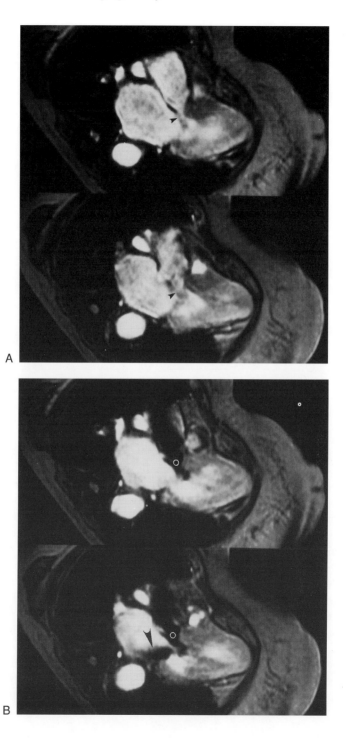

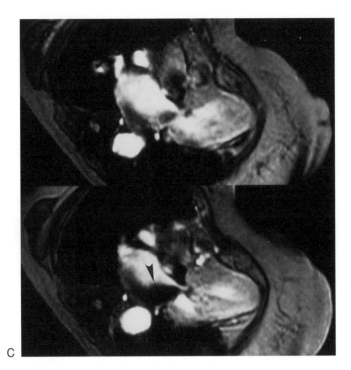

C

FIGURE 4. *(continued)*

A stenotic lesion may be assessed by measuring the flow velocity in the jet of blood passing through that stenosis; with a given flow, an increasing stenosis leads to a higher flow velocity at the orifice. The relation between the velocity of the flow jet and the difference in pressure across the stenosis can be approximated, assuming negligible proximal velocity, by the modified Bernoulli equation. This approach can be used to determine the peak instantaneous gradient across the stenosis.

On cine MRI, signal loss found in the presence of stenosis-related turbulence generally indicates that there may be insufficient signal in the turbulent volume for accurate velocity measurement by phase-velocity mapping. Accurate phase-velocity mapping of jets through stenoses requires the use of short-TE gradient-echo sequences.[24] Using this technique, quantification of jet velocity has been accurate when correlated with invasive hemodynamics, but has not yet been successfully applied to the evaluation of subaortic stenosis in hypertrophic CM. Semiquantitative assessment of resting left ventricular outflow tract obstruction in hypertrophic CM has, however, been successfully accomplished based on the duration or degree of signal void (Figure 5).[21,23]

When applied to hypertrophic CM, the wall stress construct has the following important limitations: (1) it assumes homogeneity of ventricular function and symmetric geometry, neither of which apply to ventricles inhomogeneously configured or damaged; and (2) it represents a global estimate of average midwall stress, rather than regional pathophysiology.[10] Whereas stress at a particular locus can be estimated using local geometric determinants, all simplified LaPlace approaches overlook the complexity of the material properties of the myocardium, which is composed of individual fibers that have different longitudinal and cross-fiber mechanical properties. Fiber orientation varies across the wall, and the distribution of fiber orientation varies from region to region so that myocardium is anisotropic in its mechanical properties.

In addition, conventional wall thickening analysis has the following limitations: (1) thickening is not uniform across the wall, with a maximum in the subendocardium; (2) fiber angle differs across the wall, so that the principal direction of shortening may also vary transmurally; (3) cardiac motion is complex relative to any single imaging plane, with in-plane deformation, rotational and nonrotational translation, through-plane deformation, and complex translation causing the location of a given segment to change over the cardiac cycle.[10] Therefore, transmural heterogeneity within a wall segment and relocation of the myocardium present in the image plane from end diastole to end systole is an important confounding factor in analyzing regional dysfunction, such as in hypertrophic CM.

With MRI myocardial spin-tagging or phase-tracking techniques, the relative patterns, amplitudes, and rates of displacement of myocardial elements during the cardiac cycle can be used to identify regional abnormalities in myocardial mechanics.[10,12,25,26] In the normal LV, one-dimensional analysis of tag stripe separations has been used to demonstrate that circumferential shortening has a transmural gradient in which subendocardial shortening exceeds subepicardial shortening by a 2:1 ratio[27]; in addition, the absolute area of two-dimensional triangular subendocardial elements markedly decreases during systole, probably reflecting phasic alterations in myocardial blood volume, which may be a marker of tissue perfusion.[10] There is also a long-axis gradient in circumferential shortening, with shortening greater at the apex than base. For longitudinal shortening, however, there is no transmural gradient; shortening is uniform along the length of the septum and lateral walls.[28]

By tagging analysis of left ventricular hypertrophy due to hypertension, reduced circumferential and longitudinal shortening, with no

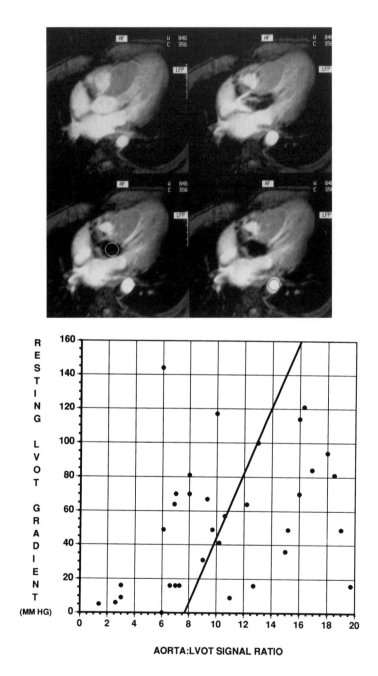

[LVOT GRADIENT = (2.9 x RATIO) + 22.8: R2 = 0.15, p=0.022]

change in transmural gradient of circumferential shortening, has been observed. These changes were found even though ejection fractions remained normal, suggesting that analysis of segment shortening is more sensitive to altered myocardial function than are global chamber indices of ventricular pump function.[28] The coexistence of reduced intramural segment shortening with normal chamber pump function probably relates to the increased ratio of wall thickness to chamber diameter; thus, less shortening per unit from more myocardium results in normal ejection fraction.[10]

Pronounced heterogeneous reductions in circumferential and three-dimensional shortening, with the septal impairment exceeding the free-wall impairment, have been described in hypertrophic CM (Figure 6).[29–32] Accentuated heterogeneity in strain rate, increasing in diastole, has also been demonstrated in hypertrophic CM.[33] The degree of contractile dysfunction has been correlated with both its abnormal geometry (eg, flattened to negative septal curvature)[34] and the severity of internal histopathology (ie, myocardial fibrosis and myofiber disarray).[35]

Although not yet fully assessed for its ability to differentiate between the primary causes of diastolic dysfunction, cine MRI is useful in defining the basic pathophysiology.[12] Because of good temporal resolution associated with this technique, the uniformly delayed diastolic filling pattern of the ventricles due to restrictive physiology can be identified. Using cine MRI to evaluate RV time-volume curves in hypertrophic CM, abnormally depressed peak filling rates and filling fractions have been demonstrated; these changes suggested diastolic dysfunction from associated restrictive physiology.[36]

By treating commercially available MRI contrast agents (eg, gadolinium-DTPA) mainly as extracted tracers, it is possible to measure myocardial perfusion from the pattern of myocardial enhancement; while the model assumes a linear relation between tracer concentration and signal enhancement, this is only true for these extracelluler agents at low concentrations, as normally applied in clinical practice.[37,38] Ultrafast MRI (eg, turbo FLASH) can provide at least one image for each cardiac cycle during the passage of the tracer for measurement of myocardial perfusion.[39,40] Bolus-contrast-enhanced ultrafast MRI has been

---

FIGURE 5. Hypertrophic CM. Relation between degree of signal void from subaortic post-stenotic flow and resting gradient in the left ventricular outflow tract by Doppler echocardiography. The descending aorta-to left ventricular outflow tract signal ratio, determined from regions of interest on the cine gradient-echo image showing the maximal subaortic signal loss (**top**), correlates directly with the resting gradient (**bottom**). (Reproduced with permission from Reference 23).

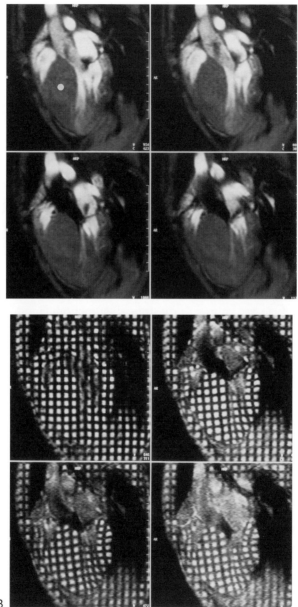

FIGURE 6. Hypertrophic CM (cine gradient-echo in standard form then with myocardial grid-tagging; consecutive horizontal long-axis). Asymmetric hypertrophy of interventricular septum (closed circle) with subaortic stenosis (**A**) and relatively impaired (compared with the free wall) septal grid deformation from altered mechanics (**B**) developing during systole.

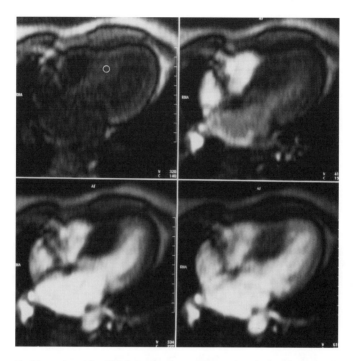

FIGURE 7. Hypertrophic CM (ultrafast gradient-echo during bolus administration of gadolinium-DTPA; cycle-to-cycle horizontal long-axis). Decreased diastolic first-pass enhancement of the hypertrophic septal myocardium (open circle).

used to study cases of hypertrophic CM; decreased diastolic first-pass enhancement of the septal myocardium (Figure 7) characteristic and it correlated with increased amounts of characteristic histopathology (eg., intramyocardial small-vessel narrowing) [41].

Restrictive Cardiomyopathy

In cases of diastolic dysfunction due to restrictive CM, rather than to constrictive pericarditis, MRI is valuable for demonstrating the absence of abnormal pericardial thickening in the presence of indirect findings of impaired ventricular filling (eg, dilatation of inferior vena cava and right atrium).[42] MRI of cardiac amyloidosis (Figure 8), a classic cause of restrictive physiology, has revealed increased thickness of the left ventricular wall without cavity dilatation.[43,44] Similar anatomic findings, in combination with slightly increased myocardial signal intensity, have been observed in some deposition diseases (eg, Fabry

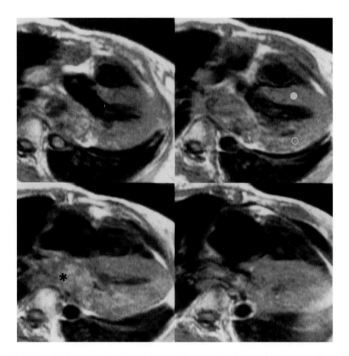

FIGURE 8. Restrictive CM (spin-echo; adjacent horizontal long-axis). Uniformly increased wall thickness and preserved configuration of the interventricular septum (closed circle) and free wall (open circle) and abnormal intra-atrial signal (asterisk) due to diastolic dysfunction related to cardiac amyloidosis.

disease) resulting in diastolic dysfunction.[45] However, for the most part, the myocardium of restrictive CM has normal MRI properties (eg, T2).[46] There are notable exceptions; in the setting of hemochromatosis, prominent susceptibility-related loss of signal within the myocardium due to iron deposition, especially on gradient-echo images, has been demonstrated using MRI.[47–49] Sarcoid heart disease, another potential cause of restrictive CM, is manifested on MRI in its acute inflammatory phase as discrete areas of high signal intensity, associated with increased wall thickness, within the left ventricular septal and free wall myocardium (Figure 9)[50] but chronically as focal areas of pronounced wall thinning, possibly with aneurysm formation, in the same left ventricular wall regions (Figure 10).

An abnormally delayed pattern of ventricular filling due to diastolic dysfunction associated with restrictive CM can be evaluated qualitatively or quantitatively using cine MRI.[51,52] In the initial stages of restrictive CM, sluggish early ventricular filling is noted with or without mild impairment of systolic function; late restrictive CM, however,

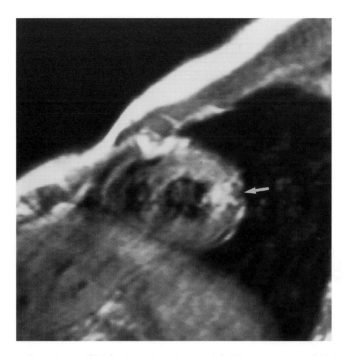

FIGURE 9. Restrictive CM (spin-echo; short-axis). Discrete area of high signal intensity within the myocardium (arrow) due to acute inflammatory changes related to sarcoid heart disease.

is characterized by rapid early, but abruptly terminated late filling of the ventricles, like constrictive pericarditis, but with significantly impaired systolic emptying of the ventricles, unlike constrictive pericarditis (Figure 11). While phase-velocity mapping of ventricular myocardium has been used to demonstrate reduction in mean peak early-diastolic velocity related to left ventricular stiffening with aging,[53] it has not been used to show alteration of myocardial velocity in restrictive CM.

By measuring the rate of flow across the tricuspid and mitral annuli in diastole, phase-velocity mapping has been proposed as a method for assessing diastolic dysfunction, as found in restrictive CM.[54] Venous flow velocity is a reflection of the pressure gradients between the pulmonary and system veins and their receiving atria and changes in these gradients under pathological conditions affect their normal biphasic forward-flow pattern (the larger surge during ventricular systole and the smaller during diastole). Using phase-velocity mapping, abnormal flow patterns in the superior vena cava have been demonstrated in restrictive CM; progressively decreasing ratio of peak flow in systole

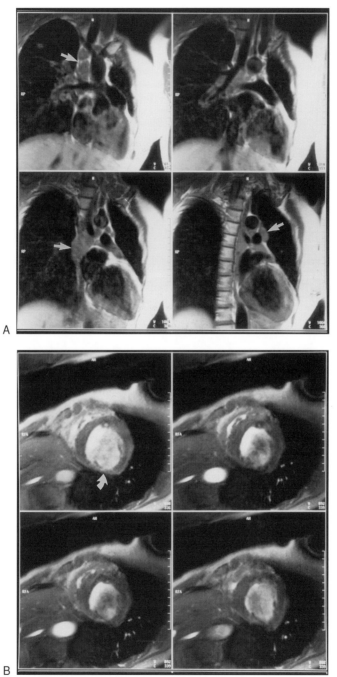

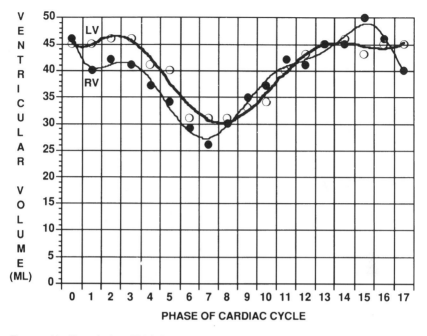

FIGURE 11. Restrictive CM (cine gradient-echo for time-vs.-ventricular volume curve analysis). Sluggish early ventricular filling with significantly impaired systolic emptying of the LV and RV indicate myocardial disease with restrictive physiology.

relative to that in diastole is found with worsening restrictive physiology (Figure 12), but such ratios do not differentiate restrictive CM from constrictive pericarditis.[55]

Right Ventricular CM

Along with dilatation of the cavity of the RV (Figure 13) thinning of its wall in regions of fibrosis (Figure 14) and increased signal inten-

FIGURE 10. Restrictive CM (spin-echo and cine gradient-echo; adjacent paracoronal and consecutive short-axis, respectively). Enlarged nodes (straight arrows) of mediastinum and hila (**A**) and posterolateral free-wall left ventricular aneurysm formation (curved arrows) with end-diastolic thinning, impaired systolic wall thickening, and end-systolic bulging (**B**) reflect long-term changes of sarcoid heart disease.

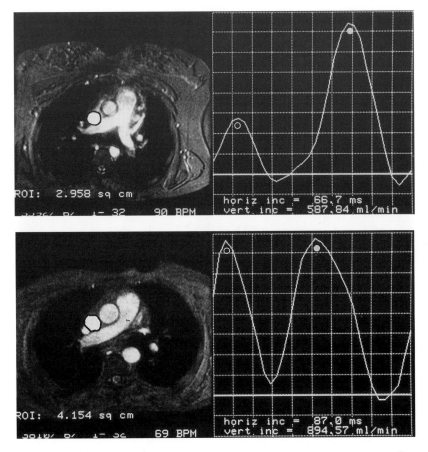

FIGURE 12. Restrictive CM (phase-velocity mapping for systemic venous flow analysis). In the superior vena cava, greater decrease in ratio of peak flow in systole (open circle) relative to that in diastole (closed circle) is found in severe (**top**) compared to mild (**bottom**) restrictive disease.

sity in regions of replacement of its myocardium with fat (Figure 15) have been well demonstrated in advanced cases of right ventricular CM (a.k.a. arrhythmogenic right ventricular dysplasia) using MRI.[56–59] Greater reduction in right ventricular ejection fraction and more pronounced structural and histological changes in the RV, including evidence of fatty replacement of the myocardium, have been more often demonstrated in right ventricular CM with than without inducible ventricular tachycardia.[59] Regional wall motion abnormalities (Figure 16), compatible with milder focal dysplasia, have been observed using cine

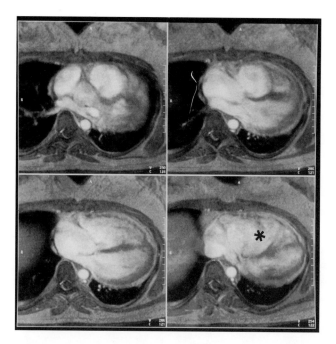

FIGURE 13. Right ventricular CM (cine gradient-echo; adjacent transaxial). Significant dilatation of the RV cavity (asterisk).

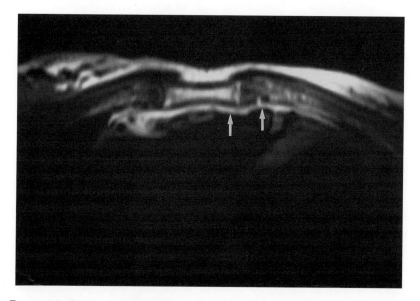

FIGURE 14. Right ventricular CM (spin-echo; transaxial). Pronounced thinning (arrows) of anterior right ventricular wall in regions of fibrosis.

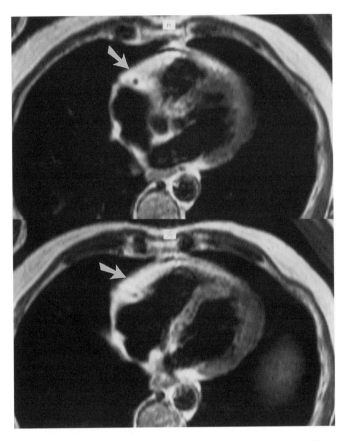

Figure 15. Right ventricular CM (spin-echo; adjacent transaxial). Increased signal intensity (arrows) in regions of replacement of right ventricular myocardium with fat near right atrioventricular groove. Usually, there is substantial epicardial fat adjacent to the right ventricular free wall. Thus, one must be careful in differentiating between epicardial and intramural increase in fat.

MRI in patients with the diagnosis of idiopathic right ventricular cut-flow tract tachycardia.[60]

Pericardial Diseases

The ability of the pericardial sac to react to disease is limited. It responds to an acute injury with one of the following: (1) congestion; (2) increased exudation of fluid into the sac; (3) exudation of both fibrin and acute inflammatory cells into the sac; or (4) a combination of these

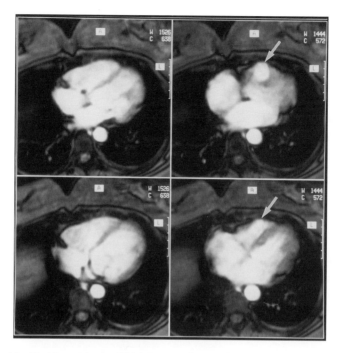

FIGURE 16. Right ventricular CM (cine gradient-echo; adjacent transaxial). Regional wall motion abnormality (arrows), with impaired systolic wall thickening and inward motion from end diastole (left) to end systole (right), compatible with mild dysplasia.

reactions.[61,62] The composition of the pericardial fluid that results depends on the cause of pericardial insult. Pericardial effusions almost always range from serous to purulent to sanguinous; rarely, pericardial effusion is composed of lymph or chyle. Serous effusions are usually related to a decreased return of pericardial fluid or to decreased serum osmolality, as in hypoproteinemia. Inflammatory effusions are often purulent. Sanguinous effusions are usually related to trauma (eg, surgery), myocarditis, myocardial or great vessel rupture, or pericarditial insult from uremia, infections, inflammation, or tumor.

Pericarditis, an inflammation of the pericardial surfaces, has many infectious and noninfectious causes.[61,62] It is generally associated with an inflammatory infiltrate in the layers of tissue and an exudate, usually composed of fibrin and inflammatory cells. Many cases of inflammatory pericarditis resolve without residual effects. In other instances, the fibrin deposits organize and form pericardial adhesions without causing constriction, but if the processes of injury and repair continue, constrictive pericarditis may result. Constrictive pericarditis is associated with pericardial thickening and adhesions with progression to the point of limitation of diastolic return to the ventricles, resulting in a gradual rise in pulmonary and systemic venous pressures; the abnormal pericardium may be soft and spongy (effusive constrictive) in the early stages and firm and fibrotic and/or calcified (fibrotic or calcific constrictive) in the later stages.

Pericardial Effusion

The normal pericardium and the contained physiologic fluid appears on MRI as only a thin (usually 2 mm or less) curvilinear line situated between the epicardial and pericardial fat.[63] MRI has an advantage over computed tomography in differentiating a small pericardial effusion from pericardial thickening because different acquisition schemes may be used in MRI to appreciate and characterize fluid.[64]

Simple pericardial effusions are visualized on spin-echo MRI as low-intensity regions between the cardiac surface with its epicardial fat and the outwardly displaced pericardial fat (Figure 17).[64–66] Because

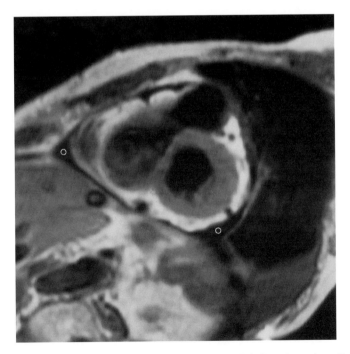

FIGURE 17. Pericardial effusion (spin-echo; short-axis). Simple pericardial effusion represented by low-intensity regions (open circles) between the cardiac surface with its epicardial fat and the outwardly displaced pericardial fat.

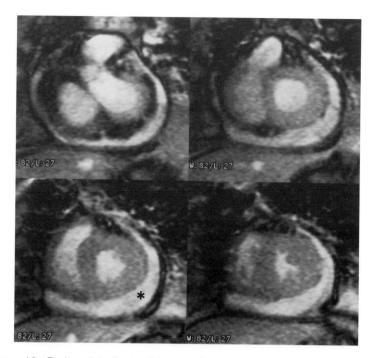

FIGURE 18. Pericardial effusion (cine gradient-echo; adjacent short-axis). Simple pericardial effusion characterized high signal intensity in the pericardial space (asterisk).

of cardiac motion, the signal intensity from simple pericardial effusions is less than that from concurrent simple pleural effusions.[64] While characterized by low signal intensity on T1-weighted images, its signal intensity may increase on more T2-weighted images; this is particularly true of the most dependent portions of the pericardial effusion. On the other hand, simple pericardial effusions produce high signal intensity on gradient-echo MRI (Figure 18) and when imaged in the form of cine gradient-echo MRI, they demonstrate mobility and changing distribution of the bright pericardial fluid during the cardiac cycle.[67]

Assessment of the distribution and general size of a simple pericardial effusion using MRI has shown good overall correlation with that of two-dimensional echocardiography.[65] However, when fluid volume has been quantitated by both techniques, the pericardial effusion has tended to measure larger by MRI.[68] In fact, MRI has been shown to detect small pericardial effusions not visualized by echocardiography and to be better for detecting fluid located superiorly in the aortic pericardial reflection or superior pericardial recess, medially at the border of the right atrium, and posteriorly at the left ventricular free wall.[65,68]

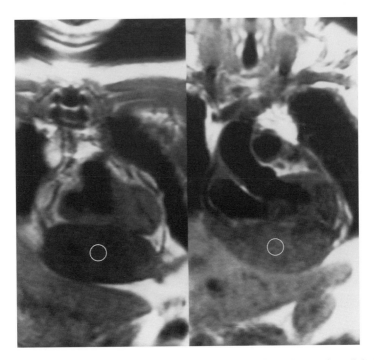

FIGURE 19. Pericardial effusion (spin-echo; coronal). Complex pericardial effusion exhibiting moderately increased signal intensity (open circles).

Because of T1 shortening from their high protein or cell content,[62] complex pericardial effusions typically exhibit greater signal intensity than simple pericardial effusions on T1-weighted spin-echo MRI (Figure 19).[65,69] Thus, on spin-echo MRI, regions of moderately increased signal within complex effusions probably represent exudate made relatively immobile by fibrinous material that has adhered to the pericardium. With exudative pericardial effusions, both the pericardium and pericardial adhesions may have greater signal intensities than a normal pericardium.[65,66]

Hemopericardium and pericardial hematoma can generally be distinguished from other types of effusion because of the high, at times extremely intense, signal of the paramagnetic blood products on spin-echo MRI.[65,70] However, these hemorrhagic pericardial effusions often contain areas of both medium and high signal intensity, reflecting the variable age of the bloody material (Figure 20).[65,66] In vitro MRI examination of human blood has shown that the signal intensity of the serum itself varies, but the signal intensity of the clot is more stable over time; during the first few hours the signal intensity of the serum is lower

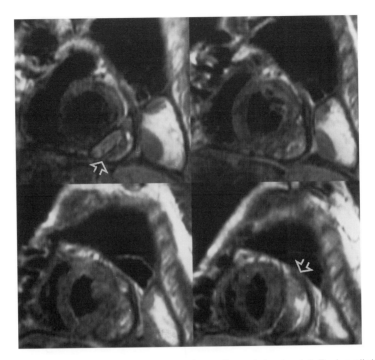

FIGURE 20. Pericardial effusion (spin-echo; adjacent short-axis). Pericardial he-matoma presenting as paracardiac mass (open arrows) compressing the left ventricular free wall and containing areas of low, medium, and high signal intensity, reflecting the variable age of the bloody material.

than that of the clot, but the serum becomes more intense than the clot after 2 to 3 weeks.[68] Whereas hemorrhagic effusions have been shown to have significantly greater effusion-to-myocardial signal intensity ratios than nonhemorrhagic effusions on T1-weighted spin-echo MRI, differences in hematocrit are not reliably appreciated.[71]

MRI appears to be superior to echocardiography in defining the nature and extent of processes causing clinical signs of cardiac chamber compromise from hemopericardium.[65,66,72] Compression of the cardiac chambers by hematoma indicates pericardial tamponade.

Pericarditis

The low intensity of the pericardium on spin-echo MRI is explained partly by the presence of a phase discontinuity artifact; the shearing action between the visceral and parietal pericardium presumably results in a large local velocity variation, causing a reduction in signal

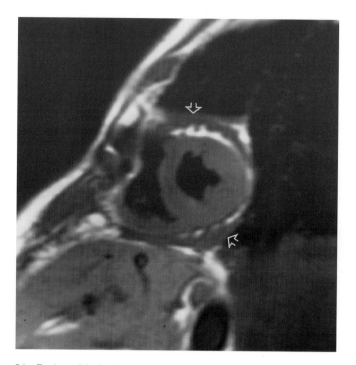

FIGURE 21. Pericarditis (spin-echo; short-axis). Abnormally thickened pericardium (open arrows).

intensity in the voxels spanning the pericardium.[73] Absence of the low-intensity pericardial line on spin-echo MRI implies that the normal transpericardial shearing motion is also absent in that region[66]; this change is caused by primary or secondary abnormalities of the pericardium (eg, inflammatory disease).

Because MRI provides excellent direct visualization of the pericardium, it can readily define the presence and extent of pericardial thickening (Figure 21). Measuring pericardial thickness is of great value in the diagnosis of constrictive pericarditis, however, the presence of pericardial thickening does not by itself indicate constriction. Pericardial thickening has been noted on MRI in several clinical settings.[65] A thickened pericardium is present for a variable time after cardiac surgery. Both pericardial thickening and effusion have been demonstrated in uremic or infectious pericarditis; because of inflammatory changes associated with both of these conditions, the pericardial signal is generally increased on spin-echo MRI, and adhesions between the irregularly thickened visceral and parietal pericardium may be detected (Figure 22). Nevertheless, MRI can be used effectively in the differentiation

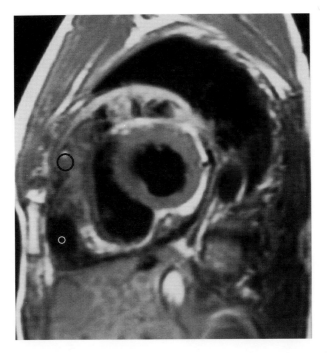

FIGURE 22. Pericarditis (spin-echo; short-axis). Acute inflammatory pericarditis with adhesions (black open circles) between the irregularly thickened visceral and parietal pericardium and intermixed with collections of simple fluid (white open circle).

between constrictive pericarditis and restrictive cardiomyopathy[65,66,74] both of which may result in similar clinical presentations due to hindered diastolic filling of the ventricles[72]; whereas restrictive cardiomyopathy could demonstrate pericardial effusion, it would not generally reveal significant pericardial thickening.

Whereas in constrictive pericarditis increased thickness of the pericardium is evident on MRI,[42,65,66,74] the associated conical or tubular narrowing of the generally nonhypertrophied ventricles, resulting from compression and confinement by the thick pericardium is more specific for the diagnosis (Figure 23). Secondary changes such as atrial enlargement, systemic vein dilatation, hepatomegaly, ascites, and occasionally pleural effusion, may also be noted on MRI. When found in association with the appropriate clinical syndrome, these abnormal anatomic findings are strongly supportive of the diagnosis of constrictive pericarditis, with 93% accuracy documented.[42] Unfortunately, MRI has not been able to differentiate reliably between fibrous tissue and calcification and is consequently of limited value, compared with computed tomog-

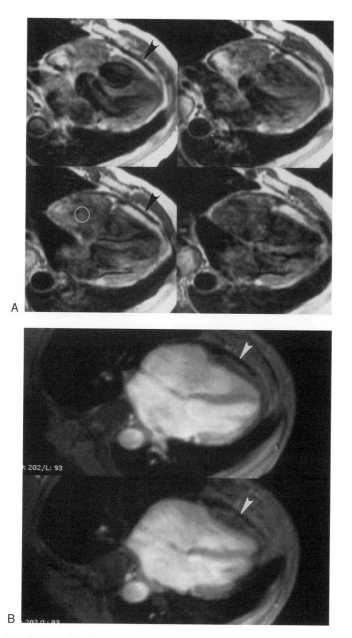

FIGURE 23. Pericarditis (spin-echo and cine gradient-echo; adjacent horizontal long-axis). Constrictive pericarditis with spin-echo (**A**) and gradient-echo (**B**) proof of the fibrotic and/or calcified nature of the abnormally thickened pericardium (arrowheads), resulting in conical narrowing of the LV and RV and enlargement of the atria containing abnormal signal (open circle) due to diastolic dysfunction.

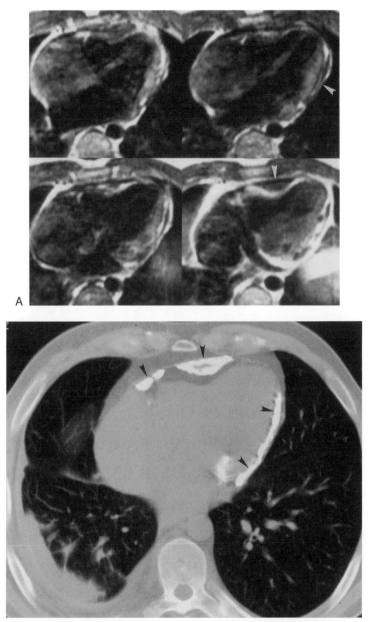

FIGURE 24. Pericarditis (spin-echo and computed tomography; adjacent horizontal long-axis and transaxial, respectively). Constrictive pericarditis with spin-echo (**A**) evidence of an abnormal pericardium (arrowheads), but clear confirmation on computed tomography (**B**) of its extensively calcified nature.

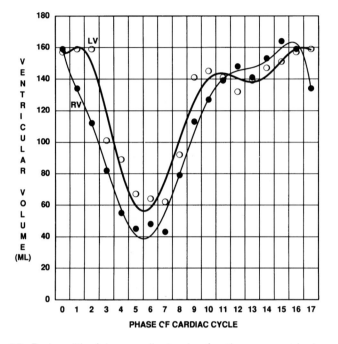

FIGURE 25. Pericarditis (cine gradient-echo for time-vs.-ventricular volume curve analysis). Rapid early ventricular filling followed by abrupt limitation of late-diastolic filling of the ventricles, in the setting of preserved systolic emptying of the LV and RV, indicate constrictive pericarditis.

raphy, in the evaluation of calcification of the pericardium in the setting of calcific pericarditis (Figure 24).[64]

Cases of constrictive pericarditis may be evaluated functionally with MRI. Absolute and relative systolic wall thickening of the LV, measured with multiphasic spin-echo MRI, has not been found to be significantly different from that in normal volunteers.[75] Cine MRI is more useful than spin-echo MRI techniques in functionally evaluating cases of diastolic dysfunction and in qualitatively or quantitatively defining the specific pathophysiologic abnormalities associated with constrictive pericarditis.[67,76] Because of the higher temporal resolution provided with this technique, the abrupt limitation of late-diastolic filling of the ventricles due to the abnormally thickened and confining pericardium in constrictive pericarditis (Figure 25) is distinguishable from the delayed diastolic filling patterns of the ventricles due to restrictive cardiomyopathy in the absence of significant pericardial thickening.

Using phase-velocity mapping, abnormal flow patterns in the superior vena cava have been demonstrated in cases of constrictive peri-

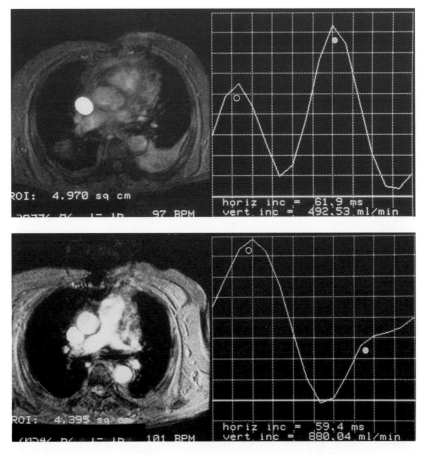

FIGURE 26. Pericarditis (phase-velocity mapping for systemic venous flow analysis). In the superior vena cava, the decrease in ratio of peak flow in systole (open circle) relative to that in diastole (closed circle) due to constrictive pericarditis (**top**) is improved after surgical pericardial stripping (**bottom**).

carditis[55]; improvement in diastolic return with pericardial stripping can be documented (Figure 26). In both normals and patients with right-sided disease, systemic venous flow measured without respiratory gating closely resemble its flow at end-expiration.[77]

Conclusion

Because of the ability of MRI to provide valuable information about the structural, histological, and functional (contraction, relax-

ation/filling, and hemodynamic) manifestations of nonischemic myocardial diseases and pericardial diseases, MRI has unique capabilities
compared with other imaging modalities.

References

1. Wynne J, Braunwald E. The cardiomyopathies and myocarditides: Toxic,
   chemical, and physical damage to the heart. In: Braunwald E, ed: *Heart
   Disease: A Textbook of Cardiovascular Medicine.* Philadelphia: WB Saunders
   Co; 1992:1394–1450.
2. Abelman WH, Lorell BH. The challenge of cardiomyopathy. *J Am Coll Cardiol.* 1989;13:1219–1239.
3. Keren A, Popp RL. Assignment of patients into the classification of cardiomyopathies. *Circulation.* 1992;86:1622–1633.
4. Gaudio C, Tanzilli G, Mazzarotto P, et al. Comparison of left ventricular
   ejection fraction by magnetic resonance imaging and radionuclide ventriculography in idiopathic dilated cardiomyopathy. *Am J Cardiol.* 1991;67:
   411–415.
5. Doherty NE, Fujita N, Caputo GR, Higgins CB. Measurement of right ventricular mass in normal and dilated cardiomyopathic ventricles using cine
   magnetic resonance imaging. *Am J Cardiol.* 1992;69:1223–1228.
6. Buser PT, Aufferman W, Holt WW, et al. Noninvasive evaluation of global
   left ventricular function with use of cine nuclear magnetic resonance. *J Am
   Coll Cardiol.* 1989;13:1294–1300.
7. Wagner S, Auffermann W, Buser P, et al. Functional description of the
   left ventricle in patients with volume overload, pressure overload, and
   myocardial disease using cine magnetic resonance imaging. *Am J Card Imaging.* 1991;5:87–97.
8. Doherty NE, Seelos KC, Suzuki J-l, et al. Application of cine nuclear magnetic resonance imaging for sequential evaluation of response to angiotensin-converting enzyme inhibitor therapy in dilated cardiomyopathy. *J Am
   Coll Cardiol.* 1992;19:1294–1302.
9. Fujita N, Hartiala J, O'Sullivan M, et al. Assessment of left ventricular
   diastolic function in dilated cardiomyopathy with cine magnetic resonance
   imaging: Effect of an angiotensin converting enzyme inhibitor, benazepril.
   Am Heart J. 1993;125:171–178.
10. Reichek N. Magnetic resonance imaging for assessment of myocardial func-
    tion. *Magn Reson Q.* 1991;7:255–274.
11. Pattynama PMT, Lamb HJ, van der Veide EO; et al. Left ventricular mea-
    surements with cine and spin-echo MR imaging: A study of reproducibility
    with variance component analysis. *Radiology.* 1993;187:261–268.
12. Holt WW, White RD. Noninvasive assessment of left ventricular function.
    Am J Card Imaging. 1991;5:305–317.
13. Dulce MC, Higgins CB. Evaluation of ventricular dimensions and function
    with magnetic resonance imaging. *Am J Card Imaging.* 1994;8:168–180.
14. Higgins CB, Holt W, Pflugfelder P, et al. Functional evaluation of the heart
    with magnetic resonance imaging. *Magn Reson Med.* 1988;6:121–139.
15. Fujita N, Duerinckx AJ, Higgins CB. Variation in left ventricular regional
    wall stress with cine magnetic resonance imaging: Normal subjects versus
    dilated cardiomyopathy. *Am Heart J.* 1993;125:1337–1345.

16. Higgins CB, Byrd BF, Stark D, et al. Magnetic resonance imaging in hypertrophic cardiomyopathy. *Am J Cardiol.* 1985;55:1121–1126.
17. Webb JG, Sasson Z, Rakowski H, et al. Apical hypertrophic cardiomyopathy: Clinical follow-up and diagnostic correlates. *J Am Coll Cardiol.* 1990; 15:83–90.
18. Park JH, Kim YM, Chung JW, et al. MR imaging of hypertrophic cardiomyopathy. *Radiology.* 1992;185:441–446.
19. Casolo GC, Trotta F, Rostagno C, et al. Detection of apical hypertrophic cardiomyopathy by magnetic resonance imaging. *Am Heart J.* 1989;117: 468–472.
20. Been M, Kean D, Smith MA, et al. Nuclear magnetic resonance in hypertrophic cardiomyopathy. *Br Heart J.* 1985;54:48–52.
21. Sardanelli F, Molinari G, Petillo A, et al. MRI in hypertrophic cardiomyopathy: A morphofunctional study. *J Comput Assist Tomogr.* 1993;17:862–872.
22. Scheffknecht BHB, Bonow RO, Dwyer AJ, et al. Functional assessment of left ventricular ejection dynamics by cine-magnetic resonance imaging in hypertrophic cardiomyopathy. *Am J Cardiol.* 1994;73:981–984.
23. White RD, Obuchowski NA, Gunawardena S, et al. Left ventricular outflow tract obstruction in hypertrophic cardiomyopathy: Pre- and post-operative evaluation by computed tomography magnetic resonance imaging. *Am J Card Imaging.* 1996;1:1–13.
24. Rebergen SA, van der Wall EE, Doornbos J, et al. Magnetic resonance measurement of velocity and flow: Technique, validation, and cardiovascular applications. *Am Heart J.* 1993;126:1439–1455.
25. Axel L, Dougherty L. MR imaging of motion with spatial modulation of magnetization. *Radiology.* 1989;171:841–845.
26. Pelc NJ, Herfkens RJ, Pelc LR. Three-dimensional analysis of myocardial motion and deformation with phase contrast cine MRI. *Magn Reson Med.* 1992;11:18–26.
27. Clark NR, Reichek N, Bergey P, et al. Circumferential myocardial shortening in the normal human left ventricle: Assessement by magnetic resonance imaging using spatial modulation of magnetization. *Circulation.* 1991;84: 67–74.
28. Palmon L, Reichek N, Clark N, et al. Long axis myocardial shortening in hypertensive left ventricular hypertrophy. *Circulation.* 1991;84.(suppl II): 371.
29. Maier SE, Fischer SE, McKinnon G, et al. Evaluation of left ventricular segmental wall motion in hypertrophic cardiomyopathy with myocardial tagging. *Circulation.* 1992;86:1919–1928.
30. Kramer CM, Reichek N, Ferrari V, et al. Regional heterogeneity of function in hypertrophic cardiomyopathy. *Circulation.* 1994;90:186–194.
31. Young AA, Kramer CM, Ferrari VA, et al. Three-dimensional left ventricular deformation in hypertrophic cardiomyopathy. *Circulation.* 1994;90: 854–867.
32. Dong SJ, MacGregor JH, Crawley AP, et al. Left ventricular wall thickness and regional systolic function in patients with hypertrophic cardiomyopathy: A three-dimensional tagged magnetic resonance imaging study. *Circulation.* 1994;90:1200–1209.
33. Beach GM, Wedeen VJ, Weisskoff RM, O'Gara PT, et al. Intramural mechanics in hypertrophic cardiomyopathy: Functional mapping with strain-rate MR imaging. *Radiology.* 1995;197:117–124.
34. Nakatani S, White RD, Powell KA, Lever HM, Thomas JD. Dynamic mag-

netic resonance imaging assessment of the effect of ventricular wall curvature on regional function in hypertrophic cardiomyopathy. *Am J Cardiol.* 1996;77:618–622.

35. White RD, Lever HM, Murphy DJ, et al. MRI-tagging measurements of impaired regional LV-midwall contractility correlate with histopathology in hypertrophic obstructive cardiomyopathy. *J Am Coll Cardiol.* 1993; 21(suppl A):266A.

36. Suzuki JI, Chang JM, Caputo GR, et al. Evaluation of right ventricular early diastolic filling by cine nuclear magnetic resonance imaging in patients with hypertrophic cardiomyopathy. *J Am Coll Cardiol.* 1991;18:120–126.

37. Wilke N, Simm C, Zhang J, et al. Contrast-enhanced first pass myocardial perfusion imaging: Correlation between myocardial blood flow in dogs at rest and during hyperemia. *Magn Reson Med.* 1993;29:485–497.

38. Van Rugge FP, Boreel JJ, Van Der Waal, et al. Cardiac first pass and myocardial perfusion in normal subjects by subsecond GD-DTPA enhanced MR imaging. *J Comput Assist Tomogr.* 1991;15:959–965.

39. Manning WJ, Atkinson DJ, Grossman W, et al. First-pass nuclear magnetic resonance imaging studies using gadolinium DTPA in patients with coronary artery disease. *J Am Coll Cardiol.* 1991;18:959–965.

40. Wilke N, Jerosch-Herold M, Stillman AE, et al. Concepts of myocardial perfusion imaging in magnetic resonance imaging. *Magn Reson Q.* 1994;10: 249–286.

41. White RD, Chow KC, Hardy PA, et al. Improved characterization of myocardial histopathology in hypertrophic obstructive cardiomyopathy with bolus-first-pass ultrafast MRI. *Circulation.* 1993;88 (suppl 1):1–83.

42. Masui T, Finck S, Higgins CB. Constrictive pericarditis and restrictive cardiomyopathy: Evaluation with MR imaging. *Radiology.* 1992;182:369–373.

43. Wilson JH, Moodie DS. Cardiac amyloidosis in a patient with Ehlers-Danlos syndrome type IV. *Cleve Clin Q.* 1986;53:205–211.

44. von Kemp K, Beckers R, Vandenweghe J, et al. Echocardiography and magnetic resonance imaging in cardiac amyloidosis. *Acta Cardiol.* 1989;1:29–35.

45. Matsui S, Murakami E, Takekoshi N, et al. Myocardial tissue characterization by magnetic resonance imaging in Fabry's disease. *Am Heart J.* 1989; 117:472–474.

46. Sechtem U, Higgins CB, Sommerhoff BA, et al. Magnetic resonance imaging of restrictive cardiomyopathy. *Am J Cardiol.* 1987;59:480–482.

47. Steudel A, Krahe T, Becher H, et al. Kardiomyopathie bei idiopathischer hamochromatose. *Dtsch Med Wschr.* 1987;112:590–592.

48. Blankenberg F, Eisenberg S, Scheinman MN, et al. Use of cine gradient echo (GRE) MR in the imaging of cardiac hemochromatosis. *J Comput Assist Tomogr.* 1994;18:136–138.

49. Jensen PD, Bagger JP, Jensen FT, et al. Heart transplantation in a case of juvenile hereditary haemochromatosis followed up by MRI and endomyocardial biopsies. *Eur J Haematol.* 1993;51:199–205.

50. Riedy K, Fisher MR, Belic N, et al. MR imaging of myocardial sarcoidosis. *AJR.* 1988;151:915–916.

51. Soldo SJ, Norris SL, Gober JR, et al. MRI-derived ventricular volume curves for the assessment of left ventricular function. *Magn Reson Imaging.* 1994; 12:711–717.

52. Hoff FL, Turner DA, Wang JZ, et al. Semiautomatic evaluation of left ventricular diastolic function with cine magnetic resonance imaging. *Acad Radiol.* 1994;1:237–242.

53. Karwatowski SP, Mohiaddin R, Yang GZ, et al. Assessment of regional left ventricular long-axis motion with MR velocity mapping in healthy subjects. *J Magn Reson Imaging.* 1994;4:151–155.
54. Hartiala JJ, Mostbeck GH, Foster E, et al. Velocity-encoded cine MRI in the evaluation of left ventricular diastolic function: Measurement of mitral valve and pulmonary vein flow velocities and flow volume across the mitral valve. *Am Heart J.* 1993;125:1054–1066.
55. White RD, Hardy PA, VanDyke CW, et al. Diastolic dysfunction: Dynamic MRI velocity-mapping of related flow patterns in the superior vena cava. *J Magn Reson Imaging.* 1993;3(P):65.
56. Blake LM, Scheinman MM, Higgins CB. MR features of arrhythmogenic right ventricular dysplasia. *AJR.* 1994;162:809–812.
57. Casolo GC, Poggesi L, Boddi M, et al. ECG-gated magnetic resonance imaging in right ventricular dysplasia. *Am Heart J.* 1987;113:1245–1248.
58. Ricci C, Longo R, Pagnan L, et al. Magnetic resonance imaging in right ventricular dysplasia. *Am J Cardiol.* 1992;70:1589–1595.
59. Auffermann W, Wichter T, Breithardt G, et al. Arrhythmogenic right ventricular disease: MR imaging vs angiography. *AJR.* 1993;161:549–555.
60. Carlson MD, White RD, Trohman RG, et al. Right ventricular outflow tract ventricular tachycardia: Detection of previously unrecognized anatomical abnormalities using cine magnetic resonance imaging. *J Am Coll Cardiol.* 1994;24:720–727.
61. Butany J. The pericardium and its diseases. In: Silver MD, ed: *Cardiovascular Pathology.* 2nd Edition. New York: Churchill Livingstone; 1991:847–894.
62. Roberts WC, Ferrans VJ. A survey of the causes and consequences of pericardial heart disease. In: Reddy PS, Leon DF, Shaver YA, eds: *Pericardial Disease.* New York: Raven Press, 1982:49–75.
63. Sechtem U, Tscholakoff D, Higgins CB. MRI on the normal pericardium. *AJR.* 1986;147:239–244.
64. Olson MC, Posniak HV, McDonald V, et al. Computed tomography and magnetic resonance imaging of the pericardium. *RadioGraphics.* 1989;9:633–649.
65. Sechtem U, Tscholakoff D, Higgins CB: MRI of the abnormal pericardium. *AJR.* 1986;147:245–252.
66. Stark DD, Higgins CB, Lanzer P, et al. Magnetic resonance imaging of the pericardium: Normal and pathologic findings. *Radiology.* 1984;150:469–474.
67. White RD, Zisch RJ. Magnetic resonance imaging of pericardial disease and paracardiac and intracardiac masses. In: Elliott LP, ed: *The Fundamentals of Cardiac Imaging in Children and Adults.* Philadelphia: J.B. Lippincott; 1991:420–433.
68. Mulvagh SL, Rokey R, Vick GW, et al: Usefulness of nuclear magnetic resonance imaging for evaluation of pericardial effusions, and comparison with two-dimensional echocardiography. *Am J Cardiol* 1989;64:1002–1009.
69. Brown JJ, van Sonnenberg E, Gerber KH, et al. Magnetic resonance relaxation times of percutaneously obtained normal and abnormal body fluids. *Radiology.* 1985:154:727–731.
70. Bradley WG: MRI of hemorrhage and iron in the brain. In: Stark DD, Bradley WG, eds: *Magnetic Resonance Imaging.* St. Louis: CV Mosby; 1988:359–374.
71. Rokey R, Vick GW III, Bolli R, Lewandowski ED. Assessment of experimental pericardial effusion using nuclear magnetic resonance imaging techniques. *Am Heart J.* 1991;121:1161–1169.

72. Shabetai R, Fowler NO, Guntheroth WG. The hemodynamics of cardiac tamponade and constrictive pericarditis. *Am J Cardiol.* 1970;26:480–489.
73. Henkelman RM, Bronksill MJ: Artifacts in magnetic resonance imaging. *Rev Magn Reson Med.* 1987;2:77–88.
74. Soulen RL, Stark DD, Higgins CB: Magnetic resonance imaging of constrictive pericardial disease. *Am J Cardiol.* 1985;55:480–484.
75. Sechtem U, Sommerhoff BA, Markiewicz W, et al. Regional left ventricular wall thickening by magnetic resonance imaging: Evaluation in normal persons and patients with global and regional dysfunction. *Am J Cardiol.* 1987;59:145–151.
76. White RD, Paschal CB, Tkach JA, et al. Functional cardiovascular evaluation by magnetic resonance imaging. *Top Magn Reson Imaging.* 1990;2:31–48.
77. Mohiaddin RH, Wann SL, Underwood R, et al. Vena caval flow: Assessment with cine MR velocity mapping. *Radiology.* 1990;177:537–541.

Chapter 6

Magnetic Resonance Imaging in Thoracic Aortic Disease

Christoph A. Nienaber, MD, Yskert von Kodolitsch, MD, and Rolf P. Spielmann, MD

Magnetic resonance imaging (MRI) noninvasively provides information on anatomy, function, and blood flow with no exposure to ionizing radiation. Its information content may greatly overlap with established methods such as echocardiography, computed tomography (CT), or angiography, but MRI is more accurate and comprehensive. Although the cost effectiveness of MRI has not been proven in all areas,[1] MRI is the preferred modality in selected areas including diseases of the aorta, such as aneurysm, dissection and its precursors, congenital and inherited heart diseases and, in particular for postoperative follow-up of aortic repair and cardiac malformations.[2-4] MRI can demonstrate the anatomy of both the proximal and distal anastomoses and serve as a measure of quality control after corrective surgery[4,5] including complex operations such as aortic reconstruction and the Jatene or Norwood procedures.[5]

Technical Aspects of Magnetic Resonance Imaging/Angiography

Throughout the 1980s, many of the computing advances that proved essential in the development of CT found a second life in MRI. Rather than producing a transmission image of x-rays (CT), MRI relies on the magnetic properties of protons in water and the influence on these protons of their immediate chemical environment. After protons are excited by a pulse of radiofrequency energy, they "relax" by emitting a radiofrequency signal. In the case of hemorrhage (ie, leaking

From: Higgins CB, Ingwall JS, Pohost GM, (eds). *Current and Future Applications of Magnetic Resonance in Cardiovascular Disease.* Armonk, NY: Futura Publishing Company, Inc.; © 1998.

aneurysm), local chemical effects become more important. Current MRI exists in two basic forms, eg, spin-echo and gradient-echo or cine-MRI. While the spin-echo technique shows lack of signal intensity in vascular compartments with rapid blood flow (black blood imaging), the cine-MRI technique depicts flowing blood as a bright signal (white blood imaging).

Magnetic resonance angiography (MRA) represents an extension of MRI. The two methods to image flowing blood are called time-of-flight MRA and phase-contrast MRA. Time-of-flight MRA applies a radiofrequency pulse to the tissue volume being sampled, then detects the unexcited, flowing protons of blood that enter the imaging field. Phase-contrast MRA depends on differences in phase of mobile (flowing) protons compared with stationary (nonflowing) protons. Both techniques have been used successfully to generate clinically useful images of the normal and diseased aorta. By acquiring the proton signals within a volume of tissue, then using a computer to "collapse" the multiple sections into one image, an angiography-like image of all vessels containing flowing blood can be produced (maximum intensity projection). MRA shows tremendous promise in evaluation of the carotid and cerebral vasculature; its ultimate role in aortic imaging, however, is not yet known.

Normal Anatomy

The cornerstone of thoracic MRI is two-dimensional spin echo (anatomic) imaging. Because the ascending and descending aorta are parallel to the long axis of the thorax, this portion of the vessel will appear circular when imaged in transverse cross section, and as two parallel walls when imaged in a longitudinal plane. Tomograms obtained in intermediate planes yield an oval aortic image. At the level of the aortic root, the ostia of the coronary arteries (particularly the left) are frequently visualized (Figure 1). Anatomic (spin-echo) and flow velocity mapping are essential parts of a complete MRI study of the thoracic aorta. Blood in the descending aorta tends to spiral as it flows toward the bifurcation, causing a characteristic flow velocity pattern. Normal aortic blood flow velocity measurement is 1.7 m/s or less.[6,7]

MRI has become increasingly useful for evaluating suspected aortic dissection, aneurysm, and congenital anomaly. With no radiation or intravascular contrast agents, MRI can image differential flow in the true and false channels of an aortic dissection. MRI, however, is not available in all hospitals, and may not be offered as an emergency service. For patients with stable or chronic aortic processes, MRI provides comprehensive superior imaging of the aortic lumen, wall, and periaortic tissues simultaneously.

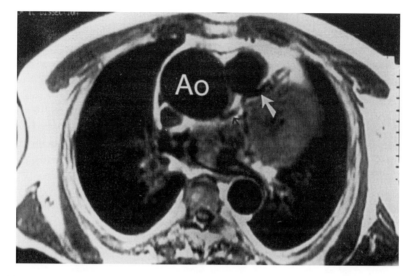

FIGURE 1. Transverse spin-echo MR image of the ascending aorta (aortic root) just above the valve; the tomogram visualizes the ostium and the proximal section of a normal left coronary artery (arrow).

Aortic Dissection

Acute dissection of the aorta is a medical emergency requiring immediate attention and therapy, with an estimated mortality rate of 1% to 2% per hour[8,9] in the first 24 to 48 hours after onset of dissection. Dissections can occur throughout the length of the aorta, and two described classification systems exist. De Bakey's nomenclature is based on the anatomic site of the intimal tear and the extent of the resulting dissection.[10] In a type I dissection, the intimal tear originates in the ascending aorta and the dissecting hematoma extends past the origin of left subclavian artery. Type II dissections are confined to the ascending aorta. Type III dissections begin after the origin of the left subclavian artery and extend distally. The Stanford classification is conceptually founded on prognostic grounds. Type A dissections involve the ascending aorta, regardless of the intimal tear's location, and type B dissections spare the ascending aorta and often imply a more favourite prognosis.[11] In general, acute dissections involving the ascending aorta require emergency surgery, yet descending aortic dissections may be successfully managed with medical therapy alone.[9,12] Thus, rapid detection and accurate diagnosis and anatomic assessment are critical in guiding successful management.

The gold standard for diagnosis of aortic dissection has been aortography, which has a reported sensitivity of 80% to 90%, specificity of 90% to 100%, and positive predictive value of approximately 95%.[12-16] Unfortunately, aortography is an invasive procedure that carries a small but real risk of complications. In addition, it requires a fully equipped catheterization laboratory and may be delayed by patient transportation and laboratory preparation. In the past several years, three less invasive diagnostic techniques, CT, echocardiography (including transesophageal echocardiography [TEE]), and MRI, have been studied and compared.[16] CT is noninvasive, usually easy to perform, and widely available; it requires intravascular contrast and provides little information on coronary anatomy, great vessels and thrombus formation in the false lumen, and none on aortic insufficiency. CT is relatively accurate for the diagnosis of dissection, with sensitivities ranging from 67% to 85% and specificities from 95% to 100%.[15,17-20]

Transthoracic ultrasound is reasonably accurate for diagnosing proximal aortic dissection. It is unreliable, however, for detecting distal thoracic dissection and is a poor screening test for diseases of the descending thoracic aorta.[15,21] TEE, however, is both a sensitive and specific diagnostic tool for aortic dissection. In a multicenter trial, Erbel et al[20] reported an overall sensitivity and specificity of 90% and 98%, respectively, for echocardiography (including both the transesophageal and transthoracic approach) in 164 consecutive patients with suspected dissection; in this study, TEE was more accurate than CT or aortography and took less time to perform. Ballal et al[19] studied a selected group of patients with proven dissection and confirmed the high diagnostic sensitivity of TEE (97%). TEE also detected coronary artery involvement in several cases and was superior to aortography in delineating aortic valvular function and pathology. Nienaber et al[22] compared TEE and MRI for the diagnosis of dissection. Overall, monoplane TEE was quite sensitive (100%), but had a lower specificity than MRI in a clinically blinded evaluation, especially in cases of dissection confined to the ascending aorta or the proximal aortic arch. MRI was as accurate as TEE in detecting pericardial effusions and was more sensitive in demonstrating false lumen thrombosis. Expanding on this observation, echocardiography was compared with MRI and CT in 110 patients with suspected dissection.[15] The sensitivities of MRI and TEE (100% and 96%, respectively) for diagnosing type A dissections were significantly higher than that of CT, although the sensitivities of all three techniques were similar for type B dissections. False-positive findings occured in only one patient by MRI, four by CT, and six by TEE (specificities of 98%, 87%, and 77%, respectively (Table 1). The low specificity of monoplane TEE in this study was mainly due to false-positive findings in the ascending aorta, where asymmetric atherosclerosis and ultrasound "reverberation" artifacts can lead to erroneous interpretation.[23]

TABLE 1

Sensitivity of Imaging Procedures in Subgroups of Aortic Dissections

Sensitivity (%)	TTE	TEE	XCT	MRI	Angio
Acute type A:	78.3*	95.2	94.1	100	81
Subacute type A:	87.5	100	80.0	100	80
Acute type B:	40.0#	100	100	100	92
Subacute type B:	29.4#	100	93.3	94.4	100

* P < .05 versus TEE, XCT, and MRI; # P < .01 versus TEE, XCT, and MRI.
TTE indicates transthoracic echocardiography; TEE, transesophageal echocardiography; XCT, X-ray computed tomography; angio, contrast angiography. Adapted from Reference 15.

Interestingly, in these trials[15,20] diagnostic test results were binary, either positive or negative; although this certainly is appropriate for investigative studies, it excludes diagnoses of probable or possible dissection. These types of TEE results may be helpful as well because they raise clinical suspicion and lead to further diagnostic testing.

Thus, MRI is emerging as the most accurate method for detecting aortic dissection. Unlike CT, MRI technology can construct images in multiple planes, thereby enhancing its diagnostic capabilities. Also, no contrast is needed, and newer techniques now permit detection and semiquantitation of aortic insufficiency,[20,24] identification of communications and thrombus formation (Table 2).

While the sensitivity and specificity of MRI approach 100%, there are, however, several important limitations. First, MRI used to be time-consuming and requires patient immobility for image acquisition. Second, metallic objects cannot be used near the MRI scanner. Finally, coronary artery involvement, which occurs in 10% to 20% of proximal dissections,[8] is not yet definable by routine MRI. The technology of MRA is advancing rapidly, and coronary arterial imaging may soon become available on a routine basis.[25,26]

In our experience, MRI has been extremely useful for rapid detection of both type A and type B aortic dissection. The procedure requires no contrast or arterial access and can take as little as 15 minutes to perform irrespective of the location of dissection (Figure 2). Longer examination times, when including gradient-echo or flow velocity imaging, may be necessary for proximal dissections and complicated cases. As part of a complete MRI examination, regional left ventricular function pericardial effusion and regurgitation can be assessed. MRI can identify intramural hemorrhage, luminal tears, stagnant blood flow

TABLE 2

Diagnostic Potential of TTE, TEE, XCT and MRI for the Detection of Thoracic Aortic Dissection in Forty-Seven Patients Who Underwent All Imaging Procedures

Dissection		Sensitivity (%)	Specificity (%)	Accuracy (%)	pos.PV (%)	neg.PV (%)
Ascending aorta	TTE	94.7	81.5	86.9	78.2	95.6
	TEE	100	82.1	89.4	79.2	100
	XCT	78.9	100*	91.5	100	85.5
	MRI	100	100*	100	100	100
Aortic arch	TTE	26.1	93.5	79.5	75.0	80.5
	TEE	92.3	93.9	93.5	85.7	96.9
	XCT	92.8	93.9	93.6	86.7	96.9
	MRI	92.8	100	97.9	100	97.0
Descending aorta	TTE	41.7†	100	66.7	100	56.2
	TEE	100	95.4	97.9	96.1	100
	XCT	88.0	86.4	87.2	88.0	86.4
	MRI	100	100	100	100	100

Percentages are calculated on the basis of all included individuals with assessable findings; PV = predictive value; * $P < .05$ versus TTE and TEE; † $P < .01$ versus TEE, XCT and MRI. Adapted from Reference 15.

versus thrombosis, and periaortic blood, eg, features to determine prognosis and guide early therapy. Moreover, MRI appears as an excellent method for long-term patient follow-up after medical or surgical treatment for ascending or descending dissections with costs varying from $1000 to $1900. This compares favorably with CT but is still substantially more expensive than TEE; an analysis of cost-effectiveness is certainly required. MRI has some potential drawbacks in a clinical scenario. Most evidently, MRI requires transportation and movement of a potentially unstable patient. With continuous electrocardiogram (ECG), pressure monitoring and voice communication, however, and with a cardiologist present no patient is in fact isolated and no side effects or substantial risks have been encountered.[15] Yet, patients with pacemakers, implanted cardioverters, or other metal devices, and/or claustrophobia cannot undergo MRI scanning. Thus, similar to TEE and CT, although both semi-invasive, MRI should be considered safe and certainly associated with less stress, blood pressure fluctuations and no risk of hypotension and nephrotoxicity from contrast material.[15,16,27]

Although MRI appears at least as safe as other methods, is usually both more accurate and comprehensive, and less prone to artifact, it lacks the portability of TEE and the widespread availability of CT.

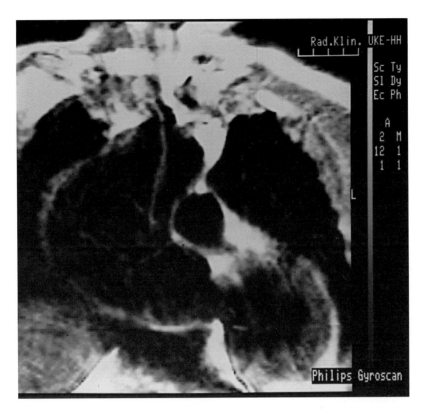

FIGURE 2. Coronal spin-echo MR image of a type A aortic dissection. A dissecting membrane clearly separates the true from the false lumen in both the ascending and descending thoracic aorta; the ascending aorta is markedly enlarged as a result of longstanding arterial hypertension

However, all methods are useful to define the specific lesions that may require surgical intervention such as proximal involvement, great vessel dissection and partial or transmural rapture.[16] Although MRI and TEE detect aortic incompetence and pericardial effusion, they cannot yet define distal coronary anatomy in an emergency situation. Some surgeons still require coronary angiography before proximal repair of a dissected aorta; we clearly feel that this time-consuming and potentially dangerous procedure is not justified in acute proximal dissection considering the urgency of repair and the possibility of visual inspection of the coronary ostia by the surgeon.[15,28]

In principle, with improving technology, coronary arteries will be routinely imaged by both MRI and TEE.[19,26] In our view distal coronary artery disease does not constitute a real problem in the setting of acute aortic dissection. Coronary artery disease is well amenable to medical treatment or elective angioplasty at follow-up. These options may render coronary angiography obsolete in the routine work-up of aortic dissection. The optimal approach to detecting dissection of the thoracic aorta should be a noninvasive strategy using MRI in all hemodynamically stable patients and TEE in patients too unstable for transportation.[16] Comprehensive and detailed evaluation can thus be reduced to a single noninvasive imaging modality in the evaluation of suspected aortic dissection.[15]

Intramural Hemorrhage of the Aorta

Along these lines, and unlike angiography, the noninvasive tomographic modalities (such as MRI, CT, and TEE) may even identify precursors of dissection such as intramural hemorrhage (IMH) with no luminal component.[29,30] IMH was first described in 1920 as "dissection without intimal tear" and was originally considered a distinct entity at necropsy.[31] However, with high-resolution tomographic imaging, the in vivo diagnosis of IMH is now feasible[29,30,32] and suggest that IMH is a precursor of dissection, particularly with the high (>30%) rate of progression to overt dissection. In our experience, both MRI and CT imaging identified IMH in 12.8% of patients with acute aortic syndromes; this percentage is almost identical to autopsy results from 204 patients with aortic dissection, 27 of whom (13.2%) had no identifiable intimal tear.[33] With clinical signs and symptoms virtually identical to classic aortic dissection IMH appears more likely to be a precursor of dissection than a separate entity.[30,34] Typical epiphenomena of dis-

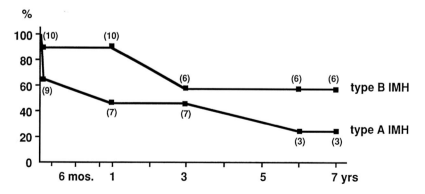

FIGURE 3. Survival analysis of patients with IMH as a function of IMH location. In analogy to the Stanford classification type A, IMH is considered to involve the ascending aorta, whereas type B IMH involved only the descending aorta.

TABLE 3

True Positive and True Negative Findings of Various Imaging Modalities for the Diagnosis of Intramural Hemorrhage (IMH) in Patients with Suspected Aortic Dissection

Findings	TEE	XCT	MRI	P
n [%]	3/25	14/25	12/25	n.s.
IMH [true positive]	3/3	14/14	12/12	n.s.
True positive findings				
ascending aorta	2/2	6/6	5/5	n.s.
aortic arch	0/1	6/6	2/2	n.s.
descending aorta	—	11/12	9/9	n.s.
True negative findings				
ascending aorta	1/1	7/8	7/7	n.s.
aortic arch	1/2	7/7	10/10	n.s.
descending aorta	2/2	2/2	3/3	n.s.

* IMH indicates intramural hemorrhage; TEE, transesophageal echocardiography; XCT, X-ray computed tomography; MRI, magnetic resonance imaging.

section such as aortic insufficiency, pericardial or pleural effusion may also occur in IMH.[32,35] Moreover, arterial hypertension is the most frequent predisposing factor for IMH as well as for overt dissection with an incidence of 67% to 84%.[35–37]

As the initiating event of IMH, spontaneous rupture of aortic vasa vasorum, especially of nutrient vessels to the media layer, was suggested to cause aortic desintegration without an intimal tear.[38,39] With a pathogenesis that explains the high rate of progression to overt aortic dissection, and prognosis and survival patterns also similar to aortic dissection urgent diagnosis by use of sensitive imaging modalities is of utmost importance (Figure 3 and Table 3).

Diagnostic Approach to IMH

With a clinical presentation similar to dissection, the diagnosis of IMH relies on the visualization of intramural blood and/or evidence of localized increased wall thickness (Figure 4A). The high density of fresh hematoma on CT scans appears specific for IMH. MRI techniques, however, not only visualize blood sequestration, but also allow the assessment of the age of the hematoma based on the formation of methemoglobin.[40] TEE has also been emphasized as diagnostic tool; however, the differentiation from severe atherosclerosis with local wall thickening may be difficult, and IMH may only be diagnosed retrospectively

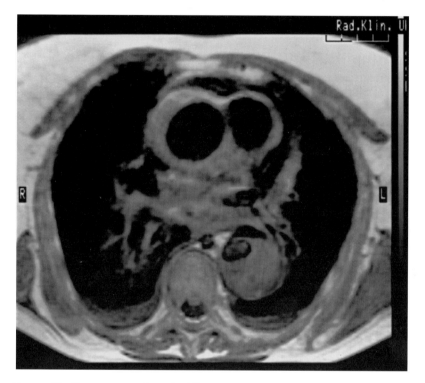

FIGURE 4A. Transverse spin-echo MR tomogram with the typical feature of IMH involving both the ascending and descending thoracic aorta after traumatic impact. The aortic wall is homogeneously thickened and no intimal laceration is identified.

with serial evaluation (resolution or progression of IMH). Moreover, false-positive findings of local thickening on tangential scans and around the hemiazygos vein may be more likely with TEE. Both TEE and CT resulted in one false-positive and one false-negative segmental finding each (pathological wall thickness without hematoma), whereas the segmental extent of IMH was correctly assessed with MRI (Table 4). Although TEE has an excellent sensitivity to detect aortic dissection,[15,16,20] the definite distinction between IMH and normal findings may require a second tomographic modality such as CT or MRI because a false-negative result (or false exclusion of IMH) is more likely to be avoided with independent morphological information. Contrast angiography is rarely diagnostic because a luminal component is a missing feature in IMH. Our own series of MRI findings in 22 cases of IMH consistently revealed abnormal thickness of the aortic wall up to 30

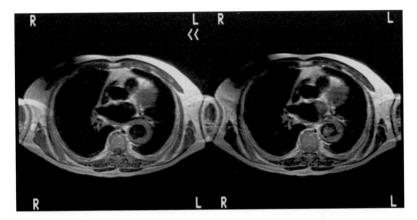

FIGURE 4B. Transverse MR tomogram of a patient with suspected dissection revealing evidence of IMH in the descending aorta 24 hours after onset of symptoms. The left side depicts a T2-weighted image, the right side represents the corresponding T1-weighted image; intramural blood is characterized by high signal intensity (arrows) on both spin echo images. Pleural effusion is also present as evidence of fluid extravasation.

TABLE 4

Survival of Intramural Hemorrhage (IMH)

	Type A IMH		Arch IMH		Type B IMH	
	Surgical	Medical	Surgical	Medical	Surgical	Medical
30 day	7/7 (100)[#]	1/5 (20)	—	1/2 (50)	5/5 (100)	5/6 (83)
1 year	5/7 (71.4)*	1/5 (20)	—	1/2 (50)	4/5 (80)	5/6 (83)

* $P < .05$; [#] $P < .01$; numbers denote surviving patients per subgroup; numbers in parentheses are percentages; type A IMH involves the ascending aorta; type B IMH involves the descending aorta only. Adapted from Reference 30.

mm both asymmetrical or symmetrical in circumference with an extent of 3 to 30 cm (Figure 4a).

Some patients revealed high-signal intensity within the aortic wall on T1 spin-echo images consistent with subacute IMH, whereas acute IMH (early stages of hemorrhage) may be overlooked on T1 images due to the isodense appearance of blood and aortic wall.[30,32,41,42] Acute IMH (early stages) are depicted on T2 images due to high initial signal intensity of blood, whereas blood of 1 to 5 days of age has lower signal intensity on T2 images (Figure 4B).

In conclusion, as a potential precursor of dissection, IMH requires careful diagnostic attention by use of high-resolution tomographic imaging; due to its physical properties MRI may play a prominent role not only to diagnose IMH, but also to assess its age and differentiate IMH from mural thrombosis. Angiography certainly is not diagnostic; given the poor experience with medical treatment, early surgical repair should be considered for all patients with ascending aortic involvement (type A IMH) and for any patient with recurrent pain. Conversely, surgery may not be required in patients with IMH of the descending aorta (Figure 4A and 4B). Moreover, patients may benefit from serial follow-up by MR imaging to rule out progression regardless of treatment strategy, due to new lesions or spontaneous relapses even after surgical repair.[42a]

Aortic Ulcers

Aortic ulcers are a complication of aortic atherosclerosis and may mimic subacute distal aortic dissection or may develop without major symptoms. In contrast to IMH, aortic ulcers are characterized on angiography by focal contrast enhancement beyond the confines of the aortic lumen but communicating with the lumen[39,43]; no consensus has been achieved on prognosis and outcome of aortic ulcers. Both IMH and ulcers are unrelated to intimal lacerations, as in acute aortic dissection.[44] Lacerations and IMH usually occur at points of greatest aortic wall stress (right lateral ascending aorta or adjacent to the ligamentum arteriosum), whereas penetrating ulcers are typically found in the descending or abdominal aorta. Conversely, discrete penetrating atheromatous ulcers (giant ulcers) have been suspected as one cause of intramural bleeding.[42] In such a setting, the hematoma, however, is confined to the rim adjacent to the ulcer. Both MRI and TEE have helped to elucidate the pathogenetic background and the complex anatomic peculiarities of these important features.[29,30,41,45,46] Accurate diagnosis of penetrating ulcers is sometimes difficult and no test is ideal.[46] CT may demonstrate the surrounding hematoma and displaced calcifications in most cases[39]; in addition to this, MRI scanning can differentiate sub-acute intramural hematoma from chronic intraluminal thrombus.[45] No large-scale studies of MRI and aortic ulcers are currently available, but due to its versatility and imaging features, magnetic resonance scanning appears best suited to characterize this form of aortic pathology as a constellation of diffuse aortic atherosclerosis, an ulceration with focal wall thickening and no evidence of aortic dissection.

Thoracic Aortic Aneurysm

Optimal treatment of thoracic aneurysms requires accurate definition of size, anatomy, rate of growth, presence of dissection or thrombus, and involvement of adjacent structures including the aortic valve. Except for MRI, no single test consistently supplies all this information.

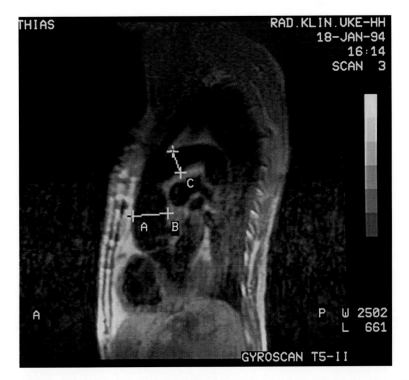

FIGURE 5A. Sagittal spin-echo MR image with beginning ectasia of the ascending aorta in a young patient with Marfan's syndrome scheduled for annual follow-up studies to identify progression and the need for surgical repair at a diameter of >5.5 cm.

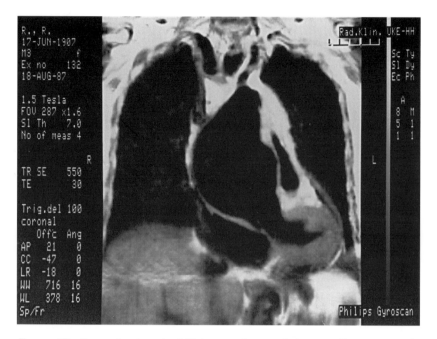

FIGURE 5B. Coronal spin-echo MR image of an end-stage aortic aneurysm in a patient with Marfan's syndrome; the ascending aneurysm has reached a diameter > 6 cm and surgical repair is advised.

Aortography may underestimate the size of aneurysms if significant intra-aortic thrombus is present and may fail to fully define saccular structures because of stagnant intra-aneurysmal blood flow.[47] CT scanning is noninvasive and suitable for serial examinations, but requires contrast and provides only axial images. Transthoracic echocardiography usually visualizes the ascending aorta adequately but may not optimally image the arch and is useless for the descending aorta.

Both TEE and MRI seem well suited for serially evaluating thoracic aortic aneurysms and almost always provide excellent images (Figures 5A and 5B). In addition to measuring aneurysm dimensions, both TEE and MRI can also detect fistulas, false channels, intraluminal thrombosis, and aortic valvular insufficiency.[48] At present, however, there are no large trials testing the value of MRI and TEE for thoracic aneurysms, and much of the literature exists in case reports.[49-52] MRI is accurate and versatile but may be to a certain degree limited by the financial expenses of serial studies. Although MRI promises to play an optimal role in the diagnosis and management of thoracic aortic aneurysms, cost considerations of multiple follow-up studies of aneurysm dimen-

sion have to be evaluated before recommending widespread use of
MRI scanning to follow stable patients with subcritical aneurysms.

Aortic Trauma

MRI has promising potential for comprehensive and accurate evaluation of suspected aortic trauma. Aortic rupture often results from
blunt thoracic trauma or deceleration injury and causes death in the
majority of affected patients (Figure 6).[53,54] Of those who survive until
hospital admission, expedient evaluation is critical. Chest roentgenog-
raphy shows abnormalities in 90% of patients with aortic rupture but
lacks specificity[55] in stabilized, even mechanically ventilated patients.
Both CT and MRI are not too difficult to perform in this setting. Aortography remains the accepted standard for the diagnosis and evaluation

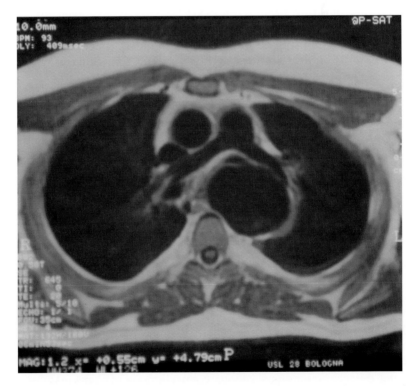

FIGURE 6. Horizontal (axial) spin-echo MR image after deceleration trauma in
a young male patient. The descending aorta shows a complete circumferential
rupture; only the integrity of the advential layer prevented from sudden exsan-
guination. (Courtesy of Dr. R. Fattori, Ospedale Policlinico S. Orsola, Bologna,
Italy.)

of aortic trauma, but requires transport of the injured patient to the angiographic laboratory for a procedure that often lasts longer than an hour and has a 10% complication rate.[56,57]

TEE can also rapidly visualize the aorta in an injured patient. The examination can proceed at the bedside or in the operating room, often during other diagnostic or therapeutic procedures. At present, there are several case reports documenting successful identification of aortic dissection and rupture in the posttraumatic setting.[58,59] Studies comparing TEE with other diagnostic modalities in small patient groups, however, have produced mixed results.[60,61] In the largest trial to date, 69 patients with suspected aortic trauma underwent both TEE and aortography soon after admission.[62] TEE revealed thoracic aortic injury in seven patients, and these injuries were all confirmed either at surgery or autopsy. Aortography in this group yielded two false-negative results and had an overall sensitivity of 67%. Both the sensitivity and specificity of TEE were 100%. TEE, however, has several limitations in the setting of aortic trauma. Protocols for airway management and cervical spine precautions have not been fully addressed, and the procedure could conceivably worsen a preexisting or unstable neck injury. Disruption of the small portion of the ascending aorta obscured by the bronchus may escape detection, and small intimal tears may also be missed. Finally, pneumothorax (which is not uncommon in thoracic trauma) can limit evaluation of the descending aorta.[14,63] TEE may help screen patients with thoracic aortic trauma to identify those who require angiography (and could perhaps replace aortography as the sole preoperative test in some cases), but long-term, large-population studies are necessary to assess the technique's best use in this setting.

Congenital and Inherited Aortic Disease

In children, transthoracic echocardiography does not always provide adequate imaging of cardiac and aortic pathology, including valvular abnormalities, subvalvular and supravalvular aortic stenosis, and right-sided aortic arch. In certain young patients with congenital cardiovascular disease, however, surface ultrasonography may be incomplete, and recently developed pediatric transesophageal probes have proven useful. Transesophageal imaging in young patients, as in adults, is especially helpful for imaging posterior structures, including atrial septal defects, anomolous venous connections, and abnormalities of the great vessels.[62] As the age and size of patients with congenital heart disease increases, the likelihood of complete and optimal transthoracic imaging gradually declines, and both MRI and TEE in selected cases assume a more important role. Both techniques detect aortic coarcta-

tion, right-sided aortic arch, congenital bicuspid aortic valve, supravalvular and subvalvular aortic stenosis, patent ductus arteriosus, aorticopulmonary window, transposition of the great vessels, and truncus
arteriosus.[5,63–67] Figures 7A and 7B demonstrate a typical case of aortic
coarctation on a spin-echo (anatomic) and gradient-echo (functional)
MR image.

Of the inherited connective tissue diseases, Marfan syndrome,
which results from mutations in genes coding for the glycoprotein fibrillin, is an autosomal dominant trait with numerous manifestations
affecting the cardiovascular, skeletal, and ocular systems.[68] Those patients with cardiovascular involvement have a decreased life expec-
tancy, primarily from progressive aortic root dilation (Figures 5A and
5B) and subsequent aortic insufficiency, dissection, and rupture.[69] In
early asymptomatic stages of aortic root dilatation chronic β-blockade
has been established as an effective means of slowing the progressive
enlargement and delaying the associated morbidity[67a] as depicted in
Figures 8A and 8B. Transthoracic echocardiography provides adequate
detail of the heart and aortic root in most instances, but occasionally,
images are suboptimal and TEE or MRI becomes necessary. In cases
of suspected dissection, TEE (or MRI) should be performed quickly
because aortic rupture, acute valvular regurgitation, and hemopericardium occur in a high proportion of patients.[70,71] Even after a successful
surgical intervention, experienced centers suggest a baseline postsurgical MRI or CT scan, followed by serial imaging in 6 months and eventually annual intervals to screen for new focal aneurysms or dissections.

Ehlers-Danlos syndrome encompasses at least 10 distinct disor-
ders, most of which affect the skin and little else. In one of the exceptions, type IV Ehlers-Danlos syndrome, the gene coding for type III
procollagen is abnormal. The resulting deficiency of this collagen component causes decreassed strength of arterial connective tissues.[72,73]
Spontaneous aortic or arterial rupture is the most common cause of
death in these patients. Arteriography is quite hazardous because of
vascular fragility, and less invasive vascular imaging is preferable.
Therefore, MRI and TEE may be helpful in cases of suspected aortic
dilatation or disruption. As yet, to our knowledge there are no large
studies of both TEE and MRI in Ehlers-Danlos syndrome or Marfan
syndrome.

Para-aortic Disease

Thoracic MRI is used mainly to visualize cardiac and vascular
structures, but it can also detect other intrathoracic pathology such
as paracardiac and pericardial tumors, pleural effusions, collapsed or

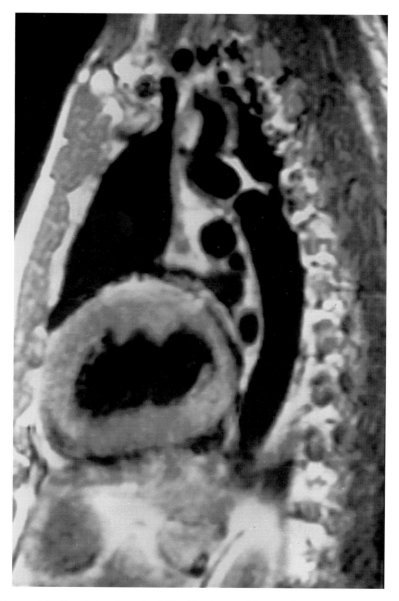

FIGURE 7A. Sagittal spin-echo MR with clear evidence of aortic coactation at the typical location distal to the great arch vessels.

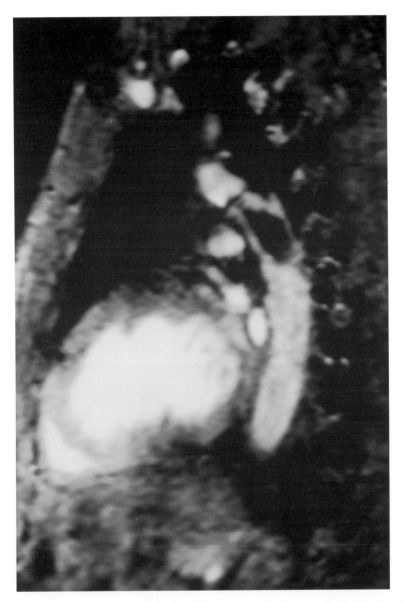

FIGURE 7B. The corresponding cine-MR image reveals a marked signal void distal to the coarctation in the direction of the bloodstream indicating accelerated blood flow velocity and turbulence.

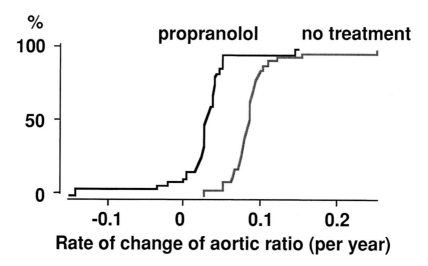

FIGURE 8A. Empirical distribution functions of the rate of change in the aortic ratio. The height of each curve at any point shows the proportion of patients with values at or below the value on the x axis. (Adapted from Reference 67a with permission.)

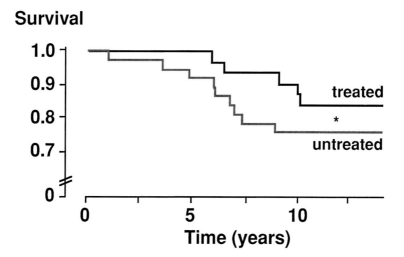

FIGURE 8B. Kaplan-Meier survival analysis based on clinical endpoints such as death, congestive heart failure, aortic regurgitation, aortic dissection or cardiovascular surgery. Adopted from reference 67b with permission of the New England Journal of Medicine.

consolidated lungs, hiatal hernias, and para-aortic masses. Fluid-filled structures are easily distinguished from solid masses, and cardiac or vascular tumor invasions can sometimes be demonstrated. Although TEE may provide useful images of such para-aortic masses, it is relatively undertested and clearly has not displaced CT or MRI. Tissue characterization techniques may provide information about tumors and other structures, but it is too early to predict whether TEE will be consistently useful in this area.[74-76]

Summary and Outlook

In the scenario of suspected aortic dissection two-dimensional echocardiography should include the transesophageal approach to improve sensitivity and assess the anatomic extent of the lesion. Both TEE and MRI as tomographic noninvasive imaging techniques proved feasible, reliable and safe even in severely ill and potentially unstable patients with acute or chronic thoracic aortic dissection. MRI yielded optimal reliability and may emerge as the future gold standard of sensitivity and specificity of thoracic aortic dissection irrespective of its location and possibly for many other diseases involving the aorta. MRI provides exact anatomic mapping of the entire aorta and adjacent tissues due to free choice of representative planes within reasonable time and at no risk. Disadvantages of current MRI technology such as patient transportation, limited patient access and longer examination time than TEE (especially in acute cases) are unlikely to result in an increased individual risk, but may be considered a limitation at the present time. Technical improvement such as open MRI scanners with better patient access and more rapid acquisition may alleviate two of these drawbacks. The use of faster and stronger gradient coils and superior surface coils may improve spatial resolution and the signal-to-noise ratio in the future, and significantly shorten the examination time. As a clinical routine we recommend TEE for immediate diagnostic evaluation of unstable and clinically deteriorating patients prior to immediate surgical intervention. MRI appears to be the method of choice in stable patients with suspected acute or subacute dissections and certainly the best method for serial follow-up studies after surgical repair or in chronic cases.

The comprehensive information from anatomic mapping using TEE or MRI may not only render invasive angiographic techniques obsolete in the clinical scenario of suspected aortic dissection, but could eventually enable surgical interventions solely guided by noninvasive imaging modalities.

Acknowledgment

The authors want to express their thanks to Mrs. Jeanette Hoffmann for preparation of the manuscript and Miss Dörte Oestreich for art and phototechnical support.

References

1. Abernethy LJ, Szczepura AK, Fletcher J, et al. Cost effectiveness of magnetic resonance imaging. *Br Med J.* 1992;304:183.
2. Parsons JM, Baker EJ, Hayes A, et al. Magnetic resonance imaging of the great arteries in infants. *Int J Cardiol.* 1990;28:73.
3. Soulen RL, Fishman EK, Pyeritz RE, et al. Marfan syndrome: Evaluation with MR imaging versus CT. *Radiology.* 1987;165:697.
4. Sampson C, Martinez J, Rees S, et al. Evaluation of Fontan's operation by magnetic resonance imaging. *Am J Cardiol.* 1990;65:819.
5. Kersting-Sommerhoff BA, Seelos KC, Hardy C, et al. Evaluation of surgical procedures for canotic congenital heart disease by using MR imaging. *AJR* 1990;155:259.
6. Mitchell MM. Evaluation of arotic disease. In: Dittrich HC, ed. *Clinical Transesophageal Echocardiography.* St. Louis: Mosby-Year Book; 1992:97–107.
7. Waggoner AD, Perez JE. Principles and physics of Doppler. *Cardiol Clin.* 1990;8:173–190.
8. Hirst AE, Johns VJ, Kime SW Jr. Dissecting aneurysm of the aorta: a review of 505 cases. *Medicine.* 1958;37:217–279.
9. Nienaber CA, von Kodolitsch Y. Meta-analysis of changing mortality pattern in thoracic aortic dissection. *Herz.* 1992;17:398–416.
10. DeBakey ME, McCollum CH, Crawford ES, et al. Dissection and dissecting aneurysms of the aorta. *Surgery.* 1982;92:1118–1134.
11. Daily PO, Trueblood W, Stinson EB, et al. Management of acute aortic dissections. *Ann Thorac Surg.* 19770, 10:237–247.
12. Eagle KA, DeSanctis RW. Aortic dissection. *Curr Probl Cardiol.* 1989;14: 231–278.
13. Erbel R, Mohr-Kahaly S, Renollet H, et al. Diagnosis of aortic dissection: the value of transesophageal echocardiography. *Thorac Cardiovasc Surg.* 1987;35:126–133.
14. Enia F, Ledda G, Lo Mauro R, et al. Utility of echocardiography in the diagnosis of aortic dissection involving the ascending aorta. *Chest.* 1989; 95:124–129.
15. Nienaber CA, von Kodolitsch Y, Nicolas V, et al. The diagnosis of thoracic aortic dissection by noninvasive imaging procedures. *N Engl J Med.* 1993; 328:1–9.
16. Cigarroa JE, Isselbacher EM, De Sanctis RW, Eagle KA. Diagnostic imaging in the evaluation of suspected aortic dissection. *N Engl J Med.* 1993;328: 35–43.
17. Singh H, Fitzgerald E, Ruttley MST. Computed tomography: The investigation of choice for aortic dissection? *Br Heart J.* 1986;56:171–175.
18. White RD, Lipton MJ, Higgins CB et al. Noninvasive evaluation of suspected thoracic aortic disease by contrast-enhanced computed tomography. *Am J Cardiol.* 1986;57:282–290.

19. Ballal RS, Nanda NC, Gatewood R, et al. Usefulness of transesophageal echocardiography in assessment of aortic dissection. *Circulation.* 1991;84: 1903–1914.
20. Erbel R, Engberding R, Daniel W, et al. Echocardiography in diagnosis of aortic dissection. *Lancet.* 1989;1:457–461.
21. Granato JE, Dee P, Gibson RS. Utility of two-dimensional echocardiography in suspected aortic dissection. *Am J Cardiol.* 1985;56:123–129.
22. Nienaber CA, Spielmann RP, von Kodolitsch Y, et al. Diagnosis of thoracic aortic dissection: Magnetic resonance imaging versus transesophageal echocardiography. *Circulation.* 1992;85:434–447.
23. Applebe AF, Walker PG, Yeoh JK, et al. Clinical significance and origin of artifacts in transesophageal echocardiography of the thoracic aorta. *J Am Coll Cardiol.* 1993;21:754–760.
24. Feilcke G, Münster F, Siglow V, et al. Dynamic magnetic resonance imaging of aortic regurgitation: Comparison with contrast aortography and color Doppler echocardiography. *Z Kardiol.* 1993;82:585–597.
25. Manning WJ, Li W, Edelman RR. A preliminary angiography with conventional angiography. *N Engl J Med.* 1993;328:828–832.
26. Paulin S, von Schulthess GK, Fossel E, Krayenbuehl HP. MR imaging of the aortic root and proximal coronary arteries. *AJR.* 1987;148:665–670.
27. Brabant SD, Eisenberg MJ, Schiller NB. The diagnostic value of imaging techniques for aortic dissection. *Am Heart J.* 1992;124:541–543.
28. Cheitlin MD. Commentary on: Anderson MW, Higgins CB. Should the patient with suspected acute dissection of the aorta have MRI, CAT scan, or aortography as the definitive study? In: Cheitlin MD, Brest AM, eds. Dilemmas in cardiology. Philadelphia: F. A. Davis, 1990:293–306.
29. Mohr-Kahaly S, Erbel R, Kearney P, et al. Aortic intramural hemorrhage visualized by transoesophageal echocardiography: Findings and prognostic implications. *J Am Coll Cardiol.* 1994;23:658–664.
30. Nienaber CA, von Kodolitsch Y, Petersen B, et al. Intramural hemorrhage of the thoracic aorta. Diagnostic and therapeutic implications. *Circulation.* 1995;92:1465–1472.
31. Krukenberg E, Beiträge zur Frage des Aneurysma dissecans. *Beitr Pathol Anat Allg Pathol.* 1920;67:329–351.
32. Wolverson MK, Crepps LF, Sundaram M, et al. Hyperdensity of recent hemorrhage at body computed tomography: Incidence and morphologic variation. *Radiology.* 1983;148:779–784.
33. Wilson SK, Hutchins GM. Aortic dissecting aneurysms: Causative factors in 204 subjects. *Arch Pathol Lab Med.* 1982;106:175–180.
34. Robbins RC, McManus RP, Mitchel RS, et al. Management of patients with intramural hematoma of the thoracic aorta. *Circulation.* 1993;88(suppl 11): II-1-II-10.
35. Kodolitsch Y, Spielmann RP, Petersen B, et al. Intramural hemorrhage as a precursor of aortic dissection. *Z Kardiol.* 1995;4:939–946.
36. Larson EW, Edwards WD. Risk factors for aortic dissection: A necropsy study of 161 patients. *Am J Cardiol.* 1984;43:849–855.
37. Sütsch G, Jenni R, von Segesser L, Turina M. Predictability of aortic dissection as function of aortic diameter. *Eur Heart J.* 1991;12:1247–1256.
38. Gore I. Pathogenesis of dissecting aneurysm of the aorta. *Arch Pathol Lab Med.* 1952;53:142–153.
39. Kazerooni EA, Bree RL, Williams DM. Penetrating atherosclerotic ulcers of the descending thoracic aorta: evaluation with CT and distinction from aortic dissection. *Radiology.* 1992;183:759–765.

40. Wolff KA, Herold CJ, Tempany CM, et al. Aortic dissection: Atypical patterns seen at MR imaging. *Radiology.* 1991;181:489–495.
41. Yamada T, Tada S, Harada J. Aortic dissection without intimal rupture: Diagnosis with MR imaging and CT. *Radiology.* 1988;168:347–352.
42. Stanson AW, Welch TJ, Ehman RL, Sheedy II PF. A variant of aortic dissection: computer tomography and magnetic resonance findings. *Cardiovasc Imaging.* 1989;1:55–59.
42a. Nienaber CA, Röttig K, Brockhoff CJ, et al. Noninvasive follow-up (F/U) in thoracic aortic dissection: transesophageal echocardiography versus magnetic resonance imaging. *Circulation.* 1994;90:I–585.
43. Hussain S, Glover JL, Bree R, Bendick PJ. Penetrating atherosclerotic ulcers of the thoracic aorta. *J Vasc Surg.* 1989;9:710–717.
44. Murray CA, Edwards JE. Spontaneous laceration of the ascending aorta. *Circulation.* 1973;47:848–858.
45. Yucel EK, Steinberg FL, Egglin TK, et al. Penetrating aortic ulcers: diagnosis with MR imaging. *Radiology.* 1990;177:779–781.
46. Cooke JP, Kazmier FJ, Orszulak TA. The penetrating aortic ulcer pathologic manifestations, diagnosis and management. *Mayo Clin Proc.* 1988;63: 718–725.
47. Eagle KA. De Sanctis RW. Disease of the aorta. In: Braunwald E, ed. *Heart Disease: A Textbook of Cardiovascular Medicine.* 4th ed. Philadelphia, Pa: WB Saunders Co: 1992;1533–1535.
48. Kamp O, van Rossum AC, Torenbeek R. Transesophageal echocardiography and magnetic resonance imaging for the assessment of saccular aneurysm of the transverse thoracic aorta. *Int J Cardiol.* 1991;33:330–333.
49. McKenney PA, Shemin RJ, Weigers SE. Role of transesophageal echocardiography in sinus of Valsalva aneurysm. *Am Heart J.* 1992;123:228–229.
50. Dorsa FB, Tunick PA, Culliford A, Kronzon I. Pseudoaneurysm of the thoracic aorta due to cardiopulmonary resuscitation: diagnosis by transesophageal echocardiography. *Am Heart J.* 1992;123:1398–1400.
51. Kronzon I, Demopoulos L, Schrem SS, et al. Pitfalls in the diagnosis of thoracic aortic aneurysm by tansesophageal echocardiography. *J Am Soc Echocardiog.* 1990;3:145–148.
52. Taams MA, Gussenhoven WJ, Bos E, Roelandt J. Saccular aneurysm of the transverse thoracic aorta detected by transesophageal echocardiography. *Chest.* 1988;93:436–437.
53. Delrossi AJ, Cernaianu AC, Madden CD, et al. Traumatic disruptions of the thoracic aorta: Treatment and outcome. *Surgery.* 1990;108:864–870.
54. Sturm JT, Biliar TR, Dorsey JS, et al. Risk factors for survival following surgical treatment of traumatic aortic rupture. *Ann Thorac Surg.* 1985;39: 418–421.
55. Marsh DG, Sturn JT. Traumatic aortic rupture: Roentgenographic indications for angiography. *Ann Thorac Surg.* 1976;212:337–340.
56. Eddy AC, Nance DR, Goldman MA, et al. Rapid diagnosis of thoracic aortic transection using intravenous digital subtraction angiography. *Am J Surg.* 1990;159:500–503.
57. Kram HB, Wohlmuth DA, Appel PL, Shoemaker WC. Clinical and radiographic indications for aortography in blunt chest trauma. *J Vasc Surg.* 1987; 6:168–176.
58. Galvin IF, Black IW, Lee CL, Horton DA. Transesophageal echocardiography in acute aortic transection. *Ann Thorac Surg.* 1991;51:310–311.
59. Goarin JP, Le Bret F, Riou B, et al. Early diagnosis of traumatic thoracic

aortic rupture by transeosphageal echocardiography. *Chest.* 1993;103: 618–620.

60. Fyfe DA, Kline CH. Transesophageal echocardiography for congenital heart disease. *Echocardiography.* 1991;8:573–586.

61. Parsons JM, Baker EJ, Anderson RH, et al. Double-outlet right ventricle: Morphologic demonstration using nuclear magnetic resonance imaging. *J Am Coll Cardiol.* 1991;18:168.

62. Kearney PA, Smith W, Johnson SB, et al. Use of transesophageal echocardiography in the evaluation of traumatic aortic injury. *J Trauma.* 1993;34: 696–703.

63. Blanchard DG, Dittrich HC, Mitchell M, McCann HA. Diagnostic pitfalls in tansesophageal echocardiography. *J Am Soc Echocardiogr.* 1992;5:525–540.

64. Ryan K, Sanyal RS, Pinheiro L, Nanda NC. Assessment of aortic coarctation and collateral circulation by biplane transesophageal echocardiography. *Echocardiography.* 1992;9:277–285.

65. Mohiaddin RH, Kilner PJ, Rees RSO, Longmore DB. Magnetic resonance volume flow and jet velocity mapping in aortic coarctation. *J Am Coll Cardiol.* 1993;22:1515–1521.

66. Simpson IA, Chung KL, Glass RF, et al. Cine magnetic resonance imaging for evaluation of anatomy and flow relations in infants and children with coarctation of the aorta. *Circulation.* 1988;78:142.

67. Bank ER, Aisen AM, Rocchini AP, Hernandez RJ. Coarctation of the aorta in children undergoing angioplasty: Pretreatment and posttreatment MR imaging. *Radiology.* 1987;162:235.

67a. Shores J, Berger KR, Murphy EA, Pyeritz RE. Progression of aortic dilation and the benefit of long-term β-adrenergic blockade in Marfan's syndrome. *N Engl J Med.* 1994;330:1335–1341.

68. Lee B, Godfrey M, Vitale E, et al. Linkage of Marfan syndrome and a phenotypically related disorder to two different fibrillin genes. *Nature.* 1991;352:330–334.

69. Pyeritz RE, McKusick VA. The Marfan syndrome: Diagnosis and management. *N Engl J Med.* 1979;300:772–777.

70. Kersting-Sommerhoff BA, Sechtem UP, Schiller NB, et al. MR imaging of the thoracic aorta in Marfan patients. *J Comput Assist Tomogr.* 1987;11:633.

71. Schaefer S, Peshock RM, Mallot CR, et al. Nuclear magnetic resonance imaging in Marfan's syndrome. *J Am Coll Cardiol.* 1987;9:70.

72. Steinmann B, Superti-Furga A, Joller-Jemelka HI, et al. Ehlers-Danlos syndrome type IV: A subset of patients disinguished by low serum levels of the amino-terminal propeptide of type III procollagen. *Am J Med Genet.* 1989;34:68–71.

73. Byers PH. Ehers-Danlos syndrome. In: Scriver CR, Beaudet AL, Sly W, Valle D, eds. *The Metabolic Basis of Inherited Disease.* 6th ed. New York, NY: McGraw-Hill Inc; 1989;2824–2833.

74. Lund JT, Ehman RL, Julsrud PR, et al. Cardiac masses: Assessment by MR imaging. *AR.* 1989;152:469.

75. Freedberg RS, Kronzon L, Rumanick WM, et al. The contribution of magnetic resonance imaging to the evaluation of intracardiac tumors diagnosed by echocardiography. *Circulation.* 1988;77:96.

76. Mügge A, Daniel WG, Haverich A, et al. Diagnosis of noninfective cardiac mass lesions by two-dimensional echocardiography: Comparison of the transthoracic and transesophageal approach. *Circulation.* 1991;83:70–78.

## Chapter 7

Morphological Evaluation in Congenital Heart Disease Using Magnetic Resonance Imaging

Mark A. Fogel, MD

Introduction

The use of magnetic resonance imaging (MRI) in the morphological evaluation of congenital heart disease[1–10] is complementary to other imaging modalities such as echocardiography and angiography. In most instances, all anatomic data necessary for diagnosis may be obtained via MRI, and may in fact add information that could not have been acquired otherwise. This is especially true in older children, adolescents, and adults, where echocardiographic windows are poor and adequate imaging can sometimes be impossible.[9] Echocardiography is also inherently limited by acoustic windows and the interposition of lung or bone, whereas MRI can acquire data in complex planes or create these complex planes offline using multiplanar reconstruction (also called oblique sectioning,[11] see below). This is extremely important in congenital heart disease, as the presence of cardiovascular abnormalities with bizarre shapes, extra or missing vascular structures, and cardiac malposition all require nonstandard views. Furthermore, unlike echocardiography, MRI is not subject to artifacts of calcification or patch materials used for surgical reconstruction, which is important in the surgical intensive specialty of pediatric cardiology.

The misshapen cardiovascular structures in congenital heart disease may not lend themselves to viewing in one plane. Echocardiography performs "sweeps" from various windows[12,13] to view the entire heart and great vessels, leaving the echocardiographer to integrate the

From: Higgins CB, Ingwall JS, Pohost GM, (eds). *Current and Future Applications of Magnetic Resonance in Cardiovascular Disease.* Armonk, NY: Futura Publishing Company, Inc.; © 1998.

data into a three-dimensional structure in the mind, which then needs to be communicated to the patient's physician and surgeon. Cardiac MRI takes advantage of it's unique ability to acquire images in contiguous parallel slices to obtain a full volume data set of the heart and great vessels that can then generate a three-dimensional shaded surface display[8,10,11] on the screen of a computer or as a hardcopy. This three-dimensional shaded surface display can be viewed from any angle desired, sectioned in any plane, and individual structures may be removed to reveal the salient points of the anatomy. This allows the three-dimensional anatomy to be viewed by physician and surgeon in a familiar way, and does not require the ability to integrate the three-dimensional data "in your head."

Using MRI to determine morphology is a necessary stepping stone in the functional analysis of the heart and determining the physiology of the specific lesion. Indeed, the anatomic data can yield evidence that the functional and physiologic analysis is correct (eg, ventricular hypertrophy in the presence of semilunar valve stenosis). Similarly, functional and physiologic analysis must be interpreted in light of the prevailing anatomy.

MRI does have its limitations in congenital heart disease.[14] Many patients are young and require sedation in order to remain still for long periods of time. Even if being still is not a problem in a given patient, cooperation may be problematic (eg, asking the child to hold his breath in a breath-hold pulse sequence). A number of patients who undergo surgery for congenital heart disease have arrhythmias that may not allow proper data acquisition, and others have bundle branch blocks or bizarre T waves that may not gate properly. Still others may not be able to be placed in the scanner because they have implanted cardiac pacemakers. Large artifacts are produced by intravascular coils, and artifacts from wires and clips may be a problem if it is near the structure of interest. Finally, MRI cannot compete with echocardiography in imaging rapidly moving leaflets of valves and chordae, as well as its portability to the bedside. Having listed all these negatives, it must be pointed out that MRI has an invaluable place in imaging morphology in congenital heart disease.[1–10]

Scanning Protocol

After the patient is sedated and lying still in the scanner, initial localizers are performed to locate the heart in the chest. Coronal localizers that are not gated to the QRS are adequate for this task using a 128 × 128 matrix and 1 excitation. Some manufacturers offer *software* that allow localizers to be performed in 3 orthogonal planes, and although it is convenient at times to obtain, it is rarely necessary. If the manufacturer does not offer this option, it's not worthwhile spending the time acquiring 3 separate localizer runs.

The next set of scans are gated, T1-weighted, contiguous axial (transverse) images throughout the entire thorax. Occasionally, the upper abdomen needs to be included if heterotaxy or anomalous pulmonary venous connections below the diaphragm is being considered. Technically, this is performed using the following parameters: 3 excitations, 128 × 256 matrix, slice thickness of 3 to 10 mm (depending on patient size), field of view of 140 to 450 mm (again, depending on patient size). The effective repetition time (TR) is the R-R interval (ranges 300 to 1000 ms) and the echo time (TE) is usually 15 ms. Some manufacturers allow the user to limit the time the computer scans the electrocardiogram (ECG) for a QRS after initiating the radiofrequency pulse. If this is done, it is usually set from 80% to 90% of the R-R interval, which ensures that every other heartbeat is not skipped. Of course, all parameters must be combined optimally to yield the desired resolution and signal-to-noise ratio.

The contiguous axial images are used as an initial, high-resolution evaluation of the cardiovascular anatomy and will be used themselves as localizers to obtain further imaging in the region of interest. If the study is terminated prematurely because of patient instability (eg, cardiopulmonary) or awakening from sedation, by obtaining this set of images first, a full volume data set has been acquired. Further evaluation of the areas of interest may then be performed offline using multiplanar reconstruction (at the cost of a lower resolution). Because all that is absolutely necessary for a three-dimensional reconstruction is a full axial volume data set, this too may be performed offline in cases of premature termination of the study.

The next set of images concentrate on the areas of interest. If nothing is previously known about the patient's diagnosis, or the axial images are unclear, a set of contiguous coronal images (more commonly) and sagittal images (less commonly) are extremely useful. This allows the physician to confirm the findings on the axial views in an orthogonal plane. For example, if a double aortic arch is found on the axial images, a set of coronals not only allows for confirmation of the diagnosis but also yields excellent views for determining which arch is larger. This is important clinically because the surgeon will ligate the smaller of the two. If discontinuous branch pulmonary arteries are suspected in a patient, for example, with hypoplastic left heart syndrome after a hemi-Fontan procedure, viewing the discontinuity in minimally 2 and optimally 3 orthogonal views are necessary to clinch the diagnosis. The golden rule to remember is always confirm the diagnosis in an orthogonal view.

Gradient-echo sequences (cine MRI) are then run to confirm the diagnosis from the spin-echo images. If, for example, stenosis of a semi-lunar valve is suspected from hypoplasia of the annulus and hypertrophy of the ventricular mass, a gradient-echo sequence is performed parallel to the path of flowing blood along the long axis of the outflow tract and great artery to observe the loss of signal secondary to turbulence across the valve. This is also useful in determining the minimum and maximum annular size when balloon valvuloplasty of the valve is contemplated. If a small ventricular septal defect (VSD) is suspected, a cine MRI perpendicular to the ventricular septum at the level of the VSD is performed to confirm the diagnosis and measure the size of the hole. This may be missed by the spin-echo images.

Finally, functional imaging is performed. The anatomy determined in the morphological part of the examination is used not only as localizers for functional imaging (magnetic myocardial tagging, magnetic blood tagging, velocity mapping, cine MRI), but as mentioned earlier, to help confirm the functional findings and allows proper interpretation of the study.

Approach to the Patient With Congenital Heart Disease

Usually, a patient with congenital heart disease is referred for cardiac MRI with a known diagnosis and specific details are addressed by the study. Sometimes, the patient's diagnosis is unclear, and the physician needs to sort *everything* out by cardiac MRI. In either case, the golden rule to follow in congenital heart disease is that no anatomic detail should be taken for granted and a standardized, systematic approach to the cardiovascular system is in order (the second golden rule, as mentioned earlier, is to always make a diagnosis from at least two orthogonal views). When performing a cardiac MRI, this author uses the segmental approach,[15,16] which necessitates the identification of all cardiac segments and intersegmental connections, and the various anomalies that occur in these segments and connections. The chamber's name is assigned based on its gross morphological features, not its spatial orientation.[17] The following section is a short, description of the segmental approach as used in cardiac MRI. The interested reader is referred to more definitive works on the subject.[15,16] Regardless of whether the diagnosis is known prior to the study, the following needs to be sorted out by MRI during the study.

Cardiac Segments

The three major cardiac segments are the atria, ventricles, and great arteries. Evaluation of the atria consists of identifying the morphological right atrium (RA) and left atrium (LA) and determining which side of the body it is on. Morphology is determined by examination of the atrial appendages[18] on MRI and identifying which chamber the inferior vena cava drains to (as most commonly, it drains to the RA). The flap of the foramen ovale is not generally seen well on MRI. The RA appendage has a wide base and a broad based triangular appearance and the LA appendage has a narrow base with a long, finger-like appearance to it.

Examination of the ventricles consists of identifying the morphological right ventricle (RV) and left ventricle (LV) and determining the inherent geometric organization to it (right- or left-handed geometry to the ventricles[14,15]). The morphological LV has a smooth septal surface, and two papillary muscles while the morphological RV has coarse septal trabeculations and one large papillary muscle (chordal attachments to the ventricular septum and morphology of the atrioventricular valves cannot be used in identifying morphology of ventricles with MRI because these are not visualized well). The inherent geometric organization to the ventricles is determined by placing the thumb in the inlet portion of the ventricle parallel to the path of flowing blood, the pointer finger in the outlet portion of the ventricle parallel to the path of flowing blood, and the palm facing the ventricular septum. A right hand fitting into an RV is termed a "D" loop and the left hand fitting into a RV is termed an "L" loop. Usually, a D-looped RV is on the right side of the body and an L-looped RV is on the left side of the body.

Inspection of the great arteries must consist of at least the following: identifying which ventricles the great arteries originate from; which side of the body the aorta is relative to the pulmonary artery; which pulmonary artery and bronchus the aortic arch goes over; the branching pattern of the aorta (including double aortic arch); the presence or absence of aortic interruption, stenosis or hypoplasia of the great vessel or anomalous origin of one of its branches. If the aorta is in fibrous continuity with the mitral valve (eg, by MRI, the aortic annulus is nearly attached to the mitral annulus) it is assigned to the LV and if the pulmonary artery is mostly over the RV, the great arteries are either solitus (aortic arch goes over the left pulmonary artery) or inversus (aortic arch goes over the right pulmonary artery). Any other arrangement of the great arteries is termed "malposition" and is identified by whether the aorta is to the left ("L" malposition) or the right ("D" malposition) of the pulmonary artery. An aortic arch that crosses the left bronchus is termed a left aortic arch and one that crosses the right bronchus is termed a right aortic arch. Branching patterns can either be normal, mirror image (in cases of a right aortic arch) or with an aberrant subclavian artery.[18]

Intersegmental Connections

Technically, the connection between the atria and ventricles must be divided into atria-to-atrioventricular valve (AVV) and AVV-to-ventricle connection. In the absence of the ability to identify the AVVs by MRI, these two connections are inferred by identifying the AVV annulus. If, for example, both atria are emptied by one AVV, the diagnosis of common atrioventricular canal is made (an atria-to-AVV lesion), but if a common AVV or both AVVs drain to one ventricle in the absence of the sinus portion of the other ventricle, the diagnosis of single ventricle is made (an AVV-to-ventricle lesion).

Connection between ventricle and great vessels are dependent on the presence or absence of conus underneath the aortic valve as alluded to earlier (aorta in fibrous continuity with the mitral valve implies no conus) and over which ventricle the great artery sits. Normally related great arteries (solitus and inversus) have been defined earlier. If the aorta has conus underneath it and is aligned with the LV and the pulmonary artery is aligned with the RV, anatomically corrected malposition is the diagnosis. If both great arteries are aligned over the RV, double-outlet RV is diagnosed, and if both great arteries are aligned over the LV, double-outlet LV (a rare lesion) is the diagnosis. When the aorta is aligned with the RV and the pulmonary artery is aligned with the LV, transposition of the great arteries is present.

Venous Connections and Situs

Systemic and pulmonary venous connections are an important diagnostic feature that should be evaluated in any patient undergoing cardiac MRI, especially when heterotaxy is being considered. The right superior vena cava most often connects to the right-sided morphological RA but can connect to a right-sided morphological LA, can on occasion connect to the *left-sided LA* (see below), or can be totally absent. A persistent left-sided superior vena cava should also be noted along with the presence or absence of a bridging vein between the two superior vena cavae. The persistent left-sided superior vena cava can connect with a left-sided LA, a left-sided RA, or the coronary sinus. The inferior vena cava usually ascends to the right of the spine and connects to the right of the spine and connects to the right-sided RA, but may ascend on the left. The inferior vena cava may connect to either atria, there may be absence of the hepato-renal segment (interrupted inferior vena cava) with azygous continuation to either superior vena cava (in which case the azygous is dilated), or there may be a double inferior vena cava.

Pulmonary veins are also a variable feature, especially in heterotaxy, and at least four need to be definitively identified as entering the LA before diagnosing normal pulmonary venous connection. The pulmonary veins may all connect to the RA or the coronary sinus. They may enter a confluence that can drain either superiorly to either superior vena cavae or innominate vein, drain inferiorly below the diaphragm to the inferior vena cava, portal vein, or any other venous structure in the abdomen, or may enter a blind sac (atresia of the common pulmonary vein), with only collaterals to drain the lung. To complicate matters further, any combination of these drainage patterns may be seen with any combination of the four pulmonary veins (anomalous pulmonary venous connection of the mixed type).

Finally, situs is an important feature to note in the cardiac MRI, espcially in heterotaxy. This is one of MRI's strongest suits in that many questions about situs can be answered in one study. In situs solitus, the liver and cecum are on the right, the stomach on the left, the left-sided bronchus has a left bronchus branching pattern with the left pulmonary artery *crossing over it* (hyparterial), and the right-sided bronchus has a right bronchus branching pattern with the right pulmonary artery *crossing in front of it* (eparterial). In situs inversus, each structure is on the opposite side (eg, liver on the left). In situs ambigous, any combination of sidedness can occur (eg, bilateral right-sided bronchi that are eparterial, liver and sotmach on left) along with a midline liver. The presence or absence of a spleen is an important finding as it may help diagnose asplenia or polysplenia in the heterotaxy syndromes and lead to clues as to the cardiovascular anatomy.

Major Uses of MRI in Morphological Evaluation of Congenital Heart Disease

Cardiac MRI has distinct advantages over other imaging modalities as noted above. However, in morphological evaluation of congenital heart disease, the images generated by cardiac MRI are so vastly superior that they are steadily becoming the standard of care. There are five broad categories for which cardiac MRI has found an increasing important role in the morphological evaluation of congenital heart disease. They are: (1) great artery anatomy both preoperative and postoperative; (2) venous connections both preoperative and postoperative; (3) imaging extracardiac conduits and intracardiac baffles; (4) complex spatial relationships; and (5) general morphological evaluation and miscellaneous, but important individual diseases not included in the other categories.

Great Artery Anatomy—Preoperative and Postoperative

Aorta

Lesions of the aorta that are commonly evaluated by MRI are classified as either (a) vascular ring or (b) nonvascular ring abnormalities.

A vascular ring is an aortic malformation where the vascular structures or former vascular structures completely surround the trachea and esophagus.[19] There can be further compromise of the trachea and esophagus by a saccular outpouching of the proximal descending aorta termed a diverticulum of Kommerell.[18-20] An advantage of cardiac MRI, imaging the trachea and bronchi as it relates to the vascular ring, allows the physician to examine the bronchoarterial relations, and find the reason for and assess the amount of airway compression.

In the MRI evaluation of a vascular ring, the initial axial images can almost always make the diagnosis. A set of contiguous coronal images are run that not only visualizes the diverticulum well, but also yields an orthogonal view to the axial images to assess the diameter of the vascular structures (which may ultimately affect the surgical management of the patient, see below). Sometimes, a three-dimensional reconstruction is useful in assessing the size of the various components of the vascular ring and in the evaluation of tracheal or bronchial compression.

Patients can be asymptomatic or they can manifest esophageal (dysphagia) or respiratory symptoms (stridor and/or wheezing).[19] Typically, a vascular ring may be suspected from chest x-ray by the presence of tracheal indentation, or by barium esophogram. Which structures make up the various components of the ring is a function of the lesion itself.

In a double aortic arch (Figure 1), the ascending aorta splits into two arch vessels that cross over both bronchi and branch pulmonary arteries coalescing behind the trachea and esophagus to form the descending aorta.[18-22] The aorta totaly surrounds the trachea and esophagus and surgical management entails ligation and division of the smaller of the two arches, which is more commonly the left one. Because this is performed by thoracotomy, cardiac MRI is crucial in determining the surgical management by assessing which arch is the smaller of the two so the surgeon knows which hemithorax to enter (Figure 1).

Right aortic arch complexes may form rings, depending on where regression in the embryonic aortic arches occurs.[18,19] The following discussion assumes a left ligamentum arteriosum and total regression of the right ductus arteriosus in fetal life. A right arch with mirror image branching most commonly does not form a ring (ductus arteriosus attaches to the innominate artery) and is usually associated with cyanotic congenital heart disease such as tetralogy of Fallot and truncus arteriosus.[18,19] On a rare instance, it can form a ring (ductus arteriosus attaches to the descending aorta with diverticulum formation).[18] A right aortic arch with an aberrant left subclavian artery can either have a retroesophageal diverticulum of Kommerell (Figure 1) or a retroesophageal left subclavian artery.[18-20] The components of the ring are as follows (in

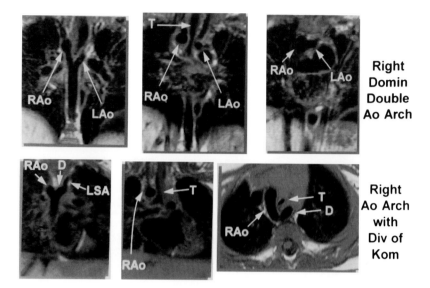

FIGURE 1. Ring aortic abnormalities. The upper panels are coronal images of a right dominant (domin) double aortic (Ao) arch and the lower panels are two coronal (left and middle panels) and one axial image of a right aortic arch with a diverticulum of Kommerell (div of Kom) (D). Coronal images progress anteriorly from left to right. In the double aortic arch, note how the amalgamation of the right (RAo) and left aortic arches (LAo) into ascending and descending aorta can be visualized. In the right aortic arch, note how the div of Kom can be visualized and that the arch passes over the right bronchus. In both examples, note how the trachea (T) is compressed.

diverticulum of Kommerell): anterior and right lateral portions formed by the aorta, posterior portion from the diverticulum and left lateral portion formed by the left ligamentum arteriosum and left pulmonary artery. A right aortic arch with an aberrant innominate artery does occur in nature (rare) and it does form a ring.[18] A left aortic arch with an aberrant right subclavian artery does not form a ring.

Nonring aortic arch abnormalities is the second group that is commonly seen by the physician performing MRIs. For most abnormalities that fall into this subgroup, as with the ring abnormalities, the initial axial images can generally yield the diagnosis or at least lead one in the correct direction. In most instances, a set of oblique sagittal images (angled sagittal to coronal) are obtained parallel to the path of flowing blood, which is generally set up on the axial image at the level of the bifurcation of the pulmonary artery. This set-up involves aligning both ascending and descending aorta, and paging through the axial images during the set-up allows for the optimal angle to be obtained. These

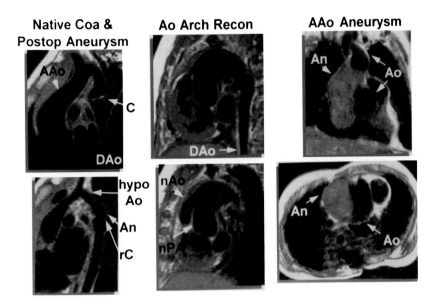

FIGURE 2. Nonring aortic abnormalities. The left panels display off-axis sagittal images of a native coarctation (C) (Coa) (upper panel) and a repaired coarctation with three residual defects (lower panel): a hypoplastic aortic arch (hypo Ao), aneurysm formation (An) and a residual coarctation (rC). The middle panels are also off-axis sagittal images separated by 4 mm, but of a patient who underwent an aortic to pulmonary anastomosis with aortic augmentation. Note how well it can be visualized and the mild residual narrowing in the proximal descending aorta (DAo). The two right images are a coronal (upper panel) and axial (lower panel) image of a patient with Marfan's syndrome who had aortic root and ascending aortic (AAo) dilatation and required a "wrap" of homograft around the AAo. The native AAo ruptured into the potential space between the native AAo and the homograft, resulting in the aneurysm (An) in these images. The signal intense region is because of stagnant blood. Ao indicates aorta; nAo, native ascending aorta; nPA, native pulmonary artery; Recon, reconstruction.

images serve as orthogonal images to the axial ones, and allow the whole arch to be visualized in one picture. Occasionally, these oblique sagittal images must be angled slightly toward the axial plane (a compound angle), generally between 5° and 15°, in cases of a tortuous aorta.

Of the nonring aortic arch abnormalities, assessment of the aortic arch for coarctation[18] (Figure 2) is one of the most frequent referrals seen. Four extremity blood pressures and an image of the coarctation by MRI is all that is necessary for the diagnosis and referral for surgery. Postoperatively, MRI is used to assess the presence of coarctation in patients with aortic arch reconstruction or may be used as follow-up in patients who have had coarctation repair, monitoring for recurrence of coarctation or aneurysm formation (Figure 2). A gradient-echo sequence parallel to the path of flowing blood may be useful in assessing the severity of coarctation by visualizing the turbulent flow caused by the coarctation or bicuspid aortic valve.

Other nonring aortic abnormalities include interruption of the aortic arch[18] as well as assessment of aortic root dilation secondary to such diseases as Marfan's syndrome,[23] cystic medial necrosis of the aorta, and annular aortic ectasia. Supravalvar aortic stenosis caused by for example, Williams syndrome,[24] also fall into this category. Postoperative nonring aortic assessment includes such situations as evaluation of the adequacy of an aortic to pulmonary anastamosis[25] or aortic aneurysm formation, such as after a "wrap" procedure (where the aorta is wrapped by homograft for support) (Figure 2).

Pulmonary Artery

Initial assessment of the pulmonary arteries is performed from the axial images. In the following discussion, the short axis of a blood vessel refers to the view that is perpendicular to the path of flowing blood, while the long axis refers to the view that is parallel to the path of flowing blood. The short axis of the pulmonary annulus and a small proximal section of the main pulmonary artery, the long axis of the main pulmonary artery running anteroposterior, the pulmonary artery bifurcation and the long axis of the individual branch pulmonary arteries (the right pulmonary artery running left to right and the left pulmonary artery running mostly anteroposterior with a slight skew right to left) can all be identified and measured accurately in axial views (Figures 3 and 4). Usually, this is followed by two separate long-axis runs in the superoinferior plane, one for each of the branch pulmonary arteries, based on the axial images. The set of right pulmonary artery images should extend to the left pulmonary artery yielding a series of short-axis views of the left pulmonary artery. Similarly, the set of left pulmonary artery images should extend to the right pulmonary artery yielding a set of short-axis images of the right pulmonary artery. Depending on the anatomy, the set of long-axis left pulmonary artery images may yield another long-axis view of the main pulmonary artery and the ventricular outflow tract. If it does not, and the long-axis view of the main pulmonary artery is crucial to visualize (eg, tetralogy of Fallot or an RV to pulmonary artery conduit), a separate run should be obtained.

Pulmonary artery lesions that are usually imaged by MRI fall into three basic categories. Stenosis or hypoplasia of one or both branch pulmonary arteries or main pulmonary artery may be a feature of multiple congenital heart lesions (Figure 3, upper panels). Tetralogy of

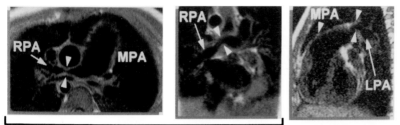

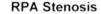

RPA Stenosis   LPA Stenosis

RPA   MPA

TOF
with
APV

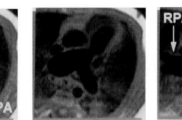

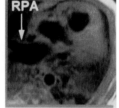

FIGURE 3. Pulmonary artery abnormalities-Stenosis, hypoplasia, dilatation. The upper left and upper middle panels are axial and off-axis coronal images respectively of a patient with tetralogy of Fallot who underwent repair and now has right pulmonary artery (RPA) stenosis, visualized in 2 orthogonal views (arrowheads). The upper right panel is an off-axis sagittal image of a patient who underwent truncus repair who has left pulmonary artery (LPA) stenosis (arrowheads). The lower panels are three axial images (progress inferiorly from left to right) of an infant with tetralogy of Fallot (TOF) with absent pulmonary valves (APV). Note the dilatation of both the RPA and LPA. MPA indicates main pulmonary artery.

Fallot, tricuspid atresia, or any right sided hypoplastic lesion can have this feature present preoperatively or postoperatively.[26] Pulmonary artery size is thought to be one of multiple prognosticators of surgical outcome in patients with single ventricle lesions leading to Fontan reconstruction.[9] Stenosis or hypoplasia of one or both branch pulmonary arteries (Figure 3, upper panels) is important to know preoperatively to help predict outcome and may affect the conduct of the surgery as pulmonary artery augmentation may be necessary.[9] The goals of the MRI examination of the pulmonary arteries in these lesions are to characterize the geometry and size of the arteries, determine branch pulmonary artery discontinuity (ideally imaging in three orthogonal planes), the amount of collaterals present from the aorta, and if pulmonary atresia is present, to determine how far the main pulmonary artery extends to the base of the heart.

Aneurysmal dilatation of the pulmonary arteries is the second category. This occurs classically in the patient with tetralogy of Fallot with

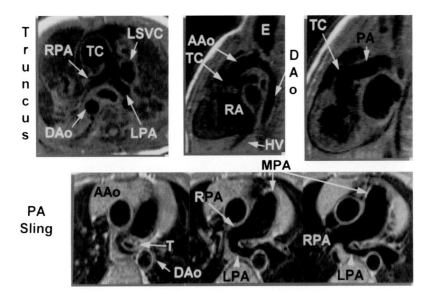

FIGURE 4. Pulmonary artery abnormalities: anomalous origin. The upper panels display an axial (**left**) and off-axis sagittal images (**middle** and **right**) of a patient with truncus arteriosus (TC) type A1, which visualizes the origin of the ascending aorta (AAo) and the main pulmonary artery (PA) (branching into right [RPA] and left pulmonary arteries [LPA]) from the TC. This patient also had esophageal atresia (E), and heterotaxy syndrome with the presence of a left superior vena cave (LSVC) and an interrupted inferior vena cava with azygous continuation. Hepatic veins (HV) emptied directly into the right atrium (RA). The lower panels display 3 axial images (progress inferiorly from left to right) of a patient with anomalous origin of the LPA from the RPA: a PA sling. Note how the LPA courses between trachea (T) and esophagus, compressing both structures. DAo indicates descending aorta; MPA, main pulmonary artery.

absent pulmonary valve leaflets[27] (Figure 3, lower panels). In this lesion, there is stenosis at the infundibulum and pulmonary valve annulus, but the main pulmonary artery and especially the branch pulmonary arteries may be enormous resulting in bronchial compression. MRI will yield the size and geometry of the pulmonary arteries and the amount of respiratory compromise, giving the physician an idea of the magnitude of the problem. Long-axis views of the right ventricular outflow tract will give the amount of stenosis present. Dilatation of the pulmonary arteries may also occur (albeit not to the same degree) in patients with pulmonary hypertension or with post-stenotic dilation caused by pulmonic stenosis.

The last category is anomalous origin of the pulmonary arteries (Figure 4). There is a long list of vascular structures from which the pulmonary arteries may arise. When the left pulmonary artery arises from the right pulmonary artery and crosses behind the trachea and in front of the esophagus (indenting the trachea posteriorly and the esophagus anteriorly on barium esophagram), a "sling" is present[28] (Figure 4, lower panels). When this occurs, there may be tracheal embarrassment; MRI can assess this as well. When the right pulmonary artery arises anomalously from the ascending aorta or when one great artery arises from the base of the heart and gives rise directly in its ascending portion to the systemic, pulmonary, and coronary circulations, hemitruncus[29] and truncus arteriosus[30] are present, respectively. The pulmonary arteries may arise from a patent ductus arteriosus or a systemic collateral. There are even reports of the pulmonary artery arising from the coronary arteries (in a case of tetralogy of Fallot with pulmonary atresia). There have been cases reported of branch pulmonary arteries crossing each other to reach the contralateral lung, noted in patients with truncus arteriosus. In all cases, MRI can and should be used to delineate size, geometry, and site of origin.

Venous Connections—Preoperative and Postoperative

Systemic and pulmonary venous connections play an important role in the physiology of congenital heart disease. At times, these may be difficult to visualize by echocardiography because of their position in the chest or poor echocardiographic windows. Cardiac MRI is a useful tool in delineating these connections. At times, especially with stenotic lesions, slow flow artifact may be problematic, and saturation bands may be used to "clean up the image" as much as possible.

Systemic Veins

Anomalies of the systemic venous system play a role in the preoperative and postoperative management of the patient with congenital heart disease. These may be isolated lesions and just a curiosity, such as persistent left superior vena cava draining to the coronary sinus, or an interrupted inferior vena cava with azygous continuation to the superior vena cava. Sometimes, these isolated lesions may have marked physiologic consequences, such as when the right or a persistent left superior vena cava connects to the left atrium,[31] causing cyanosis (Figure 5).

Other anomalies of the systemic veins may be associated with intracardiac lesions, and will affect the conduct of surgery, necessitating the need to be aware of these lesions preoperatively. For example, hypoplastic left heart syndrome and tricuspid atresia are associated with a

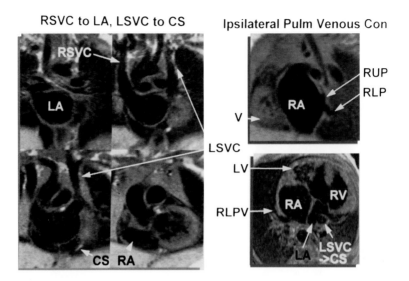

FIGURE 5. Venous anomalies. The left panel displays four coronal images (successively anterior from left to right and from top to bottom) of a patient with anomalous connection of the right superior vena cava (RSVC) to the left atrium (LA) and the presence of a left superior vena cava (LSVC) connected to the coronary sinus (CS). Note how well the RSVC to LA is visualized (top right image). The right panels are sagittal (upper) and axial (lower) images of a patient with heterotaxy syndrome and ipsilateral pulmonary (pulm) venous connections (con). Shown are the right upper (RUPV) and lower pulmonary veins (RLPV) entering the right atrium (RA), the LSVC to CS that this patient had as well, and the L-looped ventricles with the left ventricle (LV) on the right and the right ventricle (RV) on the left. V indicates ventricle.

persistent left superior vena cava that usually connects to the coronary sinus.[32] If a persistent left superior vena cava to the coronary sinus is not identified prior to Fontan reconstruction, deoxygenated blood will enter the pulmonary venous pathway, mixing with the oxygenated blood and causing cyanosis. Because the pressure is generally greater in the systemic venous pathway than the pulmonary venous pathway, if a "bridging vein" exists connecting the superior vena cava, right to left shunting of blood across this connection may occur. This not only allow deoxygenated blood to enter the pulmonary venous pathway, but will decrease the amount of deoxygenated blood entering the lungs, increasing the cyanosis. A persistent left superior vena cava can be dealt with at surgery by either a left superior vena cava to pulmonary artery anastamosis, or if a bridging vein is present, ligation of the left superior vena cava below the bridging vein. The necessity for identifying this lesion is obvious, and therefore, important to diagnose at MRI.

Because most systemic veins run in a superoinferior plane, coronal images are obtained after the contiguous axial images, delineating the vein along its long axis. This allows confirmation of the connections, assessment of the size of the vessel, and identification of any areas of stenosis.

Pulmonary Veins

The number of anomalies of pulmonary veins are myriad. In total anomalous pulmonary venous connection, all the pulmonary veins can connect to a confluence where they may drain via a vertical vein supracardiac (eg, to the innominate vein) or infradiaphragmatic (eg, to the inferior vena cava) and may be obstructive. The veins may also drain directly intracardiac; to the right atrium (Figure 5) or coronary sinus for example. They may not even all drain to the same place (eg, three to the innominate vein, one connecting infradiaphragmatic to the portal vein), the so called "mixed venous type."

Other anomalies of the pulmonary veins are important to be aware of. In partial anomalous pulmonary venous connection, some pulmonary veins may drain normally to the morphological left atrium and some may drain anomalously (for the example, the superior vena cava). There may be individual pulmonary vein atresia or stenosis, or all the pulmonary veins may drain to a confluence and end in a blind pouch with no exit, the so called atresia of the common pulmonary vein.

Axial images can delineate the pulmonary venous anatomy and can also follow the vertical vein along its course through the thorax or abdomen. Coronal images can them be obtained to confirm the diagnosis.

Extracardiac Conduits and Baffles

The postoperative assessment of these structures are important because stenosis or leaks occur and they need to be revised. Echocardiography may be hampered in imaging these structures because extracardiac conduits frequently pass immediately underneath the sternum or near the lungs and parts of the intracardiac baffle are posterior in the atria. Cardiac MRI can usually succeed where echocardiography fails, although there are caveats as well (eg, artifacts from sternal wires may hamper imaging).

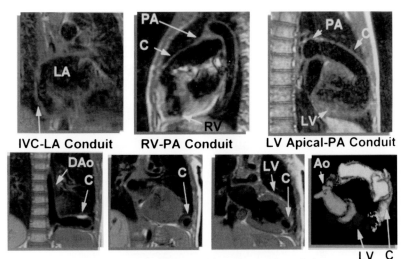

IVC-LA Conduit   RV-PA Conduit   LV Apical-PA Conduit

LV Apical to Descending Aorta Conduit   LV C

FIGURE 6. Extracardiac conduits. The top left panel is a coronal image of the inferior vena cava to left atrial (IVC-LA) conduit of a Baffes procedure for transposition of the great arteries. The top middle image is a right ventricle to pulmonary artery (RV-PA) conduit of a patient who underwent repair of tetralogy of Fallot with pulmonary atresia and now has residual stenosis (note how narrow the proximal portion of the conduit (C) is. The top right image is of a patient with situs inversus totalis, a right ventricular aorta with pulmonary atresia {I,L,L}, who underwent placement of a left ventricular (LV) apical to pulmonary artery (PA) conduit (C). The lower images are a three-dimensional shaded surface display in grayscale (right image-looking from a transverse view) and coronal images (other 3 images) of a patient with severe subaortic and aortic stenosis who underwent placement of an LV apical to descending aortic (DAo) conduit. Note how well MRI visualizes the entire extent of the conduits.

Extracardiac conduits (Figure 6) fall into a few categories. A right ventricular-to-pulmonary artery conduit such as in a Rastelli procedure,[34] an apical left ventricular-to-pulmonary artery conduit[35] such as in a patient with segments {I,L,L}, severe pulmonic stenosis and two good size ventricles, or an apical left ventricular-to-descending aorta conduit[36] in a patient with severe aortic stenosis {S,D,S} are examples of ventriculoarterial conduits. An example of a venoatrial conduit is a Baffes procedure, where the inferior vena cava is ligated and flow is channeled via a conduit to the left atrium. The right pulmonary veins are connected the right atrium in this procedure that was previously performed to palliate transposition of the great arteries. Some institutions are now performing an extracardiac venoarterial conduit for the Fontan procedure.[37] There are also occasions to perform arterio-arterial

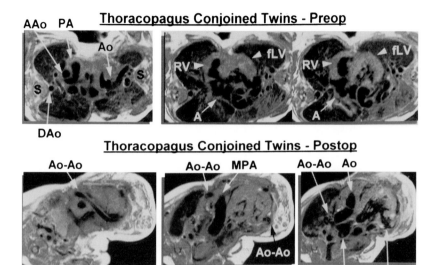

FIGURE 7. Extracardiac conduits and complex spatial relationships: thoracopagus conjoined twins. Preoperative (preop) and postoperative (postop) axial images of the fused heart (progresses inferiorly from right to left). Both infants shared a left ventricle (fLV) and the atria (A) were fused. The infant on the right had a rudimentary right ventricular outflow chamber (RVOC). Note how in the top left image, the ascending aorta (AAo) and descending aorta (DAo) are seen in cross section and the main and left pulmonary artery (PA) is seen in long axis on the left infant and the aortic (Ao) arch is visualized in the right infant. A physiologic repair of this defect required an aortic to aortic (Ao-Ao) conduit placement, visualized on the bottom 3 panels (progresses inferiorly from right to left). The Ao from the right infant originated from the RVOC which can be seen in the right lower panel. MPA indicates main pulmonary artery; RV, right ventricle; S, spine.

conduits, such as an ascending to descending aortic conduit in the case of coarctation of the aorta or an aortic to aortic conduit in the case of reconstructing the heart of thoracopagus conjoined twins (Figure 7 lower panel).

Intracardiac baffles (Figures 8 and 9) can also be categorized. Atrial baffles, which function to channel venous blood to arteries or the ventricles, include the Fontan reconstruction[37] for single ventricle complexes (Figure 8) and the Mustard[38] and Senning[39] procedures (which have been performed in the past) for the transposition of the great arteries (Figure 9). The Rastelli procedure,[34] performed for transposition of the great arteries with ventricular septal defect and pulmonic stenosis, and a component of the repair of double-outlet right ventricle are both examples of ventricular baffles (which in general, function to baffle blood

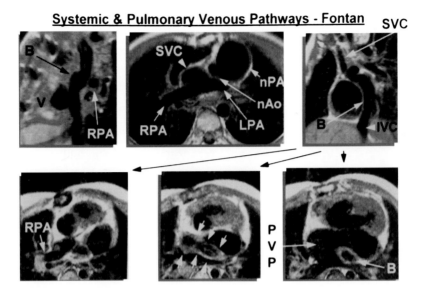

FIGURE 8. Atrial baffles: Fontan. The upper left and center images are off-axis sagittal and axial images respectively of components of the Fontan reconstruction for single ventricle complexes. The upper left image shows the long axis of the baffle (B), which creates a systemic venous (shown in long axis in the upper left image) and pulmonary venous pathway (PVP). An axial image (upper middle panel) at the level of the baffle and right pulmonary artery (RPA) shows the anastamosis of the superior vena cava (SVC) to the RPA. The proximal left pulmonary artery (LPA), native aorta (nAo) and native pulmonary artery (nPA) are also seen. Because surgeons need to be creative with Fontan reconstruction, so does the physician who performs the MRI. The upper right and lower panels are off-axis sagittal and axial images (progresses inferiorly from left to right), respectively, of a patient with a left inferior vena cava (IVC) that needed to be baffled to the RPA-SVC anastamosis. The axial images follow the baffle from the RPA-SVC anastamosis, across the atria (arrowheads) to the left inferior vena cava. A compound angle was necessary to obtain the long axis of the baffle. V indicates ventricle.

from the ventricle to the great vessels creating in this particular instance, the left ventricular outflow tract) (Figure 9). Finally, the Takeuchi operation,[40] used in the repair of anomalous left coronary artery, is an example of an intra-arterial baffle.

After contiguous axial images are performed, which can be used to follow the conduit and baffle in short-axis, double oblique angled images (coronal angled to sagittal angled to axial) are usually necessary to obtain the long axis of the conduit or baffle in one image. Sometimes, this may be impossible and the MRI physician must be satisfied with two or three images of the conduit in long axis to obtain its full extent.

Transposition of the Great Arteries, S/P Mustard

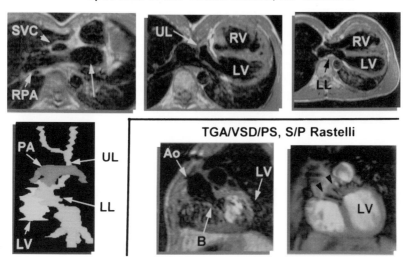

FIGURE 9. Baffles: Senning, Mustard, and Rastelli. The upper panels are axial images and the lower left panel is a three-dimensional shaded surface display of a patient with transposition of the great arteries who is after a Mustard procedure. The three-dimensional shaded surface display shows the systemic venous pathway, left ventricle (LV) and pulmonary artery (PA) from a posterior view. Note how both the upper (UL) and lower limbs (LL) of the systemic venous pathway are easily visible from the axial view and the three-dimensional course seen from the shaded surface display. These limbs baffle superior (SVC) and inferior vena cava blood to the left ventricle (LV) while pulmonary venous blood goes around the baffle into the right ventricle (RV). Arrow in the upper left image denotes the pulmonary artery posterior and the aorta (Ao) anterior. The bottom middle and right image are off-axis sagittal spin echo and cine images respectively of the left ventricular outflow tract created by the ventricular baffle (B) in a patient with transposition of the great arteries, ventricular septal defect and pulmonic stenosis (TGA/VSD/PS) who is status post (S/P) a Rastelli procedure. The left ventricular outflow tract is small and stenotic, with two jets of turbulence seen on cine MRI (black arrowheads).

Stenosis, regurgitation, or leaks across the baffle from one channel to the other can be detected by cine MRI.

Complex Spatial Relations

The orientation of various cardiovascular structures relative to each other and the rest of the body, resulting in the complex spatial relationships that exist in patients with congenital heart disease, can be sorted out by MRI easier than other imaging modalities. The ability of MRI to obtain parallel, contiguous, tomographic slices, creating three-dimensional shaded surface displays and the use of multiplanar reconstruction gives the physician a powerful tool with which to analyze the complex geometry.

As with conduits and baffles, contiguous axial images are performed that can be used to follow the various cardiovascular structures and in general, to yield a first approximation of the anatomy. Afterwards, double oblique angled images (coronal angled to sagittal angled to axial) are usually necessary to further delineate the morphology and regions of interest identified on the axial images. Confirmation of certain diagnoses can be made using cine MRI.

Superoinferior ventricles and criss-cross atrioventricular relations[41] is one example of complex spatial relationships (Figure 10). In this lesion, the two ventricles are oriented superoinferiorly instead of anteroposteriorly and right-left with the ventricular septum lying parallel to the transverse axis of the body. Further, the atrioventricular

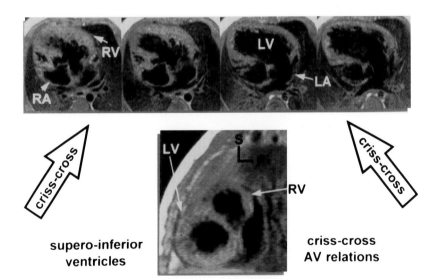

FIGURE 10. Complex spatial relations: superoinferior ventricles with criss-cross atrioventricular relations. The bottom panel is an off-axis sagittal view of the short axis of the right ventricle (RV) superiorly (S) and the left ventricle (LV) inferiorly. The upper panels display four axial images (progressing inferiorly from left to right), which depicts the criss-cross nature of the atrioventricular valves. A moderate ventricular septal defect is present (seen in the upper left panel). The right atrium (RA) which is superior and to the right, empties into the leftward and superior RV while the left atrium (LA), which is inferior and to the left, crosses the path of blood from RA to RV and empties into the rightward and inferior LV. P indicates posterior.

valves appear to cross each other connecting the atria to the ventricles, although what the valves do in reality is "wrap around" each other, giving a criss-cross appearance. To depict the ventricular relation, coronal or sagittal images are used while the criss-cross of the atrioventricular valves can be shown by the standard axial images, although off-axis coronal and sagittal images can be used to delineate the criss-cross in the superoinferior plane.

Thoracopagus conjoined twins[42] are another example of a complex spatial relation (Figure 7). The twins are joined at the thorax, and cardiac conjuncture may occur at one or multiple levels. Echocardiography is difficult postnatally because of limited acoustic windows, and in general, cannot get the entire heart at a given level on the screen. MRI is used to sort out the various cardiac structures, including the complex venous anatomy (eg, one or two inferior vena cavae, anomalous pulmonary venous return), ventricular morphology (eg, fused central (usually left ventricular morphology) ventricle, right ventricular outflow chamber and abdominal viscera; two livers or one). For all lesions in this category, three-dimensional shaded surface displays as well as multiplanar reconstruction can be extremely useful in conceptualizing the anatomy.

General Morphology and Miscellaneous Diseases

MRI can also be used for general morphological evaluation even though it is not the only imaging modality capable of doing so. Typically, echocardiography, angiography and on occasion, computerized tomography are used to delineate the anatomy. Nevertheless, MRI can be useful in the older child, adolescent, and adult for this and can add information not previously known. Furthermore, because of the wide field of view, a single MRI study may serve the purpose of multiple other studies. A typical example of this is the work-up of a patient with heterotaxy syndrome[43,44] (Figure 11), who has components of both situs solitus and situs inversus of the abdominal and thoracic viscera as well as heart disease. Sorting out the morphology and sidedness of the trachea, gastrointestinal tract, liver, and the presence or absence of a spleen (to aid in the diagnosis of asplenia or polyspenia syndromes) may all be done with MRI. A chest x-ray, echocardiogram, abdominal ultrasound, liver-spleen scan and possibly an abdominal computed tomographic scan may have to be performed otherwise.

MRI may also add another dimension to studies of lesions that have been previously performed. An example of this (Figure 12; upper left panel) is the delineation of an intracardiac myxoma or tumor.[45] The

Heterotaxy Syndrome:
**Truncus A1 with Interrupted LIVC, Az Continuation to LSVC->LA
HV & RSVC to RA, Right Aortic Arch, Mirror Image Branching,
Midline Liver**

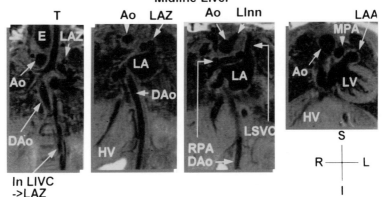

FIGURE 11. Complex spatial relations and general morphology: heterotaxy. These are four coronal images of a patient with truncus arteriosus A1 with interrupted (In) left inferior vena cava (LIVC) with azygous (Az) continuation to the left superior vena cava (LSVC) which connects to the left atrium (LA). The hepatic veins (HV) and right superior vena cava (RSVC) empty into the right atrium (RA). There is a right aortic arch (Ao) with mirror image branching and a midline liver. The patient also has esophageal atresia. MRI clearly shows the complex anatomy. Note how the Ao crosses the right bronchus and descends obliquely, crossing the diaphragm on the left. The left atrial appendage (LAA) morphology is clearly visible. DAo indicates descending aorta; E, esophagus; I, inferior; L, left; LAZ, left azygous; LInn, left innominate artery; LV, left ventricle; MPA, main pulmonary artery; R, right; RPA, right pulmonary artery; S, superior.

acoustic contrast of the lesion may be obtained by echocardiography, however, MRI can be useful by utilizing T1- and T2-weighted images, proton density images, and gadolinium-enhanced images to demarcate the extent of the tumor and its water content.

Other examples of common lesions for which I have used MRI, or have diagnosed incidentally are shown in Figure 12. Congenital left ventricular aneurysm,[46] pericardial effusion, and single ventricle lesions[47] are fairly straightforward to recognize on MRI.

An aortopulmonary window,[48] however, may not be visualized on spin-echo images. With a high index of suspicion, this may be diagnosed by cine MRI. This is done by visualizing the turbulent jet of blood shunting from aorta to pulmonary artery in the coronal view or sometimes in the axial view. Anomalous left coronary artery from the pulmonary artery may be diagnosed in a similar fashion (indirectly,

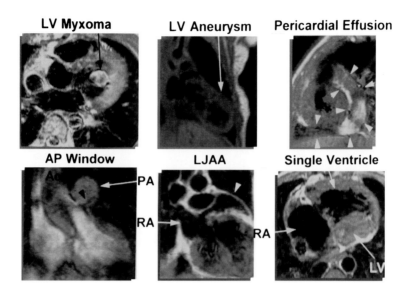

FIGURE 12. General morphology. **Upper left image** is an axial view of a left ventricular (LV) myxoma in the LV outflow tract which enhanced with gadolinium (black arrow). Upper middle image is an off-axis sagittal image of a congenital LV aneurysm. The white arrow points to the aneurysm itself whereas to the left of the arrow is the body of the LV. The **upper right panel** is a short-axis image of a patient with hypoplastic left heart syndrome, post-Fontan, who has a very large, circumferential pericardial effusion (arrowheads). The **lower left panel** is a coronal image of a patient with an aorticopulmonary (AP) window. This was missed on the spin-echo images, however, the cine MRI depicts the turbulent jet of shunting blood in systole from aorta (Ao) to pulmonary artery (PA) (black arrowhead). The **lower middle image** is also a coronal image, but of a patient with left juxtaposition of the atrial appendages (LJAA), diagnosed here by the right atrial (RA) appendage on the left side (arrowhead). This patient also had tricuspid atresia, transposition of the great arteries, and pulmonic stenosis with a hypoplastic right ventricle. The **lower right image** is an axial view patient with hypoplastic left heart syndrome who post-Fontan procedure. MRI readily depicts the hypoplastic LV, the single right ventricle and the Fontan baffle in short axis.

by visualizing the jet of blood shunting retrograde from the left coronary into the pulmonary artery), usually after 2 months of age or if the child is symptomatic. Care must be taken to distinguish the two.

Left juxtaposition of the atrial appendages[49] can be best visualized in the coronal plane (although it can be observed in the axial images), and constitute a complex of findings generally including a ventricular and/or atrial septal defect, tricuspid atresia or stenosis, a hypoplastic right ventricle, pulmonic stenosis, and bilateral infundibulum.

The Present and the Future

MRI for the morphological evaluation of congenital heart disease is an increasingly useful tool, and is gaining wide acceptance in the pediatric cardiology community. An understanding of congenital and acquired pediatric heart disease as well as knowledge of MRI physics and computers are important for the proper use of this technology. A close association between pediatric cardiologists, radiologists, and surgeons as well as computer scientists and phycisists is necessary to advance the field. Promising new technologies such as echo-planar MRI and faster pulse sequences are under development and in clinical trials, which may further aid in the future growth of this imaging modality.

References

1. Didier D, Higgins CB, Fisher M, et al. Congenital heart disease: Gated magnetic resonance imaging in 72 patients. *Radiology.* 1986;158:227–235.
2. Fletcher BD, Jacobsteink MD, Nelson AD, et al. Gated magnetic resonance imaging of congenital cardiac malformations. *Radiology.* 1984;150:137–140.
3. Higgins CB, Byrd BF, Farmer DW, et al. Magnetic resonance imaging in patients with congenital heart disease. *Circulation.* 1984;70:851–860.
4. Reed JD, Soulen RL. Cardiovascular MRI: Current role in patient management. *Radiol Clin North Am.* 1988;26:589–606.
5. Link KM, Lesko NM. Magnetic resonance imaging in the evaluation of congenital heart disease. *Magn Reson Q.* 1991;7:173–190.
6. Bank ER. Magnetic resonance of congenital cardiovascular disease. An update. *Radiol Clin North Am.* 1993;31:553–572.
7. Fogel MA. Evaluation of ventricular geometry and performance in congenital heart disease utilizing magnetic resonance imaging. In: *Proceedings SPIE-Medical Imaging, 1994: Physiology and Function from Multidimensional Images.* 1994;2168:195–217.
8. Adams R, Fellows KE, Fogel MA, Weinberg PM. Anatomic delineation of congenital heart disease with 3D magnetic resonance imaging. In: *Proceedings SPIE-Medical Imaging, 1994: Physiology and Function from Multidimensional Images.* 1994;2168:184–194.
9. Fogel MA, Ramaciotti C, Hubbard AM, Weinberg PW. Magnetic resonance and echocardiographic imaging of pulmonary artery size throughout stages of Fontan reconstruction *Circulation.* 1994;90:2927–2936.
10. Bornemeier RA, Weinberg PM, Fogel MA. Three-dimensional magnetic resonance, echocardiographic, and angiographic imaging of extracardiac conduits. *Am J Cardiol.* In press.
11. Hoffman EA, Gnanaprakasam D, Gupta KB, et al. VIDA: An environment for multidimensional image display and analysis. In: *Proceedings SPIE.* 1992; 1660:694–711.
12. Snider AR, Serwer GA *Echocardiography in Pediatric Heart Disease.* St. Louis: Mosby Yearbook; 1990:21–77.

13. Chin AJ *Noninvasive Imaging of Congenital Heart Disease.* Armonk NY: Futura Publishing Company; 1994:7–8.
14. Fogel MA. Preoperative magnetic resonance imaging: Form and function. In: Chin AJ, ed: *Noninvasive Imaging of Congenital Heart Disease.* Armonk NY: Futura Publishing Company; 1994:239–269.
15. Weinberg PM. Systematic approach to diagnosis and coding of pediatric cardiac disease. *Pediatr Cardiol.* 1986;7:35–48.
16. Van Praagh R. The segmental approach to diagnosis in congenital heart disease. *Birth Defects.* 1972;8:4–23.
17. Lev M. The pathologic diagnosis of positional variations in cardiac chambers in congenital heart disease. *Lab Invest.* 1954;3:71–82.
18. Schuford WH, Sybers RG, Hogan GB. *The Aortic Arch and Its Malformations.* Springfield, MA: Charles C. Thomas; 1974:41–244.
19. Morrow WR, Huhta JC. Aortic arch and pulmonary artery anomalies. In: Garson A, Bricker JT, McNamara DG, eds. *The Science and Practice of Pediatric Cardiology.* Philadelphia/London: Lea & Feibiger; 1990:1421–1452.
20. Knight L, Edwards JE. Right aortic arch: Types and associated cardiac anomalies. *Circulation.* 1974;50:1047–1051.
21. Edwards JE. Anomalies of the derivatives of the aortic arch system. *Med Clin North Am.* 1948;32:925–949.
22. Riker WL. Anomalies of the aortic aortic arch and their treatment. *Pediatr Clin North Am.* 1954;1:181–195.
23. Pyeritz RE, McKusick VA. The Marfan syndrome: Diagnoses and management. *N Engl J Med.* 1979;300:772–777.
24. Williams JCP, Barratt-Boyes BG, Lowe JB. Supravalvar aortic stenosis. *Circulation.* 1961;24:1311–1318.
25. Rychik J, Murdison KA, Norwood WI, et al. Surgical management of severe aortic outflow obstruction in lesions other than hypoplastic left heart syndrome: Use of a pulmonary artery-to-aorta anastomosis. *J Am Coll Cardiol.* 1991;18:809–816.
26. Nakata S, Imai Y, Takanashi Y, et al. A new method for the quantificative standardization of cross-sectional areas of the pulmonary arteries in congenital heart disease with decreased pulmonary blood flow. *J Thorac Cardiovasc Surg.* 1984;88:610–619.
27. Lakier JB, Stanger P, Heymann MA, et al. Tetralogy of Fallot with absent pulmonary valve. *Circulation.* 1974;50:167–174.
28. Gumbiner CH, Mullins CE, McNamara DG. Pulmonary artery sling. *Am J Cardiol.* 1980;45:316–320.
29. Kutsche LM, Van Mierop LH. Anomalous origin of a pulmonary artery from the ascending aorta: Associated anomalies and pathogenesis. *Am J Cardiol.* 1988;61:850–856.
30. Van Praagh R, Van Praagh S. The anatomy of common aorticopulmonary trunk (truncus arteriosus communis) and its embryologic implications. *Am J Cardiol.* 1965;16:406–425.
31. Vasquez-Perez J, Frontera-Izquierdo P. Anomalous drainage of the right superior vena cava into the left atrium as an isolated anomaly: Rare case report. *Am Heart J.* 1979;97:89–91.
32. Bharati S, McAllister HA, Tatooles CJ, et al. Anatomic variations in underdeveloped right ventricle related to tricuspid atresia and stenosis. *J Thorac Cardiovasc Surg.* 1976;72:383–400.
33. Healey JE, Jr. An anatomic survey of anomalous pulmonary veins: Their clinical significance. *J Thorac Cardiovasc Surg.* 1952;23:433–444.

34. Marcelletti C, Mair DD, McGoon DC, et al. The Rastelli operation for transposition of the great arteries. *J Thorac Cardiovasc Surg.* 1976;72:427–434.
35. Crupi G, Pillai R, Parenzan L, et al. Surgical treatment of subpulmonary obstruction in transposition of the great arteries by means of a left ventricular-pulmonary artery conduit. *J Thorac Cardiovasc Surg.* 1985;89:907–913.
36. Norwood WI, Lang P, Castaneda AR, et al. Management of infants with left ventricular outflow obstruction by conduit interposition between ventricular apex and thoracic aorta. *J Thorac Cardiovasc Surg.* 1983;86:771–776.
37. Fontan F, Baudet E. Surgical repair of tricuspid atresia. *Thorax.* 1971;26: 240–248.
38. Mustard WT. Successful two-stage correction of transposition of the great vessels. *Surgery.* 1964;55:469–472.
39. Senning A. Surgical correction of transposition of the great vessels. *Surgery.* 1959;45:966–980.
40. Takeuchi S, Imamura H, Katsumoko K, et al. New surgical method for repair of anomalous left coronary artery from pulmonary artery. *J Thorac Cardiovasc Surg.* 1979;78:7–11.
41. Anderson RH, Shinebourne EA, Gerlis LM. Criss-cross atrioventricular relationships producing paradoxical atrioventricular concordance or discordance. Their significance to nomenclature of congenital heart disease. *Circulation.* 1974;50:176–180.
42. Marin-Padilla M, Chin AJ, Marin-Padilla TM. Cardiovascular abnormalities in thoracopagus twins. *Teratology.* 1981;23:101–113.
43. Ivemark BI. Implications of agenesis of the spleen in the pathogenesis of conotruncus anomalies in childhood: An analysis of the heart malformations in the splenic agenesis syndrome, with fourteen new cases. *Acta Paed Scand.* 1955;44(suppl 104):1–110.
44. Moller JH, Nakib A, Anderson RC, et al. Congential cardiac disease associated with polysplenia. A developmental complex of bilateral "left sidedness." *Circulation.* 1967;36:789–799.
45. Nadas AS, Ellison RC. Cardiac tumors in infancy. *Am J Cardiol.* 1968;21: 363–366.
46. Long WA, Willis PW, Henry W. Childhood traumatic infarction causing left ventricular aneurysm: Diagnosis by two-dimensional echocardiography. *J Am Coll Cardiol.* 1985;5:1478–1483.
47. Van Praagh R, Ongley PA, Swan HJC. Anatomic types of single or common ventricle in man: Morphologic and geometric aspects of 60 necropsied cases. *Am J Cardiol.* 1964;13:367–386.
48. Kutsche LM, Van Mierop LHS. Anatomy and pathogenesis of aorticopulmonary septal defect. *Am J Cardiol.* 1987;59:443–447.
49. Melhuish BPP, Van Praagh R. Juxtaposition of the atrial appendages. A sign of severe cyanotic congenital heart disease. *Br Heart J.* 1968;30:269–284.

Chapter 8

Magnetic Resonance Imaging in Adult Congenital Heart Disease

Albert de Roos, MD, Willem A. Helbing, MD, R. André Niezen, MD, Sidney A. Rebergen, MD, Ernst E. van der Wall, MD, and Jaap Ottenkamp, MD

Introduction

It is estimated that there are between 500,000 and 600,000 adults with congenital heart disease in the United States, and each year another 10,000 children who have undergone surgical repair reach adulthood.[1] The largest diagnostic category among patients undergoing repair is isolated ventricular septal defect, followed by tetralogy of Fallot. Imaging techniques are required to evaluate a wide spectrum of postoperative residua and sequelae after initial repair. Magnetic resonance imaging (MRI) provides a wide array of techniques that allow the evaluation of residua and sequelae after surgery for congenital heart disease, unsurpassed by other noninvasive modalities.[2-4] The value of MRI is becoming firmly established in the follow-up of patients with a variety of congenital heart and great vessel abnormalities.[5] This is partly due to the complexity of the postoperative anatomy and function of particularly the right ventricle, as well as to the limitations of alternative imaging modalities that can be used in this category of patients. Echocardiography may be hampered in these patients by the presence

From: Higgins CB, Ingwall JS, Pohost GM, (eds). *Current and Future Applications of Magnetic Resonance in Cardiovascular Disease.* Armonk, NY: Futura Publishing Company, Inc.; © 1998.

of sternal wires and scar tissue, rib and chest deformations, and inter-posed lung tissue. The value of this approach in presurgical planning of complex cardiovascular malformations has been compared with echocardiography and cardiac catheterization in a prospective study of a series of patients with heterotaxy syndrome.[4] In that study, MRI provided excellent anatomic and functional information that was in some patients not available by echocardiography or catheterization. However, cardiac catheterization is still required when determination of pulmonary vascular resistance is necessary for decision making or when an interventional procedure is indicated.[4] In this chapter the role of magnetic resonance (MR) techniques for the evaluation of anatomy, function, and flow in patients with adult congenital heart disease is discussed.

Magnetic Resonance Evaluation of Cardiovascular Anatomy

The value of MRI for the evaluation of morphology of the heart and great vessels has been widely recognized.[6–9] An accurate diagnosis of anatomic anomalies can be achieved in more than 90% of the patients with congenital heart disease.[10] MRI appears to be effective in both simple and complex cardiovascular malformations. Analysis of the silent anatomic details in patients with complex cardiovascular malformations is accomplished to best advantage with the aid of a step-by-step analysis of the segmental anatomy.[11–13]

After initial morphological evaluation, the gradient-echo cine series are commonly obtained to assess cardiovascular flow and function tailored to the clinical situation and the malformation under investigation. The combined use of spin-echo and cine MRI in patients with complex cardiovascular malformations provides most relevant information for presurgical planning.[4]

Magnetic Resonance Evaluation of Ventricular Function

Systolic Ventricular Function

Evaluation of global ventricular function is dependent on accurate measurement of ventricular volumes. Until now, transthoracic echocardiography has been the most widely applied technique for this purpose. However, the absence of appropriate acoustic windows and the requirements of geometrical assumptions for volume measurements may limit its value. These geometrical assumptions are of special concern when measuring right ventricular volumes.

Gradient-echo MRI is a three-dimensional technique that encompasses both the left and right ventricle in multiple transverse or short-axis images. The high temporal resolution is adequate to isolate end-diastolic and end-systolic time points. Ventricular volumetrics can thus be derived without the need for geometrical assumptions.[14] Ventricular volume measurements with MRI appear to be more reproducible than those with other imaging modalities. MRI now appears to emerge as the most accurate imaging modality for measuring ventricular volumes and myocardial mass.[15] The clinical utility and accuracy of gradient-echo MRI of right and left ventricular volumes has been shown in normal children and in children with various types of congenital heart disease with abnormal loading conditions of the right ventricle.[16] MRI appears to be well suited to evaluate biventricular systolic function in children with complex cardiac morphology and abnormal loading conditions (Figure 1).

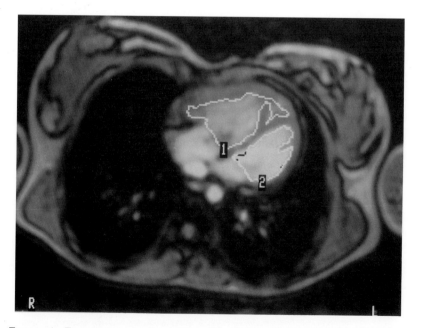

FIGURE 1. Transverse gradient-echo MR image at midventricular level in a child, illustrating the right (contour 1) and left (contour 2) ventricular tracings. MRI allows the evaluation of both systolic and diastolic biventricular function with high success rate and good reproducibility.

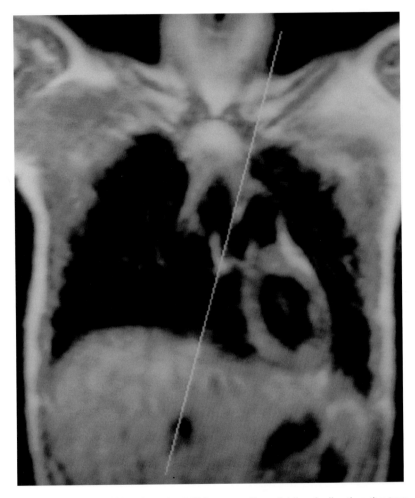

FIGURE 2. Coronal (**A**) spin-echo MR image with solid line indicating the transection of the double oblique scan plane for velocity mapping of tricuspid flow.
Gradient-echo MR image (**B**) indicates with solid line the level of the tricuspid
flow map in the transverse plane. The double oblique magnitude image (left
upper panel in **C**) is based on the previous planscans for orientation. The
resulting flow map at this level shows rapid tricuspid inflow (right upper panel
in C), diastasis (left lower panel), and flow during atrial contraction (right lower
panel). Tricuspid flow measurements provide data on right ventricular diastolic
function both in terms of flow velocity and flow volume.

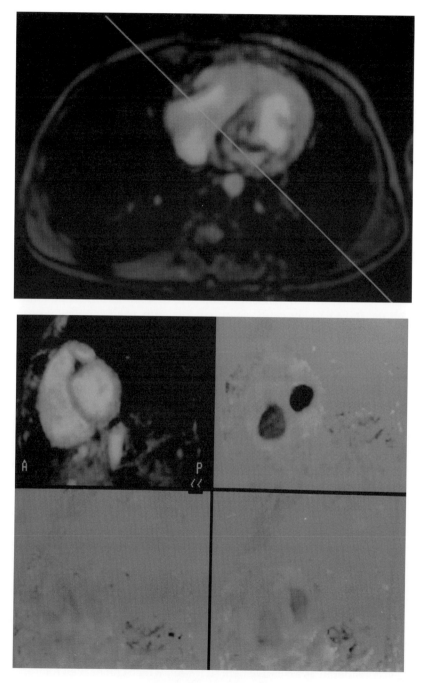

FIGURE 2. *(continued)*

Diastolic Ventricular Function

MRI techniques may also allow evaluation of diastolic ventricular function.[17] Diastolic dysfunction may be defined as the inability of the left ventricle to fill at normal end-diastolic pressure. The filling of the left or right ventricle normally has a triphasic character as defined by magnetic resonance measurement of transmitral or transtricuspid flow: [18] an initial, rapid filling phase is followed by a second phase of diastasis with very slow diastolic filling and finally by a third phase of filling during atrial contraction (Figure 2). The rapid filling phase may be characterized by parameters such as peak filling rate, time-to-peak filling rate, acceleration and deceleration slope of the early filling peak, and the duration of the rapid filling period, whereas the atrial contraction may be quantified by the atrial filling velocity. In addition, magnetic resonance velocity mapping techniques have been used to measure transmitral and transtricuspid flow as markers for diastolic ventricular function.[19] Thus, a variety of magnetic resonance derived measurements provide an opportunity to assess diastolic function of both the right and left ventricle in patients with adult congenital heart disease.

MR Evaluation of Postoperative Tetralogy of Fallot

In patients with tetralogy of Fallot, anterior displacement of the infundibular septum results in a ventricular septal defect and the development of infundibular pulmonary stenosis. Right ventricular hypertrophy is caused by right ventricular hypertension resulting from both the ventricular septal defect and pulmonary stenosis. The fourth component of tetralogy is the overriding aorta onto the right ventricle. Surgical repair is aimed at relief of the right ventricular outflow obstruction and closure of the ventricular septal defect.

Despite improved surgical methods, pulmonary stenosis and pulmonary regurgitation are common postoperative sequelae after repair of tetralogy of Fallot. Spin-echo and gradient-echo MRI are effective for the postsurgical evaluation of the anatomic and functional residua.

Pulmonary regurgitation is commonly found, especially when a transannular patch has been used for relief of outflow obstruction of the right ventricle (Figure 3). Controversy exists with regard to the significance of residual pulmonary regurgitation. On one hand, it has been considered as a relative benign lesion, which can be well tolerated over long periods of time.[20] On the other hand, others emphasize that pulmonary regurgitation-induced right ventricular volume overload

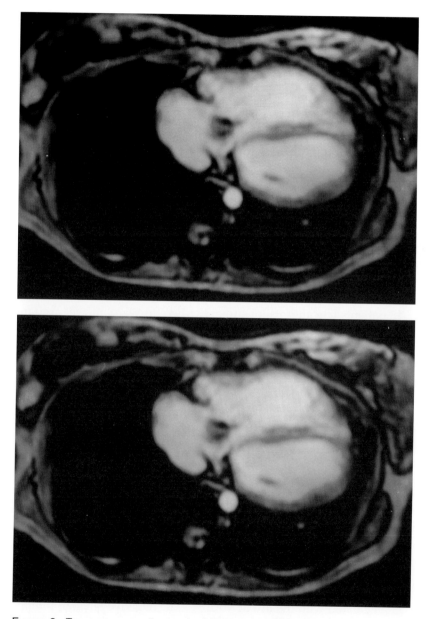

FIGURE 3. Transverse gradient-echo MR images (**A and B**) in a young patient with marked pulmonary regurgitation after Fallot repair. Note enlargement of the right ventricle due to volume overload (A). The regurgitant pulmonary flow extends far into the inflow portion of the right ventricle and is visualized as a signal void extending into the right ventricular outflow tract (B).

may predispose to the development of ventricular arrhythmia, a risk factor for sudden death.[21]

The evaluation of the clinical significance of pulmonary regurgitation after repair of tetralogy of Fallot has been hampered since there was no noninvasive modality that could accurately quantitate pulmonary volume flow. Magnetic resonance velocity mapping has been shown to be an accurate method for noninvasive, volumetric quantification of pulmonary regurgitation after surgical correction of tetralogy of Fallot.[22] In addition, multislice gradient-echo MRI is an accurate method to perform measurements of right ventricular volumes, without the limitations inherent to the complex geometry of the right ventricle.[23,24] The consequences of pulmonary regurgitation on right ventricular function in patients after repair of tetralogy of Fallot can be comprehensively evaluated by the combined use of magnetic resonance velocity mapping and gradient-echo MRI. Furthermore, the measurement of left and right ventricular stroke volume based on the tomographic method can be used as an internal reference to validate the direct measurement of pulmonary flow. This approach was explored in a study of 18 patients late after Fallot surgery, where forward and regurgitant volume flow was measured directly in the main pulmonary artery with magnetic resonance velocity mapping.[22] Pulmonary regurgitation volumes closely agreed with the difference between the corresponding right and left ventricular stroke volumes as measured tomographically by gradient-echo MRI.

Thus, magnetic resonance velocity mapping appears to be ideally suited for monitoring pulmonary regurgitation and right ventricular function, and this technique may help to plan surgical intervention for residual pulmonary regurgitation after repair of tetralogy of Fallot. MRI is also well suited to assess the effect of pulmonary regurgitation on right ventricular function.[16,23,24] Late deterioration of right ventricular function is an important determinant of clinical outcome in various forms of adult congenital heart disease. The high success rate of MRI of the right side of the heart and the accuracy of the magnetic resonance measurements illustrate the practical applicability of this technique in children.[16] The effects of pulmonary regurgitation after repair of tetralogy of Fallot on both biventricular systolic and diastolic function have been evaluated with the use of MRI.[25,26] The negative effect of pulmonary regurgitation on right and left systolic ventricular function has been demonstrated, reflected by the inverse relation between the degree of pulmonary regurgitation and ventricular ejection fractions. Diminished diastolic relaxation parameters of the right ventricle have been identified after repair of tetralogy of Fallot, whereas an association was found between diastolic dysfunction and diminished exercise performance, independent from the degree of pulmonary regurgitation and systolic ventricular function.

Thus, MRI provides complete information on adult congenital heart disease, including biventricular systolic function and mass, pulmonary flow as well as diastolic ventricular function. This evaluation may have important prognostic and therapeutic implications for management of patients with congenital heart disease.

References

1. Allen HD, Gersony WM, Taubert KA. Insurability of the adolescent and young adult with heart disease: Report form the Fifth Conference on Insurability, October 3–4, 1991. *Circulation.* 1992;86:703–710.
2. Link KM, Lesko NM. Magnetic resonance imaging in the evaluation of congenital heart disease. *Magn Reson Q.* 1991;7:173–190.
3. De Roos A, Van der Wall EE. Magnetic resonance imaging and spectroscopy of the heart. *Curr Opin Cardiol.* 1991;6:946–952.
4. Geva T, Vick W, Wendt RE, Rokey R. Role of spin echo and cine magnetic resonance imaging in presurgical planning of heterotaxy syndrome. *Circulation.* 1994;90:348–356.
5. Kersting-Sommerhoff BA, Seelos KC, Hardy C, et al. Evaluation of surgical procedures for cyanotic congenital heart disease by using MR imaging. *AJR.* 1990;155:259–266.
6. Fellows KE, Weinberg PM, Baffa JM, Hoffman EA. Evaluation of congenital heart disease with MR imaging: current and coming attractions. *AJR.* 1992; 159:925–931.
7. Kersting-Sommerhoff BA, Diethelm L, Teitel DF, et al. Magnetic resonance imaging of congenital heart disease: Sensitivity and specificity using receiver operating characteristic curve analysis. *Am Heart J.* 1989;118:155–161.
8. Baker EJ, Ayton V, Smith MA, et al. Magnetic resonance imaging of coarctation of the aorta in infants: Use of a high field strength. *Br Heart J.* 1989; 62:97–101.
9. Bank ER, Aisen AM, Rocchini AP, Hernandez RJ. Coarctation of the aorta in children undergoing angioplasty: pretreatment and posttreatment MR imaging. *Radiology.* 1987;162:235–240.
10. Didier D, Higgins CB, Fisher MR, et al. Congenital heart disease: Gated MR imaging in 72 patients. *Radiology.* 1986;158:227–235.
11. Shinebourne EA, Macartney FJ, Anderson RH. Sequential chamber localization: Logical approach to diagnosis in congenital heart disease. *Br Heart J.* 1976;41:327–340.
12. Tynan MJ, Becker AE, Macartney FJ, et al. Nomenclature and classification of congenital heart disease. *Br Heart J.* 1979;41:544–553.
13. Van Praagh R. The importance of segmental situs in the diagnosis of congenital heart disease. *Semin Roentgenol.* 1985;20:254–271.
14. Higgins CB, Sechtem UP, Pflugfelder P. Cine MR: Evaluation of cardiac ventricular function and valvular function. *Int J Cardiac Imaging.* 1988;3: 21–28.
15. Pattynama PMT, Lamb HJL, Van der Velde EA, et al. Left ventricular measurements with cine and spin-echo MR imaging: A study of reproducibility with variance component analysis. *Radiology.* 1993;187:261–268.

16. Helbing WA, Rebergen SA, Maliepaard J, et al. Quantification of right function with magnetic resonance imaging in children with normal hearts and with congenital heart disease. *Am Heart J.* 1995;130:828–837.
17. Fujita N, Hartiala J, O'Sullivan M, et al. Assessment of left ventricular diastolic function in dilated cardiomyopathy with cine magnetic resonance imaging: Effect of an angiotensin converting enzyme inhibitor, benazepril. *Am Heart J.* 1993;125:171–178.
18. Mostbeck GH, Hartiala JJ, Foster E, et al. Right ventricular diastolic filling: Evaluation with velocity-encoded cine MRI. *J Comput Assist Tomogr.* 1993; 17:245–252.
19. Hartiala JJ, Mostbeck GH, Foster E, et al. Velocity-encoded cine MRI in the evaluation of left ventricular diastolic function: Measurement of mitral valve and pulmonary vein flow velocities and flow volume across the mitral valve. *Am Heart J.* 1993;125:1054–1066.
20. Jones EL, Conti CR, Neill CA, et al. Long-term evaluation of tetralogy patients with pulmonic valvular insufficiency resulting from outflow-patch correction across the pulmonic annulus. *Circulation.* 1973;47/48(suppl III): 11–18.
21. Marie PY, Marcon F, Brunotte F, et al. Right ventricular overload and induced sustained ventricular tachycardia in operatively "repaired" tetralogy of Fallot. *Am J Cardiol.* 1992;69:785–789.
22. Rebergen SA, Chin JGJ, Ottenkamp J, et al. Pulmonary regurgitation in the late postoperative follow-up of tetralogy of Fallot: Volumetric quantitation by nuclear magnetic resonance velocity mapping. *Circulation.* 1993;88(part 1):2257–2266.
23. Markiewicz W, Sechtem U, Higgins CB. Evaluation of the right ventricle by magnetic resonance imaging. *Am Heart J.* 1987;113:8–15.
24. Møgelvang J, Stubgaard M, Thomsen C, Henriksen O. Evaluation of right ventricular volumes measured by magnetic resonance imaging. *Eur Heart J.* 1988;9:529–533.
25. Niezen RA, Helbing WA, Meinesz S, Rebergen SA, Van der Wall EE, De Roos A.: Pulmonary regurgitation in children with surgically corrected tetralogy of Fallot: follow-up with MR imaging (Abstract). Radiology, 197(P): 433, 1995.
26. Helbing WA, Niezen RA, Van der Geest RJ, et al. Right ventricular diastolic function in children with surgically corrected tetralogy of Fallot and pulmonary regurgitation: Volumetric evaluation with MR velocity mapping. *Radiology.* 1995;197(P):335.

Chapter 9

Cost-Effective Diagnostic Algorithms for the Surgical Management of Congenital Heart Disease
The Classic Approach Applied to Managed Care

James B. Kinney, MD, Vincent B. Ho, MD,
Flavian M. Lupinetti, MD, and
David J. Sahn, MD

Since the advent of extracorporeal circulation, the surgical correction of structural heart disease has become routine in children. Classically, these patients were managed by a "surgical cardiologist" who worked with the operating surgeon (personal communication with Dr. W. M. Thompson, Jr.). Utilizing clinical tools and tailored angiograms, the surgical cardiologist, a role later assumed by the pediatric cardiologist, answered the essential preoperative questions necessary for surgical intervention.

Over the years, the diagnostic tools for cardiac evaluation have dramatically improved and become more sophisticated. In particular, the noninvasive studies of transthoracic echocardiography (TTE),[1-7] transesophageal echocardiography (TEE),[8] and magnetic resonance imaging (MRI)[9-34] have revolutionized diagnostic pediatric cardiology. TTE, for example, has become the preferred modality, especially in

The opinions or assertions contained herein are the private views of the authors and are not to be construed as official or reflecting the views of the Department of the Army or of the Department of Defense.
From: Higgins CB, Ingwall JS, Pohost GM, (eds). *Current and Future Applications of Magnetic Resonance in Cardiovascular Disease.* Armonk, NY: Futura Publishing Company, Inc.; © 1998.

TABLE 1. Clinical Imaging Algorithms for the Assessment of Congenital Heart Diseases

Surgical groups	%	Conditions that need to be known	Conditions that need to be excluded	Imaging strategy
1. VSD	14.8	Location of VSD	Multiple VSDs Subaortic obstruction Prolapsed aortic valve Coarctation of the aorta	TTE → T1W MRI[a] → cine 5.MRI[b]
2. PDA	8.3	Aortic arch anatomy	Coarctation of the aorta	TTE (Include T1W MRI and cine MRI II coarctation of the aorta is suspected)
3. Aortic valve operations	7.5	Degree of aortic stenosis/insufficiency Location of any supra/subaortic pulmonic stenosis Pulmonary valve integrity and size for possible Ross procedure	Left ventricular dysfunction Occult subaortic obstruction VSD	Simple valvular aortic stenosis: TTE (emphasizing continuous-wave doppler[c]) All others: add T1W MRI → cine MRI
4. Tetralogy of Fallot	7.0	Infundibular anatomy Anatomy of the pulmonary arteries Size of the pulmonary arteries Size of the pulmonary annulus	Double outlet right ventricle Multiple VSD Large aortopulmonary collaterals (Anomalous coronary artery anatomy)	TTE (emphasizing coronary artery anatomy[d] → T1W MRI → cine MRI → (Angiography)[e]
5. Obstructed aortic arch (coarctation/interruption)	7.0	Location, length and severity of obstruction Adequacy of left ventricular inflow/outflow	VSD Aortic stenosis	T1W MRI and cine MRI (include TTE if VSD and/or aortic stenosis is suspected and Gd-3OTOF MRI angiography[g] for delineation of collateral vessels in questionable cases)
6. Atrioventricular canal	5.2	Complete versus incomplete Atrioventricular valve anatomy and their associated competence	VSD distant from canal pathology Right ventricular outflow tract obstruction ("Tetralogy canal") Straddling valve (chordae)	TTE (TEE for cleft mitral valves[f]) → T1W MRI and cine MRI (for suspected straddling valve (chordae) and "Tetralogies")

7. ASD partial anomalous pulmonary venous return	5.1	Location and number of ASD(s) Anatomy of venous return	Occult on premium ASD Scimitar syndrome Peripheral pulmonary arterial stenosis	TTE → T1W MRI (add cine MRI for ASD location and pulmonary artery anatomy and phase-contrast MRI venography[h] and cine MRI for anomalous venous connections)
8. Other "closed procedures" Bullock-Taussig shunts pulmonary artery bends vascular rings	4.7	Aortic arch anatomy Pulmonary artery anatomy	Hypoplastic pulmonary artery	T1W MRI → cine MRI
9. Transposition of the great vessels	4.4	Relation of the great vessels Presence of VSD Ventricular size and function Amount of left ventricular outflow obstruction	Coarctation of the aorta Large aortopulmonary collaterals Multiple VSDs (Anomalous coronary artery anatomy[e])	TTE → T1W MRI → cine MRI → (Angiography[e])
10. Mitral valve repair/replacement	2.9	Severity of mitral stenosis/insufficiency Mitral valve anatomy (cleft, supravalvular ring, chordae rupture...)	Poor left ventricular function	TTE and TEE

T1W, T1-weighted; MRI, magnetic resonance imaging; Gd, Gadolinium; 3D TOF, 3-dimensional time-of-fight

[a] T1-weighted MRI performed in the orthogonal planes (axial, sagittal and coronal) are excellent for the delineation of the cardiac and pericardiac structures. Axial images are especially good.[9–20]

[b] Cine MRI, both gradient-echo and phase-contrast (PC), acquires images throughout the cardiac cycle which affords dynamic evaluation of cardiac function and flow. Cine PC MRI has the added ability to quantitate flow.[15,16,21–33]

[c] Reference 7

[d] Reference 3

[e] The need for angiography for the identification of anomalous coronary artery anatomy is debatable. Please refer to the discussion in the text.

[f] Reference 8

[g] Dynamic Gd-enhanced three-dimensional time-of-flight MRA is a recently described technique that promises to provide excellent blood pool images of the thoracic aorta.[16,34]

[h] Phase-contrast MR venography can be performed to evaluate the systemic or pulmonary venous anatomy in the chest by the prescription of low velocity encoding settings (20–40 cm/sec).[16]

infants, for screening of structural cardiac anomalies.[5,6] There also have been dramatic improvements in angiographic technique and equipment that have generated the perception of enhanced safety for diagnostic catheterization and led to the frequent performance of routine preoperative cardiac catheterization using a standard "cookbook" protocol.

Today, with the establishment of managed care and cost containment environments and complex contracting arrangements, a return to a more integrated, cost-effective, and tailored approach to the preoperative evaluation of patients with congenital heart disease has been mandated. These opportunities for cost savings, furthermore, can be both revenue generating and program sustaining. With the introduction of alternative and less costly imaging options such as TTE, TEE, and MRI, the use of a standard preoperative cardiac catheterization diagnostic package is no longer fiscally tenable.

Successful preoperative management of structural heart disease still revolves around answering the essential questions related to surgical planning for the operating surgeon. We have found that the majority of these essential questions are sufficiently answered noninvasively by a combination of TTE, TEE, and MRI. Using these techniques, the pediatric cardiologist is capable of generating cost-effective information that is cost competitive, and in some cases more robust, in quality to the anatomic detail of traditional angiography. Encouraged by 3 years of MRI experience with the evaluation of over 200 cases of congenital heart disease, we have generated imaging strategies or algorithms (Table 1) for the 10 most common groups of surgically correctable congenital heart diseases. In Table 1, the essential questions that the surgeon needs answered in order to safely and successfully operate on the patient with structural heart disease are listed by surgical group in descending order of their operative frequency. These clinical questions are further divided into those concerning conditions that must be known and those that must be known and those that must be excluded. For each group, the imaging strategy we use to answer the clinical questions are listed. We have found these algorithms to be functional even when the surgeon is located remotely from the managed care contract or the administrating medical evaluation site. Information obtained by TTE, TEE, and MRI have the added benefit that they can be video recorded and easily combined onto a single videotape. The videotape, in turn, can be mailed or teletransmitted to the attending surgeon for his review and display at the surgical conference. In this age of the information superhighway and global networks, the actual raw data sets of digital information obtained by ultrasound and MRI can be sent to remote sites for further data processing.

The frequency of each surgical category listed in Table 1 is based on the tabulated operative experience of the surgical author (FML) at the Children's Hospital and Medical Center, Seattle, Washington, from September 1993 through June 1995. A typical regional or community health care entity would be less likely to have as high a frequency of unusual cases as are treated at this institution, and accordingly would be more likely to find an even higher percentage of surgical candidates that can be placed in the 10 most common categories listed. It is estimated that upwards of 85% to 95% of surgical patients would therefore be candidates to undergo operative repair without the need for angiography.

Special mention should be made regarding the need for delineation of coronary anatomy prior to surgical intervention. Although coronary anatomy is frequently abnormal in some congenital heart defects and precise intraoperative identification is mandatory, there is less compelling need for preoperative angiography than was previously the case. In tetralogy of Fallot, for example, where repair in infancy has become increasingly common,[35] the presence of an anomalous left anterior descending coronary artery arising from the right coronary artery may preclude a right ventriculotomy. This may be regarded as a justification for preoperative cardiac catheterization and angiography. When this lesion is recognized for the first time in the operating room, however, the surgeon has at least three excellent options: (1) complete repair with transatrial-transpulmonary infundibular muscle resection; (2) repair with a right ventricle to pulmonary artery allograft; or (3) a modified Blalock-Taussig shunt.[36,37] One of these three options would most likely be used in any event if the coronary anatomy is anticipated. Accordingly, the advantage of precise foreknowledge must be compared with the additional risk and expense of catheterization. In the most critically ill neonates and infants and possibly older children as well, the latter would seem to exceed the former. A similar problem may exist in patients with transposition of the great arteries, for whom an arterial switch repair has become the operative correction of choice. Coronary artery transfer remains the most critical element for the successful performance of this operation. Echocardiography has become highly reliable in determining coronary anatomy[38] and angiography may add little or nothing to the preoperative evaluation. Magnetic resonance angiography is probably even more effective than transthoracic echocardiography for evaluation of the path of anomalous coronary arteries. At present, nearly all anatomic subtypes of coronary anatomy are compatible with excellent surgical results.[39] The most difficult coronary anatomic subtypes, notably the intramural coronary anomalies, may not be well delineated even with careful angiography.

The cost of the proposed algorithms, of course, varies regionally and relies on the individual health care entity's financial arrangements and the availability of and cost of each imaging modality for the center. Of the imaging modalities, echocardiography appears to be the least expensive. In the Pacific Northwest, the cost of an MRI examination amortized over a 5-year period and including maintenance, supply and technologist expenses, is no more than 2 to 3 times that of an echocardiogram (unpublished data, the authors). Similarly calculated, a standard diagnostic pediatric catheterization is conservatively 8 to 12 times that of an echocardiogram (unpublished data, the authors). Should the contracting organization own both a comprehensive pediatric catheterization laboratory and a fully outfitted MRI unit, the cost savings to the contract is simply the difference between the cost for cardiac catheterization minus the cost of the displacing diagnostic imaging modality (TTE, TEE, and/or MRI) for each patient.

Calculating the savings becomes more complex when the contracting health care entity owns an MRI unit, but lacks the ability to perform pediatric angiography. This scenario is the most common as there are clearly more MRI units (nearly 4000 in the United States[40]) than catheterization laboratories equipped to perform pediatric cases. In addition, an increasing number of MRI units are freestanding or mobile, not necessarily affiliated with a university medical center.[41–43] For patients traditionally handled by angiography but who have essential questions answered adequately by echocardiography and/or MRI:

savings = X (subcontract debt per angiogram) − Y (cost per MRI) − Z (cost per echocardiogram)

$$X = \text{number of angiograms}$$

$$Y = \text{number of MRI exams}$$

$$Z = \text{number of echocardiograms}$$

One is quick to ask if the contracting health care entity should outfit an existing adult catheterization laboratory to do pediatric cases. The cost of subcontracting the approximately 5% to 15% of the cases will likely be less than the expense of adequately upgrading an adult catheterization laboratory. The expenses of such an endeavor depends not only on the need to upgrade or to purchase an additional C-arm unit for the angiography suite and to acquire pediatric injectors, but also to stock the laboratory with the necessary pediatric diagnostic catheters and catheter kits. The presence of a highly trained technician, access to a surgical recovery unit, and availability of surgical backup coverage are additional important management and financial issues. Should pediatric angioplasty be performed in the laboratory, the cost calculations would change somewhat. Other than simple pulmonary balloon angioplasty, however, pediatric interventions are increasingly being referred to large university medical centers to be handled by an individual with additional training and expertise in this developing new subspecialty.

Potentially, more savings to the contract might be realized if the pediatric cardiologist belonging to the contracting facility goes to the subcontracting institution and performed the angiographic studies himself, further reducing charges to the contract (for example, external CHAMPUS contract). By centralizing cardiac catheterization activities to one pediatric laboratory in a region, it becomes abundantly clear that the amortized cost per study drops precipitously, so that the charges by the subcontractor can become increasingly competitive.

In a fee-for-service setting, the pediatric cardiologist is tracked in an institution by the billing that he or she generates. In a managed care setting, particularly with a capitated contract outside of a university medical center, the pediatric cardiologist must be acknowledged for the savings realized by the use of echocardiography and MRI in place of angiography. The health care entity employing the pediatric cardiologist must measure productivity of the pediatric cardiologist against a different set of standards.

In the vast majority of surgical heart disease cases, echocardiography and MRI can adequately answer the obligate preoperative clinical questions. Sometimes the vascular anatomic detail of MRI and the gradient and flow information of echocardiography are both required for optimum diagnostic power. The quality of the echocardiographic and MRI images are essential elements for a successful diagnostic program and that quality heavily relies on the expertise of the imaging physicians. Naturally, it remains the surgeon's perogative to accept or to reject the preoperative studies as adequate for the surgical management. The collective efforts of the pediatric radiologist, radiologist and pediatric cardiothoracic surgeon cannot be overemphasized as the success of the program is impingent on their collaboration. The undertaking of this type of cost-saving endeavor requires a strong commitment by those involved. Mutual education and "cross-training" is necessary to bridge the traditional boundaries between the disciplines, namely that of radiology and cardiology. In the ideal situation, routine echocardiograms and cardiac MRI studies could be adequately performed by the same group of cardiologists and radiologists, eliminating the costly need for specific cardiovascular MRI or pediatric echocardiographic backup coverage.

Managed care is currently an accepted reality for a large segment of the American population. Its emphasis on cost effectiveness without compromise of patient care has resulted in the creative reorganization of medical resources and personnel. Using the newer, less expensive, noninvasive technology of echocardiography and MRI, we have avoided compromise of quality patient care by honoring the classic concepts that have safeguarded the surgical care of children with heart disease. In this chapter, we have stated the essential questions that traditionally must be answered to surgically manage the 10 most common groups of congenital lesions and have proposed the most cost-effective manner for their preoperative evaluation. The pediatric cardiologist, radiologist, and cardiothoracic surgeon must work together to answer the appropriate questions prior to each procedure—this is the classic approach. By using echocardiography and MRI to implement the classic approach, cost-effective quality patient care can be achieved in the managed care environment.

Acknowledgments

The authors would like to thank Dr. Norman Shumway of Stanford University and Dr. Charles B. Higgins of the University of California San Francisco for their thoughtful advice and encouragement in the preparation of this manuscript. We would also like to thank Major General James B. Peake, MC, commanding general at Madigan Army Medical Center, without whose support this chapter would not be possible.

References

1. Silverman NH, Hunter S, Anderson RH, et al. Anatomic basis of cross sectional echocardiography. *Br Heart J*. 1983;50:421–431.
2. Henry WL, DeMaria A, Gramiak R, et al. Report of the American Society of Echocardiography Committee on Nomenclature and Standards in two-dimensional Echocardiography. *Circulation*. 1980;62:212–215.
3. Sahn DJ, Anderson F. *Two-Dimensional Anatomy of the Heart*. New York John Wiley, 1982.
4. Silverman NH, Schiller NB. Apex echocardiography. A two-dimensional technique for evaluating congenital heart disease. *Circulation*. 1978;57: 503–511.
5. Lange LW, Sahn DJ, Allen HD, Goldberg SJ. Subxiphoid cross-sectional Echocardiography in infants and children congenital heart disease. *Circulation*. 1979;59:513–524.
6. Snider AR, Silverman NH. Suprasternal notch echocardiography: A two dimensional technique for evaluating congenital heart disease. *Circulation*. 1981;63:165–173.
7. Hatle L, Angelsen BA, Tromsdal A. Non-invasive assessment of aortic stenosis by Doppler ultrasound. *Br Heart J*. 1980;43:284–292.
8. Weintraub RG, Sahn DJ, Ritter SB, et al. Transesophageal echocardiography in infants and children with congenital heart disease. *Circulation*. 1992;86: 711–722.
9. Didier D, Higgins CB, Fisher MR, et al. Congenital heart disease: Gated MR imaging in 72 patients. *Radiology*. 1986;158:227–235.

10. Link KM, Lesko NM. Magnetic resonance imaging in the evaluation of congenital heart disease. *Magn Reson O*. 1991;7:173–190.
11. Gutierrez FR, Brown JJ, Mirowitz SA, eds. *Cardiovascular Magnetic Resonance Imaging*. St. Louis: Mosby-Yearbook, 1992.
12. Bank ER. Magnetic resonance of congenital cardiovascular disease: An update. *Radiol Clin North Am*. 1993;31:533–572.
13. Fellows KE, Weinberg PM, Baffa JM, et al. Evaluation of congenital heart disease with MR imaging: Current and coming attractions. *AJR*. 1992;159: 925–931.
14. Bissett GS, III. Magnetic resonance imaging of congenital heart disease in the pediatric patient. *Radiol Clin North Am*. 1991;29:279–291.
15. Higgins CB. MRI of congenital heart disease. In: Higgins CB. *Essentials of Cardiac Radiology and Imaging*. Philadelphia: JB Lippincott Company; 1992; 283–331.
16. Ho VB, Kinney JB, Sahn DJ. Contributions of newer MR imaging strategies for congenital heart disease. *RadioGraphics*. 1996;16:43–60.
17. Burrows PE, MacDonald CE. Magnetic resonance imaging of the pediatric thoracic aorta. *Semin US CT MRI*. 1993;14:129–144.
18. von Schulthess GK, Higashino SM, Higgins SS, et al. Coarctation of the aorta: MR imaging. *Radiology*. 1986;158:469–474.
19. Diethelm L, D'Cry R, Lipton MJ, Higgins CB. Atrial-level shunts: Sensitivity and specificity of MR in diagnosis. *Radiology*. 1987;162:181–186.
20. Rees RSO, Somerville J, Underwood SR, et al. Magnetic resonance imaging of the pulmonary arteries and their systemic connections in pulmonary atresia: Comparison with angiographic and surgical findings. *Br Heart J*. 1987;58:621–626.
21. von Schulthess GK, Higgins CB. Blood flow imaging with MR: Spin-phase phenomena. *Radiology*. 1985;157:687–695.
22. Mostbeck GH, Caputo GR, Higgins CB. MR measurement of blood flow in the cardiovascular system. *AJR*. 1992;159:453–461.
23. Sechtem U, Pflugfelder P, Cassidy MC, et al. Ventricular septal defect: Visualization of shunt flow and determination of shunt size by cine MR imaging. *AJR*. 1987;149:689–692.
24. Simpson IA, Chung KJ, Glass RF, et al. Cine magnetic resonance imaging for evaluation of anatomy and flow relations in infants and children with coarctation of the aorta. *Circulation*. 1988;78:142–148.
25. Pflugfelder PW, Landzberg JS, Cassidy MM, et al. Comparison of cine MR imaging with Doppler echocardiography for the evaluation of aortic regurgitation. *AJR*. 1989;152:729–735.
26. de Roos A, Reichek N, Axel L, Kressel HY. Cine MR imaging in aortic stenosis. *J Comput Assist Tomogr*. 1989;13:421–425.
27. Nayler GL, Firmin DN, Longmore DB. Blood flow imaging by cine magnetic resonance. *J Comput Assist Tomogr*. 1986;10:715–722.
28. Bogren HG, Klipstein RH, Firmin DN, et al. Quantification of antegrade and retrograde blood flow in the human aorta by magnetic resonance velocity mapping. *Am Heart J*. 1989;117:1214–1222.
29. Rees S. Firmin D, Mohiaddin R. Underwood R. Longmore D. Application of flow measurements by magnetic resonance velocity mapping to congenital heart disease. *Am J Cardiol*. 1989;64:953–956.
30. Brenner LD, Caputo GR, Mostbeck G, et al. Quantification of left to right atrial shunts with velocity-encoded cine nuclear magnetic resonance imaging. *J Am Coll Cardiol*. 1992;20:1246–1250.

31. Rebergen SA, van der Wall EE, Doornbos J. de Roos A. Magnetic resonance measurement of velocity and flow: Technique, validation, and cardiovascular applications. *Am Heart J.* 1993;126:1439–1456.
32. Steffens JC, Bourne MW, Sakuma H, et al. Quantification of collateral blood flow in coarctation of the aorta by velocity encoded cine magnetic resonance imaging. *Circulation.* 1994;90:937–943.
33. Ho VB, Kinney JB, Sahn DJ. Ruptured sinus of Valsalva aneurysm: Cine phase contrast MR characterization. *J Comput Assist Tomogr.* 1995;19: 652–656.
34. Prince MR. Gadolinium-enhanced MR aortography. *Radiology.* 1994;191: 155–164.
35. Groh MA, Meliones JN, Bove EL, et al. Repair of tetralogy of Fallot in infancy. Effect of pulmonary artery size on outcome. *Circulation.* 1991; 84(suppl III):III-206–III-212.
36. Humes RA, Driscoll DJ, Danielson GK, Puga FJ. Tetralogy of Fallot with anomalous origin of left anterior descending coronary artery. Surgical options. *J Thorac Cardiovasc Surg.* 1987;94:784–787.
37. Pacifico AD, Sand ME, Bargeron LM Jr, Colvin EC. Transatrial-transpulmonary repair of tetralogy of Fallot. *J Thorac Sardiovasc Surg.* 1987;93:919–924.
38. Pasquini L, Sanders SP, Parness IA, et al. Coronary echocardiography in 406 patients with d-loop transposition of the great arteries. *J Am Coll Cardiol.* 1994;24:763–768.
39. Lupenetti FM, Bove EL, Minich LL, Snider AR, Callow LB, Meliones JN, Crowley DC, Beekman RH, Serwer G. Dick M II, Vermilion R. Rosenthal A. Intermediate-term survival and functional results after arterial repair for transposition of the great vessels. *J Thorac Cardiovasc Surg.* 1992;103: 421–427.
40. Brice J. Industry execs respond to recessionary market. *Diagnostic Imaging.* 1994;(February):35–41.
41. Evens RG, Jost RG, Evens RG Jr. Economic and utilization analysis of magnetic resonance imaging units in the United States in 1985. *AJR.* 1985;145: 393–398.
42. Hillman AL, Schwartz JS. The diffusion of MRI: Patterns of siting and ownership in an era of changing incentives. *AJR.* 1986;146:963–969.
43. Evens RG, Evens JG Jr. Analysis of economics and use of MR imaging units in the United States in 1990. *AJR.* 1991;157:603–607.

Chapter 10

Magnetic Resonance Imaging of the Cardiovascular System: Can It Be Cost Effective?

Edward T. Martin, MD and
Gerald M. Pohost, MD

In an era of health care reform everyone is looking for strategies to reduce cost and to improve outcomes. While this may seem like an impossible task, this chapter will serve to demonstrate the way in which magnetic resonance methods might indeed allow improved diagnosis, prognostication, and outcomes. As such, it would be a diagnostic technology that would benefit the patient with cardiovascular disease under most circumstances, including those of managed care.

Magnetic resonance imaging (MRI) is already being used to evaluate patients with congenital heart disease, cardiac masses, aortic disease, valvular heart disease, and constrictive pericarditis. Because of its unique ability to image the right ventricle it is also an ideal technology to evaluate the function of both ventricles. The potential of magnetic resonance lies in its ability to assess virtually all aspects of ischemic heart disease.

This chapter reviews the current literature on magnetic resonance approaches with potential to combine morphological, functional, angiographic, perfusion, and viability imaging in a unique package whose diagnostic accuracy can compete favorably with existing technologies and that will be cost effective in an era of managed care.

Morphology

MRI can provide images with high resolution in multiple planes and is the technology of choice for defining anatomy. There has been

From: Higgins CB, Ingwall JS, Pohost GM, (eds). *Current and Future Applications of Magnetic Resonance in Cardiovascular Disease.* Armonk, NY: Futura Publishing Company, Inc.; © 1998.

substantial progress since the first suggestion that magnetic resonance methods would be useful for assessment of cardiovascular disease.[1] From the standard transverse, sagittal, and coronal planes any oblique plane can be set up and visualized. Cardiac chamber sizes can be accurately measured and volumes can be calculated using either the area-length method or Simpson's rule. Because of this high resolution and dimensional accuracy, congenital heart disease and the subsequent results of reparative surgery can be comprehensively evaluated. This is especially important because these patients often have poor echo windows. Patients with prior myocardial infarction can be assessed and followed using wall thickness and left ventricular mass.[2–8] Complications of myocardial infarction (MI) such as a left ventricular (LV) aneurysm or thrombus can also be easily viewed.[9,10] MRI has proven to be highly accurate for identifying pericardial thickening and calcium as well as pericardial effusions. Echocardiography can also detect pericardial effusions, but has limited diagnostic accuracy in identifying a thickened pericardium. Finally, the location and extent of cardiac and paracardiac masses and their relationship to other structures in the thorax can be demonstrated[11,12] more safely and accurately with MRI than with any other imaging modality.

Function

Because MRI can acquire images in any plane, global and regional wall motion assessment can be performed quickly and accurately. Using cine MRI tomograms, ejection fraction can be calculated from end-diastolic and end-systolic volumes.[13–16] Because ventricular volumes influence survival after an MI, and remodeling is also an important consideration, MRI can be used to follow patients after an MI. End-systolic volumes are also an important factor when deciding on replacing or repairing valves in aortic insufficiency and mitral regurgitation. Regional assessment of LV wall motion and thickness can be an easy way of differentiating nonviable from viable myocardium.[17,18] If low-dose dobutamine is added, such a test can examine the ability of asynergic ventricular segments to improve with adrenergic stimulation, a sign of myocardial viability.[19,20] Functional assessment can be further enhanced because magnetic resonance is uniquely capable of tagging the myocardial tissue so as to study the finer detailed movements of contractile function.[21,22]

Valvular regurgitation causes signal voids on gradient echo images of the heart most likely due to dephasing of spins of the blood in the turbulent jet. Measurement of regurgitation by signal-void size has been correlated with Doppler echo, but because multiple parameters can affect the size of the signal void, quantitative approaches, such as phase velocity mapping, have been developed and can now be used.[23-26] Quantitation has also been shown to compare favorably with cardiac catheterization.

Valvular stenosis can also be assessed using phase velocity mapping techniques. Pressure gradients and valve areas have correlated well with cardiac catheterization and echocardiography in several studies.[27-29] This area will need continued development in the future to reduce acquisition and processing times and to reduce artifact resulting from poor positioning of the velocity-encoded slice.

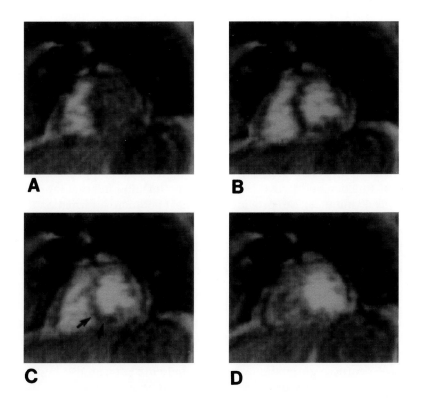

FIGURE 1. Myocardial perfusion. This figure illustrates the first pass technique at mid ventricle using gadolinium as the contrast agent. **A:** contrast (white) is seen in the right ventricle; **B:** contrast passes to the left ventricle; **C:** contrast is now seen in the myocardium of the left ventricle however there is a delay in the inferior and inferoseptal walls which suggest ischemia (black arrows); **D:** contrast is now only seen in left ventricular cavity and myocardium (all left ventricular myocardium is now of equal intensity that validated the inferior and inferoseptal walls as delayed and thus ischemic).

Assessment of Myocardial Ischemia

Currently there are two methods in use for evaluating the extent of myocardial ischemia. The first method assesses regional wall motion before and after infusions of a pharmacological agent. Some have used the stress agent dobutamine, and others have assessed wall motion with the vasodilator dipyridamole. Both agents have been shown to have sensitivities and specificities that are almost comparable to radionuclide perfusion imaging.[30-34] The second method exclusively uses the vasodilator dipyridamole combined with an MRI contrast agent, gadolinium, to directly assess myocardial perfusion (Figure 1). Presently there are good data in both humans and animals showing the utility of this method.[35-37] Previously, a limitation of this technique has been the fact that only one tomographic slice at a time could be studied. Multislice techniques are presently being studied. With the development of gadolinium-based contrast agents it is possible to bolus inject and track the gadolinium using higher speed magnetic resonance methods thus allowing a comprehensive evaluation of myocardial perfusion. Likewise, zones that do not demonstrate contrast enhancement suggest myocardial infarction. Combining function and perfusional information obviates the need for multiple technologies such as echocardiography and radionuclide imaging, as well as left ventriculography via catheter approaches. These two magnetic resonance approaches that assess function and perfusion in the same imaging interval (approximately 60 minutes), can provide the same if not more information than the other tests combined.

Vascular Imaging and Coronary Angiography

Presently MRI has become the gold standard for evaluating stable thoracic aortic disease.[38,39] Current MRI techniques can identify both the origin and the extent of aortic dissection without the use of contrast agents. Complications of dissection, such as involvement of branch vessels, aortic regurgitation or pericardial effusion can also be accurately identified and displayed in three dimensions for easy analysis (Figure 2). Aortic aneurysms can be modeled in a similar way. The cardiovascular surgeon prefers the three dimensional display since it allows formulation of an accurate approach preoperatively.

By combining the morphological, angiographic, and phase velocity mapping approaches, MRI technology has virtually unlimited application in vascular evaluation. In coarctation of the aorta one can derive accurate dimensions of narrowing as well as pressure gradients. Other

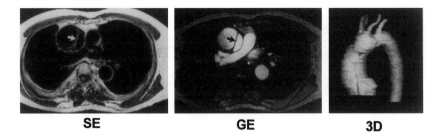

SE   GE   3D

FIGURE 2. Aortic dissection. This figure shows how aortic dissection can be diagnosed using three different magnetic resonance techniques: SE: spin echo (white arrow points to true lumen); GE: gradient echo (black arrow points to true lumen; and 3D: three-dimensional. Surgeons often prefer the three-dimensional image to help them plan operative repairs.

arterial vessels can be evaluated in a similar manner from carotids to femorals. The venous system can also be assessed just as easily.

With time, magnetic resonance coronary angiography should evolve into an approach that promises to obviate the need for diagnostic coronary angiography that currently is being done using invasive catheterization approaches. Presently, there have been good results from several groups using different imaging techniques that demonstrate high resolution images of the coronary arteries and coronary artery bypass grafts.[40-44] Magnetic resonance coronary angiography is limited by cardiac and respiratory motion and by the presence of epicardial fat that decreases artery contrast. But with the development and application of higher speed methods, resolution will be enhanced and consistent diagnostic quality coronary angiograms using non-invasive magnetic resonance angiographic methods will be generated. By combining magnetic resonance coronary angiography with assessment of function and perfusion imaging in a 90-minute time interval will address much of the information needed to assess patients with possible or definite coronary artery disease prior to an intervention.

Viability

As mentioned previously, by using MRI to assess ventricular function at rest and during infusion of dobutamine, it is possible to evaluate the viability of segments that are asynergic at rest, ie, those that contract with adrenergic stimulation.

Even more elegant is the ability to use spectroscopic imaging of molecules containing the nuclear magnetic resonance (NMR) sensitive nuclei ^{31}P and ^{1}H. ^{31}P imaging provides a strategy to assess viability using endogenous metabolically active high-energy phosphates. Hydrogen NMR spectroscopic imaging provides a potential means for assessing triglyceride content of myocardium. During the change to anaerobic metabolism, myocardium metabolizes glucose and triglycerides accumulate. If myocardium becomes nonviable, triglycerides are not formed. While substantially more development is necessary to enable application of these spectroscopic approaches clinically, it is clear progress is being made.

Cost Comparison

This section compares the equipment and start-up costs as well as hospital charges for the major noninvasive cardiovascular imaging modalities. The five current imaging modalities include echocardiography (ECHO), radionuclide imaging (RN), electron beam computed tomography (EBCT), positron emission tomography (PET), and magnetic resonance imaging (MRI). As can be seen in Table 1, MRI is the only technology that has the potential to cover all areas of cardiac evaluation. Therefore, if an initial investment of capital can compete with the other modalities MRI would be the most cost effective.

Initial equipment and start-up costs for the different imaging modalities are estimated in Table 2 (personal communications L. Tauxe, N. Nanda, MD, and J. Camaratta). Echocardiography is the least expensive at $400,000, followed by RN imaging at approximately $500,000; EBCT at $2.1 million; and PET at $4.4 million (for camera and cyclotron). MRI can be analyzed in one of two ways: (1) purchase of a new system, or (2) upgrade of an existing system with software packages.

Starting from scratch, a new magnetic resonance state-of-the-art scanner with the potential to perform the cardiovascular studies would cost about $1.8 million for the scanner and $60,000 for two technolo-

---

TABLE 1

Methods Useful for Each Evaluation

• Morphology	ECHO, EBCT, MR
• Function	ECHO, RN, EBCT, MR
• Perfusion	RN, MR
• Coronary angio	X-ray Cine (Cath), MR
• Viability	ECHO (Dobut), RN, MR

Cath indicates Catheterization; Dobut, dobutamine; EBCT, electron beam computed tomography; Echo, echocardiography; MR, magnetic resonance; RN, radionuclides.

TABLE 2

Equipment and Start-Up Costs

Echocardiogram	
Equipment	$300,000
Technical Support	$40,000
System Maintenance	$30,000/yr
Total	**$370,000**
Electron Beam Computed Tomography	
Equipment	$1.9 million
System Maintenance	$180,000/yr
Technical Support	(included)
Total	**$2.1 million**
MRI #1 (Hardware not in place)	
Equipment	$1.5–1.8 million
System Maintenance	$160,000/yr
Cryogens	$10,000/yr
Technical Support	(included)
Total	**$2.0 million**
MRI #2 (Hardware in place)	
Depreciation on Hardware	$214,000/yr
Cardiac Software Package	$60,000/yr
Technical Support	(included)
Total	**$500,000**
Positron Emission Tomography	
Camera	$1.9 million
Cyclotron	$1.5 million
System Maintenance	$300,000/yr
Technical Support	(included)
Total	**$4.4 MILLION**
Radionuclides	
Single-Photon Emission Computed	Single Head/Dual Head
Tomography (SPECT) Camera	$200,000/375,000
System Maintenance	$20,000/40,000/yr
Radiation Materials Handling	$4,000
Licensing fees	$1,000/yr
Total	**$450,000–$500,000**

gists. If a research facility is to be started, an additional cost of $1 million for the physical plant and $80,000 for a physicist would also need to be added to the above numbers. Because the new systems use helium at a relatively low rate, cryogen costs could be maintained at about the level of $10,000 per year. A maintenance contract will generally cost 10% of the price of the system or $180,000 per year. One can count on a magnetic resonance scanner lasting for at least 5 years. To make this economically optimal, the cardiovascular specialist would enter into an arrangement with other subspecialists, eg, orthopedists, neurologists, neurosurgeons, etc., or a hospital or health maintenance organization (HMO) to share in the initial equipment and start-up costs.

A more likely scenario would be that there is already an MRI system in place and a cardiovascular specialist wishes to apply MRI to his clinical practice. More often than not, an arrangement can be worked out with the physicians who are already using the magnet, ie, orthopedists, neurologists, etc., for magnet time and to share in the initial hardware costs. An equitable way to this would be to depreciate to zero dollars the initial investment of capital over a 7-year lifespan and divide this by the number of user groups (neurology, cardiology, and orthopedics would constitute three groups). This number would constitute the buy-in. The cardiovascular specialist would then collect the technical and professional fees. If a hospital or HMO owns the magnet, it can be argued that the addition of cardiovascular hardware and software could help fill magnet time and increase the referral base from outside groups. The cardiology addition may also help with cardiovascular surgery satisfaction and quality of care by providing three-dimensional reconstructions in stable thoracic aortic disease before patients go to the operating room. If this were the case, the cardiovascular specialist would get reimbursed solely for the professional fees and the purchasing facility would collect the technical fees to defray the initial investment in the facility. The cardiologist or hospital/HMO can purchase a cardiac software package for the existing magnet for approximately $60,000. Therefore, the initial start-up costs would fall from $2.0 million

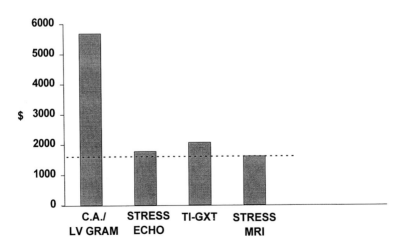

FIGURE 3. Hospital charges. CA indicates angiogram; LV GRAM, left ventriculography; ECHO, echocardiogram; TI/GXT, thallium with graded exercise test.

dollars to about $500,000 (this would include buy-in and technician retraining as well as software), which compares quite favorably to both echo and gamma counter systems. These software packages and their upgrades are important because system gradients cannot progress much further than their present state-of-the-art. They also can improve speed and signal-to-noise ratio on less powerful systems. The turbo BRISK approach developed in our laboratory[45] can be implemented on existing systems to increase acquisition speed without adding hardware.

Hospital charges for MRI and the standard imaging modalities for the assessment of ischemic heart disease are shown by the graph in Figure 3.[46] If the potential for MRI becomes reality, a single MRI session can eliminate multiple cardiac tests and substantially reduce costs.

Conclusions

With the appropriate evolution of magnetic resonance technology, it is clear that virtually all other imaging technologies will be impacted. Its ability to depict ventricular function in three dimensions should eliminate the need for a catheter-performed ventriculogram, a radionuclide cineangiogram, and an echocardiogram and also reduce risk and cost. By using the three-dimensional and high-spatial resolution characteristics of magnetic resonance together with dobutamine infusion, echocardiographic studies to assess viability will be reduced. With the ability to image the coronaries, the diagnostic coronary angiogram could be replaced. Perfusion imaging using paramagnetic contrast agents should ultimately replace radionuclide perfusion imaging methods.

Future developments with improvement in computer technology, the possibility of enhanced and automated analytical approaches to assess ventricular function, stress or dipyridamole, myocardial perfusion imaging, responses of asynergic segments to dobutamine infusion, coronary angiography and spectroscopic methods to assess viability using endogenous substrates and high energy phosphates will obviate the need for multiple tests and offer clinicians a "one-stop shop" for cardiovascular disease assessment. Finally, within the next decade, the possibility of interactive real-time imaging with a state-of-the-art MRI scanner may even allow the performance of optimal diagnostic studies and the ability to perform cardiovascular interventions.

References

1. Goldman MR, Pohost GM, Ingwall JS, et al. Nuclear magnetic resonance imaging: Potential cardiac applications. *Am J Cardiol.* 1980;46:1278–1283.

2. Byrd BF, Schiller NB, Botvinick EH, Higgins CB. Normal cardiac dimensions by magnetic resonance imaging. *Am J Cardiol.* 1985;55:1440–1442.
3. Kaul S, Wismer GL, Brady TJ, et al. Measurement of normal left heart dimensions using optimally oriented MR images. *AR.* 1986;146:75–79.
4. Semelka RC, Tomei E, Wagner S, et al. Normal left ventricular dimensions and function: interstudy reproducibility of measurements with cine MR imaging. *Radiology.* 1990;174:763–768.
5. Semelka RC, Tomei MD, Wagner S, et al. Interstudy reproducibility of dimensional and functional measurements between cine magnetic resonance studies in the morphologically abnormal left ventricle. *Am Heart J.* 1990;119:1367–1373.
6. Ostrega E, Maddahi J, Honma H, et al. Quantification of left ventricular myocardial mass in humans by nuclear magnetic resonance imaging. *Am Heart J.* 1989;117:444–452.
7. Shapiro EP, Rogers WJ, Beyar R, et al. Determination of left ventricular myocardial mass by magnetic resonance imaging in hearts deformed by acute infarction. *Circulation.* 1989;79:706–711.
8. McDonald KM, Parrish T, Wennberg P, et al. Rapid, accurate and simultaneous noninvasive assessment of right and left ventricular mass with nuclear magnetic resonance imaging using the snapshot gradient method. *J Am Coll Cardiol.* 1992;19:1601–1607.
9. Sechtem U, Theissen P, Heindel W, et al. Diagnosis of left ventricular thrombi by magnetic resonance imaging and comparison with angiocardiography, computed tomography and echocardiography. *Am J Cardiol.* 1989; 64:1195–1200.
10. Jungehulsing M, Sechtem U, Theissen P, et al. Left ventricular thrombi: evaluation with spin-echo and gradient-echo MR imaging. *Radiology.* 1992; 182:225–229.
11. Lund JT, Ehman RL, Julsrud PR, et al.: Cardiac masses: assessment by MR imaging. *AJR.* 1989;152:469–473.
12. Blackwell GG. MRI assessment of paracardiac masses. In: Ezekowitz M, ed. *The Heart as a Source of Systemic Embolization.* New York: Marcel-Dekker, 1993.
13. Buckwalter KA, Aisen AM, Dilworth LR, et al.: Gated cardiac MRI: ejection-fraction determination using the right anterior oblique view. *AJR.* 1986; 147:33–37.
14. Lawson MA, Blackwell GG, Davis ND, Roney M, Del'Italia LJ, Pohost GM.: Accuracy of biplane long-axis left ventricular volume determined by cine magnetic resonance imaging in patients with regional and global dysfunction. *Am J Cardiol.* 1996;77:1098–1104.
15. Blackwell G, Cranney G, Lotan C. Ventricular volume, function and mass. In: Blackwell G, Cranney G, Pohost G, eds. *MRI: Cardiovascular System.* New York: Gower Medical Publishing, 1992:5.2–514.
16. Cranney GB, Lotan CS, Dean L, et al. Left ventricular volume measurement using cardiac axis nuclear magnetic resonance imaging: Validation by calibrated ventricular angiography. *Circulation.* 1990;82:154–163.
17. Peschock RM, Rokey R, Malloy CM, et al. Assessment of myocardial systolic wall thickening using nuclear magnetic resonance imaging. *J Am Coll Cardiol.* 1989;14:653–659.
18. Baer FM, Smolarz K, Jungehulsing M, et al. Chronic myocardial infarction: Assessment of morphology, function, and perfusion by gradient echo magnetic resonance imaging and ^{99m}Tc-methoxyisobutyl-isonitrile SPECT. *Am Heart J.* 1992;123:636–645.

19. Baer FM, Voth E, Schneider CA, et al. Comparison of low-dose dobutamine-gradient-echo magnetic resonance imaging and positron emission tomography with [^{18}F]Flourodeoxyglucose in patients with chronic coronary artery disease: A functional and morphological approach to the detection of residual myocardial viability. *Circulation*. 1995;91:1006–1015.

20. Baer FM, Voth E, LaRosée K, et al.: Comparison of dobutamine transesophageal echocardiography and dobutamine magnetic resonance imaging for detection of residual myocardial viability. *Am J Cardiol*. 1996;78:415–419.

21. Zerhouni EA, Parish DM, Rogers WJ, et al. Human heart: tagging with MR imaging—a method for noninvasive assessment of myocardial motion. *Radiology*. 1988;169:59–63.

22. Weiss JL, Shapiro EP, Buchalter MB, Beyar R. Magnetic resonance imaging as a noninvasive standard for quantitative evaluation of left ventricular mass, ischemia, and infarction. *Ann NY Acad Sci*. 1990;601:95–106.

23. Underwood, SR, Klipstein RH, Firmin DN, et al. Magnetic resonance assessment of aortic and mitral regurgitation. *Br Heart J*. 1986;56:455.

24. Walker PG, Cape EG, Pohost GM, et al.: Regurgitant orifice isovelocity contour mapping using NMR velocity encoding (abstract.) *Circulation*. 1990; 82(Suppl. III):44.

25. Higgins CB, Caputo GR. Magnetic resonance imaging of valvular heart disease. In: Pohost, GM, ed. *Cardiovascular Applications of Magnetic Resonance*. Mt. Kisco, NY: Futura Publishing Company: 1993; pp. 91–115.

26. Hundley WG, Li HF, Willard JE, et al. Magnetic resonance imaging assessment of the severity of mitral regurgitation: comparison with invasive techniques. *Circulation*. 1995;92:1151–1158.

27. Adler RS, Chenevert TL, Fowlkes JB, et al.: Calculation of pressure gradients from MR velocity data in laminar flow model. *J Comput Assist Tomogr*. 1991;15:483.

28. Spielman RP, Schneider O, Thiele F, et al. Appearance of poststenotic jets in MRI: Dependence on flow velocity and on imaging parameters. *Magn Reson Med*. 1991;9:67.

29. Kilner PJ, Manzara CC, Mohiadin RH, et al.: Magnetic resonance jet velocity mapping in mitral and aortic valve stenosis. *Circulation*. 1993;87:1239.

30. Pennell DJ, Underwood SR, Ell PJ, et al. Dipyridamole magnetic resonance imaging: a comparison with thallium 201 emission tomography. *Br Heart J*. 1990;64:362–369.

31. Baer FM, Smolarz K, Jungehulsing M, et al. Feasibility of high-dose dipyridamole-magnetic resonance imaging for detection of coronary artery disease and comparison with coronary angiography. *Am J Cardiol*. 1992;69:51–56.

32. Pennell DJ, Underwood SR, Manzara CC, et al. Magnetic resonance imaging during dobutamine stress in coronary artery disease. *Am J Cardiol*. 1992; 70:34–40.

33. Van Rugge FP, Vander Wall EE, De Roos A, Bruschke AG. Dobutamine stress magnetic resonance imaging for detection of coronary artery disease. *J Am Coll Cardiol*. 1993;22:431–439.

34. Fung AY, Gallagher KP, Buda AJ. The physiologic basis of dobutamine as compared with dipyridamole stress interventions in the assessment of critical coronary stenosis. *Circulation*. 1987;76:943–951.

35. Manning WJ, Atkinson DJ, Grossman W, Paulin S, Edelman RR. First-pass nuclear magnetic resonance imaging studies using gadolinium-DTPA in patients with coronary artery disease. *J Am Coll Cardiol*. 1991;18:959–965.

36. Wilke N, Simm C, Zhang J, Ya X, Merkle H, Path G, Ludemann H, Bache

RJ, Ugurbil K. Contrast-enhanced first pass myocardial perfusion imaging: correlation between myocardial blood flow in dogs at rest and during hyperemia. *Magn Res Med.* 1993;29:485–497.

37. Schaefer S, van Tyen R, Saloner D. Evaluation of myocardial perfusion abnormalities with gadolinium-enhanced snapshot MR imaging in humans. *Radiology.* 1992;185:795–801.
38. Dinsmore RE, Liberthson RR, Wismer GL, et al. Magnetic resonance imaging of thoracic aortic aneurysms: comparison with other imaging methods. *AJR.* 1986;146:309–314.
39. Nienaber CA, von Kodolitsch Y, Nicolas V, et al. The diagnosis of thoracic aortic dissection by noninvasive imaging procedures. *N Engl J Med.* 1993; 328:1–9.
40. Aurigemma GP, Reichek N, Axel L, et al. Noninvasive determination of coronary artery bypass graft patency by cine magnetic resonance imaging. *Circulation.* 1989;80:1595–1602.
41. Galjee MA, van Rossum AC, Doesburg T, et al. Value of magnetic resonance imaging in assessing patency and function of coronary artery bypass grafts, an angiographically controlled study. *Circulation.* 1996;93:660–666.
42. Manning WJ, Li W, Boyle NG, Edelman RR. Fat-suppressed breath-hold magnetic resonance coronary angiography. *Circulation.* 1993;87:94–104.
43. Manning WJ, Li W, Edelman RR. A preliminary report comparing magnetic resonance coronary angiography with conventional angiography. *N Engl J Med.* 1993;328:823–832.
44. Pennell DJ, Bogren HG, Keegan J, et al. Assessment of coronary artery stenosis by magnetic resonance imaging. *Heart.* 1996:75:127–133.
45. Doyle M, Walsh EG, Foster RE, Pohost GM. Rapid cardiac imaging with turbo BRISK. *Magn Reson Med.* 1997:410–417.
46. University of Alabama at Birmingham. *Guide to Hospital Changes,* 1996.

Part 3

Magnetic Resonance Techniques

Chapter 11

Identification of Regional Myocardial Ischemia Using Function and Perfusion Assessment by Magnetic Resonance Imaging Techniques

Peter T. Buser, MD, Jens Bremerich, MD,
Christoph Grädel, MD, Risto Miettunen, MD,
Georg Bongartz, MD

Introduction

Ischemic heart disease remains the leading cause of death in highly developed countries. During the last few years, short-term mortality after acute myocardial infarction has decreased substantially due to the widespread use of thrombolytic therapy, antithrombotic regimens, early detection, and treatment of life-threatening arrhythmias and early revascularization procedures. Nevertheless, mortality and recurrent ischemic events during the first year after acute myocardial infarction remain a relevant problem in acute infarct survivors.[1,2] There is general agreement based on clinical evidence that myocardial infarction patients who are at high risk for death or nonfatal ischemic events should undergo early cardiac catheterization and, if feasible, revascularization. However, as many as 60% of patients considered clinically to be at low risk after myocardial infarction will suffer from complications during the first year.[3] In order to identify patients at increased risk in this

From: Higgins CB, Ingwall JS, Pohost GM, (eds). *Current and Future Applications of Magnetic Resonance in Cardiovascular Disease.* Armonk, NY: Futura Publishing Company, Inc.; © 1998.

clinically low-risk group and to avoid unnecessary invasive procedures in patients at very low risk for fatal and/or nonfatal events during the first year after myocardial infarction, noninvasive testing is mandatory in this group. It has been recommended that patients with extensive myocardial perfusion defects during thallium-201 scintigraphy or left ventricular wall motion abnormalities on stress echocardiography should undergo further evaluation with coronary angiography for possible percutaneous transluminal coronary angioplasty (PTCA) or coronary artery bypass grafting (CABG).[4] It has recently been shown that radionuclide angiocardiography at rest and during exercise could provide the most accurate risk prediction[5] because it allows the assessment of ischemia based on clinical observation of the patient and alterations of global and regional function of the left ventricle.

Thus, in order to stratify patients after acute myocardial infarction who are clinically judged to be at low risk for fatal and nonfatal ischemic events for the following year, a stress test with simultaneous assessment of left ventricular wall motion abnormalities and myocardial perfusion would be desirable. Magnetic resonance imaging (MRI) with its excellent temporal and spatial resolution is ideally suited for evaluation of the cardiovascular system. It has evolved as a very accurate method for the assessment of global and regional ventricular function, myocardial mass, ventricular volumes, and site and extension of jeopardized myocardial area after ischemic events.[6] MRI is considered a new gold standard for the assessment of these parameters in patients with ischemic heart disease.[7–10] Pharmacological stress testing can be applied as with other imaging methods. Alterations of regional wall motion and global ventricular function allow for the identification of normal, ischemic, or scarred myocardium in response to the stress test. In addition, it has been shown in clinical studies, that MRI is an accurate method for the assessment of myocardial perfusion in patients with ischemic heart disease.

Assessment of Global and Regional Left Ventricular Function During Rest and Pharmacological Stress Testing

During the last decade, cine gradient-echo MRI (cGRE MRI) has been used to assess volumes,[11,12] myocardial mass,[13] global,[14,15] and regional function and wall motion[16–20] of both the right and left ventricle. Functional parameters such as ventricular stroke volumes[21] or ejection fraction[22] can be derived easily. Intra- and interobserver as well as interstudy reproducibility of measurements of left ventricular function have been shown to be excellent with a percent variability for volume measurements of usually less than 6%.[23,24] Thus, a reasonable argument can be made that MRI now represents a new gold standard for the determination of ventricular mass, volumes, and global and regional function. However, whereas descriptors of global ventricular function have great importance as prognostic parameters in patients with heart disease, they may be insufficient to evaluate the consequences of significant coronary artery disease. Especially in patients after acute myocardial infarction, the assessment of diastolic segmental wall thickness and the extent of segmental systolic wall thickening during pharmacological stress testing may be of outmost importance for the differentiation of normal, ischemic, stunned or necrotic myocardium. In contrast to endocardial excursion analysis, wall thickening is directly related to myocyte shortening. The distinction between stunned but still viable myocardium from a myocardial scar may help to stratify patients after myocardial infarction in high- or low-risk groups for death and/or non-fatal ischemic events during the following year. This again will influence the decision process as to whether a specific patient should undergo coronary angiography and subsequently revascularization.

cGRE MRI is the only, widely available method for the assessment of segmental function and systolic wall thickening throughout the entire left ventricular myocardium. If segmental wall motion changes are analyzed during pharmacological stress testing either with dipyridamole or dobutamine, ischemic myocardial dysfunction can be detected. Using intravenous dobutamine infusion with increasing doses up to 20 μg/kg/min, 20 of 22 patients with significant coronary artery disease had reversible wall motion abnormalities. Comparison of abnormal segments of perfusion by dobutamine thallium tomography and wall motion by dobutamine MRI showed 96% agreement at rest, 90% agreement during stress, and 91% agreement for the assessment of functional reversibility.[25] In this study, sensitivity of MRI for the detection of individual coronary arterial stenosis was 80% for left anterior descending (LAD), 94% for left circumflex artery (LCA), and 92% for right coronary artery (RCA).

In a recently published study, sensitivity for the detection of coronary artery disease using dobutamine cGRE MRI in 35 patients with angiographically documented coronary arterial disease was 84% overall, 77% in single-vessel disease, and 89% in multivessel disease. This compared well with the sensitivity using dobutamine-MIBI-SPECT (87%, 77%, 95% respectively).[26]

In 39 consecutive patients with clinically suspected coronary artery disease referred for coronary angiography and 10 normal volunteers who underwent cGRE MRI at rest and during peak dobutamine stress, percent regional wall thickening was measured in the basal state and during dobutamine stress. The overall sensitivity of dobutamine MRI for the detection of significant coronary artery disease was 91%, specificity was 80%, and accuracy 90%. Sensitivity for identification of single-vessel disease was 88%, two-vessel disease 91%, and three-vessel disease 100%.[27] However, in 1 of 6 patients without significant coronary artery disease, abnormal stress induced wall thickening was observed, resulting in a 80% specificity. This false-positive study was found in a patient with left ventricular hypertrophy.[27]

In 35 patients with chronic myocardial infarction, viability was investigated by low-dose (10 μg/kg/min) dobutamine-cGRE MRI. Definition of viability was preserved end-diastolic wall thickness ($\geq$5.5 min) and/or systolic wall thickening $\geq$1 mm during stress test. Findings were compared with corresponding [^{18}F]fluorodeoxyglucose uptake as assessed by positron emission tomography (PET). Preserved end-diastolic wall thickness in the infarct zone was found in 48% and functional recovery during stress testing in 54%. Viability was indicated by PET in 66% yielding a diagnostic agreement between PET and myocardial morphology in 83% and between PET and functional recovery in 89%. Dobutamine-induced wall thickening was a better predictor of viability (sensitivity = 81%, specificity = 95%, positive predictive accuracy = 96%) than end-diastolic wall thickness (72%, 89%, 91% respectively).[28]

In the presence of significant coronary artery disease, dipyridamole can induce myocardial ischemia. This pharmacological stress test is used routinely as a substitute for exercise stress testing in scintigraphic myocardial perfusion imaging[29] and echocardiography.[30] Pennel et al[31,32] first reported dipyridamole-induced wall motion abnormalities and impaired systolic wall thickening using MRI in patients with coronary artery disease. Sensitivity for the detection of coronary artery disease was comparable with planar thallium-201 scintigraphy.[32] Feasibility, safety, and diagnostic accuracy of cGRE MRI with high-dose dipyridamole stress testing was assessed in 23 patients without significant wall motion abnormalities at rest but with severe angiographically documented coronary artery stenosis. Short-axis MRI images were evaluated by grading standardized segments as normal, hypokinetic, akinetic, or dyskinetic. Dipyridamole MRI was considered abnormal if segmental wall motion deteriorated by $\geq$1 grade after administration of dipyridamole. Abnormal studies during dipyridamole stress were observed in 18 of 23 (78%) patients. Sensitivity was 89% for single-vessel disease and 90% for two-vessel disease.[33]

Thus, the analysis of regional wall motion using cGRE MRI during rest and pharmacological stress testing allows for accurate detection of significant coronary artery disease and the differentiation of viable from necrotic myocardium in patients with chronic myocardial infarction. Side effects of dobutamine stress testing included angina pectoris, an increasing number of ventricular premature beats, palpitations, tingling or flushing sensations during dobutamine infusion and chest pain, headache, nausea or flushing after dipyridamole injection. However, all these side effects disappeared when dobutamine infusion was stopped or nitroglycerine was given, or in the case of dipyridamole when theophyline, a dipyridamole antagonist, was given. In all studies, side effects were not considered as an indication for premature interruption of the stress test.

Assessment of Myocardial Perfusion During Dipyridamole Stress Testing

The magnetic resonance first-pass technique in concert with the extracellular magnetic resonance contrast agent gadolinium-diethylenetriamine pentaacetic acid (Gd-DTPA) has been used to assess myocardial perfusion in patients with ischemic heart disease at rest[34,35] and during pharmacological stress.[36-39] Qualitative measurements of the myocardial Gd-DTPA inflow by ultrafast MRI have been made and the results seem promising although the experience is limited to small patient groups.

Manning et al[35] were able to demonstrate in their study of 17 patients with suspected coronary artery disease undergoing cardiac catheterization that myocardial perfusion imaging using ultrafast gradient-refocused MRI and rapid intravenous bolus injection of Gd-DTPA is clinically feasible. In a study including four healthy subjects and six patients with angiographically documented coronary artery disease a good correlation between hypoperfused myocardial segments during dipyridamole stress assessed by thallium-201 scintigraphy and Gd-MRI was found. In one patient hypoperfusion of an inferior segment was observed by both thallium-201 scintigraphy and Gd-enhanced MRI, but the corresponding coronary angiography did not show significant stenosis of the perfusion related right coronary artery.[36]

In a study of five patients with angiographically documented coronary artery disease, perfusion defects detected by Gd-enhanced MRI during dipyridamole stress testing were compared with [99m]TC-sestamibi single-photon emission computed tomography (SPECT). With SPECT as the gold standard, prospective MRI had a sensitivity of 77% and a specificity of 75%. With recent coronary angiography as the gold standard, however, MRI had a sensitivity of 81% and a specificity of 100%.[38]

In 10 patients with documented coronary artery disease a feasibility study was conducted using MRI and dynamic first-pass bolus tracking after injection of Gd-DTPA during dipyridamole stress in order to detect myocardial ischemia. Observations in three MRI planes were compared with exercise thallium scintigraphy. Detection of ischemic regions showed a sensitivity of 65%, a specificity of 76% and a diagnostic accuracy of 74%.[37] However, in this study infusion of 0.56 mg/kg/min dipyridamole for 4 minutes did not cause any change in blood pressure or heart rate. Electrocardiogram (ECG) abnormalities were detected in only 2 of 10 and 1 of 10 patients who experienced angina requiring theophyline injection. Thus, the severity of ischemia induced by dipyridamole may not have been comparable to exercise stress testing, which may explain some of the discrepancies found between MRI and thallium scintigraphy in this study.

It is therefore possible to identify hypoperfused myocardial regions using Gd first-pass MRI during dipyridamole stress testing[41] and the MRI first-pass data are in general agreement with the results of radionuclide and angiographic studies.[42]

Simultaneous Assessment of Myocardial Function and Perfusion

Diagnostic accuracy for the detection of regional ischemia by the assessment of regional myocardial function alone or perfusion alone may be limited. For example, in hypertensive patients with left ventricular hypertrophy, regional ventricular function may decrease during stress testing in the absence of coronary artery disease. Myocardial perfusion, however, may be normal in a region of a previous myocardial infarction when the infarct related vessel is patent—either due to pharmacological or spontaneous thrombolysis—and the remaining culprit lesion causes a stenosis of <75%. MRI is the only available noninvasive imaging method that has been shown to possess the potential for the assessment of both regional systolic wall thickening and perfusion of the myocardium.

A preliminary study was performed applying the simultaneous assessment of regional myocardial function and perfusion during dipyridamole stress testing using cGRE MRI and Gd-enhanced turbo FLASH MRI. Twelve male patients (age range 49–61 years) with clinically suspected coronary artery disease were included in this study. Criteria for inclusion were ability to perform stress testing, no contraindications for MRI, and the performance of myocardial perfusion scintigraphy and coronary angiography. All studies including coronary angiography were performed within 36 hours without intervening ischemic event.

For pharmacological stress testing, intravenous infusion of dipyridamole (0.56 mg/kg) was used. Patients abstained from substances containing xanthenes for 48 hours prior to the stress test. Dipyridamole was administered as a short intravenous (IV) infusion over 4 minutes; ECG was continuously monitored during pharmacological stress. The dipyridamole antidote aminophilline was available (240 mg IV in 5 minutes) but not needed, because only two patients reported mild chest discomfort.

Rest and stress dipyridamole MIBI-SPECT was performed with a standardized protocol. After fasting, stress test with dipyridamole was performed as described above and patients received 7 mCi (260 MBq)[99m]Tc-MIBI (Cardiolite, DuPont Radiopharmaceuticals) and 2 hours later 20 mCi (740 MBq) of ^{99m}Tc-MIBI was injected at rest. SPECT was performed 90 minutes after dipyridamole-stress and at-rest injection of ^{99m}Tc-MIBI. Coronary arteriography was performed in the standard manner.

For MRI, patients were placed in supine position in a 1.5 T scanner (Siemens Magnetom SP, body coil) with ECG electrodes on back or chest for prospective triggering in order to obtain optimal R-wave in the ECG. Multisection sagittal, coronal, and transverse ECG gated spin-echo images were acquired to define the cardiac axes. Midventricular short-axis planes were chosen for perfusion imaging. A turbo FLASH sequence (TR, 6.2 ms; TE, 3 ms; FA, 10^2; matrix 80 × 128; FOV 350 mm; slice thickness 10 mm) was used. Test measurements were performed with different post inversion-pulse delay times (T1). T1 with signal nulling of myocardium and intraventricular blood (= 100 ms) was chosen to provide maximal sensitivity to the Gd-DTPA induced T1-reduction. End-diastolic images were acquired with every heartbeat. Imaging was started with the bolus-injection of Gd-DTPA (0.02 mmol/kg) and repeated for 60 heartbeats. Subsequently, cGRE MRI for wall motion analysis was obtained in the same image plane (turbo FLASH with segmented k-space; TR, 660 ms; TE, 6 ms; FA, 30°, matrix 130 × 256; FOV 350 mm; slice thickness 8 mm). Dipyridamole for stress testing was applied as described above and the imaging procedure was repeated. An interval of 20 minutes was allowed between consecutive injections of Gd-DTPA to maximize washout of the contrast medium from the myocardium. Shortening of the RR interval during stress testing made it necessary to readjust T1 to minimize signal from the myocardium and blood. Total MRI time ranged from 20–30 minutes according to patients' heart rate.

The midventricular short-axis MRI and radionuclide scans were subdivided into eight corresponding sectors of 45° each. Sectors 6–8 and 1 were related to the LAD, sectors 2–5 to the left circumflex (LCA) and right coronary artery (RCA). For perfusion analysis, signal intensity was measured in every sector via operator adjustable regions of interest in pre- and postcontrast images, both at rest and under stress. Care was taken to avoid pixels in the subendocardial and subepicardial regions that might have been altered by chamber blood or epicardial fat. Signal intensity measurements were obtained of the interventricular

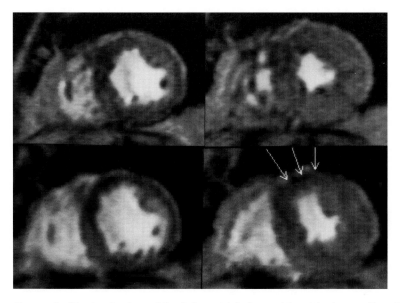

Figure 1. Short-axis view of the left ventricle in a midventricular position. Top row shows end-diastolic (left) and end-systolic (right) frames at rest. Bottom row shows end-diastolic (left) and end-systolic (right) frames during dipyridamole stress testing. During stress testing, the end-diastolic volume is increased (left bottom vs. left top) and distinct wall motion abnormality with hypo- and akinesia (arrows, right bottom vs. right top) can be detected at end systole.

wall, anterior wall, anterolateral wall, and inferior wall. The segment with highest signal enhancement was defined as normal. Relative signal intensities were calculated by dividing measured signal intensities by the intensity of the segment defined as normal. MRI data were analyzed by one cardiologist and one radiologist, both experienced in reading cardiac MRI.

Wall motion was analyzed on cGRE MRI (Figure 1) by one radiologist and one cardiologist. A segment was graded hypokinetic if systolic wall thickening was reduced but not absent, akinetic if systolic wall thickening was absent or severely reduced, or dyskinetic if systolic outward movement of the myocardial wall occurred. Normal wall motion at rest and normal/hyperkinetic wall motion pattern during dipyridamole stress was defined as normal. Segments with a wall motion pattern that was normal at rest and pathological during stress were defined as ischemic, and segments with pathological wall motion pattern at rest and during stress as scar.

Radionuclide scans were evaluated by two cardiologists and two radiologists, blinded to MRI and coronary angiography. Myocardial segments were assigned in a way corresponding to the MR studies. Segments with reversible defects in tracer uptake were defined as ischemic and those with irreversible defects were defined as scar. Segments with both components (scar with border zone ischemia) were graded as ischemia as well.

In 10 patients, 23 stenotic lesions (5 with 50% to 75%, 18 with >75% stenosis) were angiographically identified. Eight were located in the RCA, 8 in the LAD, and 7 in the LCA. Of the patients, 1 had single-vessel disease, 7 had two-vessel, and 2, three-vessel disease. A total of 80 segments were analyzed by ^{99m}Tc-MIBI-SPECT. In 15 of 80 segments, reversible hypoperfusion was observed and these segments were therefore considered ischemic during stress testing. Of 80 segments, 12 had fixed defects during stress and rest and were therefore considered as scar. Thus, in 27 of 80 (34%) segments abnormal perfusion was detected by ^{99m}Tc-MIBI-SPECT.

During dipyridamole Gd-MRI perfusion defects could be detected in 21 of 80 segments (26%). In 10 segments, reversible defects during stress testing were observed and 11 had fixed defects during stress testing and rest.

On cGRE-MRI 23 of 80 (29%) segments with abnormal wall motion were detected. Twelve had reversible abnormalities of wall motion only during stress testing and 11 showed wall motion abnormalities already at rest that did not worsen during stress testing.

When dipyridamole Gd-MRI and cGRE MRI were combined, 24 of 80 (30%) segments were found to have either perfusion defects and/or wall motion abnormalities. All 11 segments that were considered as scar were identically identified by dipyridamole Gd-MRI and cGRE MRI. However, with cGRE MRI, 3 segments were judged to be ischemic during stress testing that were not detected by dipyridamole Gd-MRI. Conversely, 1 segment with a perfusion defect was only detected by dipyridamole Gd-MRI.

Thus, using ^{99m}Tc-MIBI-SPECT as gold standard overall sensitivity to detect ischemic or necrotic segments was 78% for dipyridamole Gd-MRI, 85% for cGRE MRI, and 89% for the combined analysis of both MRI techniques. Sensitivity to detect ischemic segments was 67% with dipyridamole Gd-MRI, 80% with cGRE MRI, and 87% with the combination of both. Scar was equally detected with a sensitivity of 92% with either MRI technique. The two ischemic segments that were not detected by MRI were observed in one patient and were located posterior (segments 2 and 3). The only segment that was considered as scar and was not detected by MRI was located in segment 3 and included the border zone of a larger scar located in segment 4 and 5 (interior).

Correlation of abnormal segments during dipyridamole Gd-MRI and cGRE MRI with the anatomic location of coronary artery stenoses was good. In one vessel (LAD) with a 75% stenosis, ^{99m}Tc-MIBI-SPECT, MRI perfusion and wall motion were normal. Thus, this specific LAD lesion was considered to be hemodynamically not significant.

These preliminary data show that the combined assessment of myocardial perfusion and regional wall motion during dipyridamole stress testing using MRI is feasible and safe. With ^{99m}Tc-MIBI-SPECT as gold standard sensitivity to detect ischemia and scar is high. However, missed defects by MRI were all located posterior. In this region, false-positive test results can be observed by scintigraphic techniques due to attenuation from the diaphragm.

Conclusion

cGRE MRI with pharmacological stress testing has been shown to be an excellent tool for the analysis of regional wall motion abnormalities and the identification of ischemic and viable myocardium and scars. Using dipyridamole, Gd-MRI segmental myocardial perfusion can be assessed at rest and during stress testing with high diagnostic accuracy. MRI is an unique technique that allows simultaneous assessment of regional wall motion and perfusion of the myocardium at rest and during pharmacological stress testing. The combined analysis may further improve the diagnostic accuracy. It is therefore an ideal tool for stratification of patients after myocardial infarction to detect residual ischemia, stunned but viable myocardium or to define the extension of a scar and the impairment of global left ventricular function.

References

1. Simoons ML, Serruys PW, van den Brand M, et al. Improved survival after early thrombolysis in acute myocardial infarction: A randomized trial by the Interuniversity Cardiology Institute in the Netherlands. *Lancet.* 1985;2: 578–582.
2. Gruppo Italiano per lo Studio della Streptochinasi nell'Infarto miocardico (GISSI). Long-term effects of intravenous thrombolysis in acute myocardial infarction: final report of the GISSI study. *Lancet.* 1987;1:871–874.
3. Candell-Riera J, Permanyer-Miralda G, Castell J, et al. Uncomplicated first myocardial infarction: Strategy for comprehensive prognostic studies. *J Am Coll Cardiol.* 1991;18:1207–1219.
4. Pitt B. Evaluation of the postinfarct patient. *Circulation.* 1995;91:1855–1860.
5. Pfisterer M, Salamin PA, Schwendener R, Burkart F. Clinical risk assessment after first myocardial infarction—Is additional noninvasive testing necessary? *Chest.* 1992;102:1499–1506.
6. Reichek N. Magnetic resonance imaging for assessment of myocardial function. *Magn Reson O.* 1991;4:255–74.

7. Blackwell GG, Pohost GM. The eveolving role of MRI in the assessment of coronary artery disease. *Am J Cardiol*. 1995;75(suppl D):74D–78D.

8. Weiss JL, Shapiro EP, Buchalter MB, Beyar R. Magnetic resonance imaging as a noninvasive standard for quantitative evaluation of the left ventricular mass, ischemia and infarction. *Ann NY Acad Sci*. 1990;601:95–106.

9. Higgins CB. Which standard has the gold? *J Am Coll Cardiol*. 1992;19: 1608–1609.

10. Sayad DE, Clarke GD, Peshock RM. Magnetic resonance imaging of the heart and its role in current cardiology. *Curr Opin Cardiol*. 1995;10:640–649.

11. Cranney GB, Lotan CS, Dean L, et al. Left ventricular volume measurement using cardiac axis nuclear magnetic resonance imaging. *Circulation*. 1990; 82:154–163.

12. Sechtem U, Pflugfelder PW, Gould RG, et al. Measurement of right and left ventricular volumes in healthy individuals with cine MR imaging. *Radiology*. 1987;163:697–702.

13. Shapiro EP, Rogers WJ, Beyar R, et al. Determination of left ventricular mass by magnetic resonance imaging in hearts deformed by acute infarction. *Circulation*. 1989;79:706–711.

14. Buser PT, Auffermann W, Holt WW, et al. Noninvasive evaluation of global left ventricular function with use of cine nuclear magnetic resonance. *J Am Coll Cardiol*. 1989;13:1294–1300.

15. Wagner S, Buser P, Auffermann W, et al. Cine magnetic resonance imaging: Tomographic analysis of left ventricular function. *Cardiol Clin*. 1989;7: 651–659.

16. Buser PT, Wu S, Auffermann W, et al. Three-dimensional analysis of regional contractile performance of the normal and cardiomyopathic left ventricle using cine magnetic resonance imaging. *Z Kardiol*. 1990;79:573–579.

17. Lotan CS, Cranney GB, Bouchard A, et al. The value of cine nuclear magnetic resonance imaging for assessing regional ventricular function. *J Am Coll Cardiol*. 1989;14:1721–1729.

18. Pflugfelder PW, Sechtem UP, White RD, Higgins CB. Quantification of regional myocardial function by rapid cine MR imaging. *AJR*. 1988;150: 523–529.

19. Sechtem U, Sommerhoff BA, Markiewicz W, et al. Regional left ventricular wall thickening by magnetic resonance imaging: Evaluation in normal persons and patients with global and regional dysfunction. *Am J Cardiol*. 1987; 59:145–151.

20. Peshock RM, Rokey R, Malloy CM, et al. Assessment of myocardial systolic wall thickening using nuclear magnetic resonance imaging. *J Am Coll Cardiol*. 1989;14:653–659.

21. Kondo C, Caputo GR, Semelka R, et al. Right and left ventricular stroke volume measurement with velocity encoded cine MR imaging: In vitro and In vivo validation. *AJR*. 1991;157:9–16.

22. Stratemeier EJ, Thompson R, Brady TJ, et al. Ejection fraction determination by MR imaging: Comparison with left ventricular angiography. *Radiology*. 1986;158:775–777.

23. Semelka RC, Tomel E, Wagner S, et al. Interstudy reproducibility of dimensional and functional measurement between cine magnetic resonance studies in the morphologically abnormal left ventricle. *Am Heart J*. 1990;119: 1367–1673.

24. Benjelloun H, Cranney GB, Kirk KA, et al. Interstudy reproducibility of biplane cine nuclear magnetic resonance measurements of left ventricular function. *Am J Cardiol*. 1991;67:1413–20.

25. Penell DJ, Underwood SR, Manzara CC, et al. Magnetic resonance imaging during dobutamine stress in coronary artery disease. *Am J Cardiol.* 1992; 70:34–40.
26. Baer FM, Voth E, Theissen P, et al. Coronary artery disease: Findings with GRE MR imaging and Tc-99m-Methoxyisobutyl-Isonitrile SPECT during simultaneous dobutamine stress. Radiology 1994;193:203–9.
27. Van Rugge FP, van der Wall EE, Spanjersberg SJ, et al. Magnetic resonance imaging during dobutamine stress for detection and localization of coronary artery disease. Quantitative wall motion analysis using a modification of the centerline method. *Circulation.* 1994;90:127–138.
28. Baer FM, Voth E, Schneider CA, et al. Comparison of low-dose dobutamine gradient echo magnetic resonance imaging and positron emission tomography with [^{18}F]fluorodeoxyglucose in patients with chronic coronary artery disease. A functional and morphological approach to the detection of residual myocardial viability. *Circulation.* 1995;91:1006–1015.
29. Leppo J, Boucher CA, Okada RD, et al. Serial thallium-201 myocardial imaging after dipyridamole infusion: Diagnostic utility in detecting coronary stenosis and relationship to regional wall motion. *Circulation.* 1982; 66:649–657.
30. Picano E, Morales MA, Distante A, et al. Dipyridamole-echocardiography test in angina at rest: noninvasive assessment of coronary stenosis undelying spasm. *Am Heart J.* 1986;111:688–691.
31. Pennell DJ, Underwood SR, Longmore DB. Detection of coronary artery disease using MR imaging with dipyridamole infusion. *J Comput Assist Tomogr.* 1990;14:167–170.
32. Pennell DJ, Underwood SR, Ell PJ, et al. Dipyridamole magnetic resonance imaging: a comparison with thallium-201 emission tomography. *Br Heart J.* 1990;64:362–369.
33. Baer FM, Smolarz K, Jungehülsing M, et al. Feasibility of high-dose dipyridamole-magnetic resonance imaging for detection of coronary artery disease and comparison with coronary angiography. *Am J Cardiol.* 1992;69:51–56.
34. Wilke N, Engels A, Weiki A, et al. Dynamic perfusion studies by ultrafast MR imaging: initial clinical results from cardiology. *Electromedica* 1990;58: 102–108.
35. Manning WJ, Atkinson DJ, Grassman W, et al. First pass MR imaging studies using gadolinium DTPA in patients with coronary artery disease. *J Am Coll Cardiol.* 1991;18:959–965.
36. Schaefer S, van Tyen R, Saloner O. Evaluation of myocardial perfusion abnormalities with gadolinium-enhanced snapshot MR imaging in humans. *Radiology.* 1992;185:795–801.
37. Eichenberger AC, Schuiki E, Kochil VD, et al. Ischemic heart disease: Assessment with gadolinium-enhanced ultrafast MR imaging and dipyridamole-stress. *J Magn Reson Imaging.* 1994;4:425–431.
38. Klein MA, Collier BD, Hellman RS, Barnrah VS. Detection of chronic coronary artery disease: Value of pharmacologically stressed, dynamically enhanced turbo-fast low-angle shot MR images. *AJR.* 1993;161:257–263.
39. Walsh EG, Doyle M, Lawson MA, et al. Multisilce first-pass myocardial perfusion imaging on a conventional clinical scanner. *Magn Reson Med.* 1995;34:39–47.
40. Wilke N, Jerosch-Herold M, Stillman AE, et al. Concepts of myocardial perfusion imaging in magnetic resonance imaging. *Magn Reson O.* 1994;10: 249–286.

41. Lombardi M, Kvaemess J, Soma J, et al. Ultrafast MRI at 0.5 T to study perfusion deficits in subacute myocardial infarction in man. *Presented at 11th Scientific Meeting of the European Society for Magnetic Resonance in Medicine and Biology.* Vienna: ESMRMB, 1994:242.
42. Matheijssen NAA, van Rugge FP, Louwerenburg HW, et al. Comparison of dipyridamole magnetic resonance imaging with dipyridamole sesta MIBI SPECT for detection of perfusion abnormalities in patients with one-vessel coronary artery disease. *Presented at 11th Scientific Meeting of the European Society for Magnetic Resonance in Medicine and Biology.* Vienna: ESMRMB, 1994:244.

## Chapter 12

Quantification of Myocardial Perfusion with Magnetic Resonance: Clinical Implications and Potential

Norbert Wilke, MD and Michael Jerosch Herold, PhD

Introduction

Over the last several years magnetic resonance imaging (MRI) has been applied for the morphological, functional, and metabolic characterization of the heart. It has been recognized that MRI may be useful in assessing patients with coronary artery disease by detecting either abnormalities of left ventricular wall motion[1,2] and/or abnormalities of regional myocardial perfusion.[3–5] MR myocardial tissue tagging techniques[6,7] were developed to quantify both myocardial translation and transmural differences in wall motion in an observer-independent fashion. An at least equally compelling case can be made for the quantification of myocardial blood flow for an unbiased, observer-independent assessment of myocardial ischemia.

It was hypothesized early on that magnetic resonance (MR) contrast media could play an important role for the assessment of perfusion and for differentiating between ischemic and infarcted myocardium. This can be done by monitoring the wash-in of contrast agent (CA) with rapid MRI during the first pass of the contrast agent,[3,4,8–11], or by evaluating

Supported by NIH grant RO1HL58876-01. MJ-H gratefully acknowledges funding support through a seed grant from the RSNA Research and Education Fund. NW gratefully acknowledges support through an AHA grant-in-aid.

From: Higgins CB, Ingwall JS, Pohost GM, (eds). *Current and Future Applications of Magnetic Resonance in Cardiovascular Disease*. Armonk, NY: Futura Publishing Company, Inc.; © 1998.

the signal intensity patterns after the contrast agent has reached an equilibrium state.[12,13] The signal time course in a myocardial region observed with the first-pass technique relates primarily to blood flow and blood volume,[14] whereas investigations of late signal enhancement patterns reveal changes in compartmentalization and cell membrane integrity.[15] MR contrast agents are excluded from the intracellular fluid in normal and ischemic noninfarcted myocardium, but this is not the case in an infarct zone where cell membrane integrity has been compromised.[15,16]

The focus of this chapter is on the assessment of myocardial perfusion with first-pass imaging. Initial reports dating back to the period between 1990 and 1991[3-5] about rapid imaging during wash-in of the contrast agent gadolinium-diethylene-triamine pentaacetic acid (Gd-DTPA) demonstrated that regional myocardial perfusion in the territory of a diseased vessel coincided with a lower peak signal intensity and a lower rate of signal increase than observed in normal perfused myocardial regions. The peak signal enhancement, and the change in the rate of signal enhancement in the myocardium have been compared in patients with the results obtained with established methods, such as coronary angiography,[4,11] [201]Thallium-SPECT,[17,18] and ^{99m}Tc-MIBI.[19] More recently it was demonstrated that MR first-pass imaging with an exogenous contrast agent allows perfusion assessment with sufficient spatial and temporal resolution for the differentiation of epicardial and endocardial perfusion changes.[20] Quantitative measures of blood flow obtained from MR first-pass images have been validated in animal models with radioisotope labeled microspheres.[8,14] The focus of first-pass imaging studies of the heart has shifted since its original inception from a qualitative to a more quantitative assessment of myocardial blood flow. This chapter consequently emphasizes the quantitative assessment of myocardial perfusion as a clinical tool for treatment prognosis and treatment monitoring. The examples shown provide an overview of recent experiences with first-pass imaging in patients and animal models.

Over the years positron emission tomography (PET) has been established as the gold standard for the noninvasive quantification of myocardial blood flow.[21,22] Significant advantages of nuclear imaging techniques such as PET and single-photon emission computed tomography (SPECT) are, that they are inherently three-dimensional imaging modalities, and that they allow full coverage of the heart to determine the extent and size of ischemic lesions. Disadvantages are exposure of the patient to radiation, the borderline spatial resolution for analysis of the transmural distribution of blood flow, and a far less than single heartbeat temporal resolution. It is in this context that MRI has unique advantages for the noninvasive, patient-friendly assessment of myocardial perfusion with the first-pass technique. They are: superior temporal and spatial resolution, which can be combined with multislice coverage of the heart; absence of any radiation hazards; and the availability of highly stable and inert MR contrast agents of low toxicity. The spatial resolution is sufficient to analyze the transmural distribution of blood flow.

The Role of Magnetic Resonance Perfusion Imaging

For coronary lesions causing less than 40% to 50% narrowing, the vessel response to increased blood flow demand is not significantly impaired.[23] The resistance of a stenotic lesion can increase dramatically once the luminal diameter has been reduced by more than ~ 70%. It has been recognized that the coronary flow reserve is a better indicator than the luminal diameter, or area measurements of the functional significance of a stenotic lesion.[24,25] While the measurement of the coronary flow reserve with an intracoronary Doppler guidewire is characterized by excellent reproducibility, it is nevertheless an invasive method. Recently cine phase-phase contrast MRI has been applied in an closed-chest canine model[26] and normal volunteers[27] to determine the coronary flow reserve.

Despite the considerable attractiveness of the noninvasive MR methods for measuring the coronary flow reserve, one should bear in mind that they do not establish the degree of regional myocardial hypoperfusion, in particular in the subendocardial layer. By virtue of the tight coupling between blood flow and oxygen demand, any method that quantifies myocardial blood flow, including microvascular flow, is suitable for the assessment of myocardial ischemia. The need to assess regional myocardial blood flow is further borne out by the role collateral blood flow plays in the protection against ischemia. Thus, an indispensable component of a comprehensive study of coronary artery stenosis, both in experimental animal models and patients, is the determination of regional myocardial perfusion, possibly in an absolute sense (eg, in units of $mL \cdot min^{-1}$ per g of tissue). New treatment regimes, such as the stimulation of collateral vessel development in the ischemic myocardium with vascular endothelial growth factor,[28] or revascularization of the myocardium with laser channels,[29] call for development of such diagnostic tools to quantify perfusion changes, and assess collateral blood supply.

Requirements for Magnetic Resonance Perfusion Studies

There is a wide array of rapid MRI techniques, ranging from inversion recovery prepared FLASH to echoplanar imaging (EPI). The premise of MR first-pass studies should be the quantification of myocardial blood flow, and to a lesser degree, blood volume (changes). Therefore, some important criteria need to be met in the selection of the MRI technique. It has been shown that the ability to obtain a blood pool input function is an important requirement for modeling and quantification of myocardial blood flow.[30] Quantification of contrast agent concentration is most straightforward if based on T_1-changes, which are short-range, versus T_2^* changes produced by the magnetic susceptibility effects of the contrast agent, and that extend beyond the immediate vicinity of the spaces permeated by the contrast agent. The observed signal enhancement in the myocardium should ideally vary linearly with contrast agent concentration. This is in particular the case for an extracellular agent where the signal enhancement is a sum of the contributions from the vascular and interstitial compartments and where the respective volume fractions are *a priori* unknown. The signal in the left ventricular blood pool should increase monotonically with contrast agent concentration over a range corresponding to typical bolus dosages (eg, 0.05–0.08 mmol/kg of Gd-DTPA). Only then can the signal time course in the left ventricular (LV) blood pool be used to reconstruct an approximation to the arterial input function.

The characteristics of the contrast agent administration are of paramount importance. A power injector is recommended for reproducible and crisp contrast bolus administration. A compact bolus results in a more pronounced signal enhancement in myocardial tissue, and improved contrast to noise ratios for detection of even mild perfusion changes. Variations in the heart rate or arrhythmias during first-pass imaging should not introduce artifactual modulation of the image intensity that may mimic a different perfusion state in the myocardium.[31] In addition, as infarct size constitutes one of the present key criteria for coronary artery disease prognosis, MR first-pass imaging will only be fully embraced for clinical trials if the whole heart can be covered with multiple slices.

EPI would appear to be a good choice for ultrafast first-pass imaging of the heart (approximately 60–100 ms per image). Nevertheless EPI perfusion studies on animal models and humans suffer from the strong attenuation of the signal changes in the blood pool and tissue, due to T_2^* susceptibility effects. The inversion recovery snapshot FLASH technique[32] has previously been shown to provide a suitable blood pool input function for perfusion modeling.[8,14] To increase the number of slices that can be covered in a first-pass study with the T_1 weighted FLASH technique requires either the use of high slew rate magnetic field gradients to reduce the repetition time (TR) or sparser sampling of k-space as realized with variants of the keyhole technique such as BRISK.[33] An example of the latter approach is given by the studies of Walsh et al,[19] which included a comparison of radionuclide images with the low-pass filtered MR perfusion images, and where the blood pool signal had been subtraced to better match the radio nuclide images. It was thus found that the MR first-pass images were not only of similar appearance, but more importantly, of comparable diagnostic value as the 99mTc-MIBI images.[19]

Ultrafast, Quantitative, First-Pass Imaging

We have developed in our laboratory a novel first-pass technique with arrhythmia insensitive contrast enhancement (AICE)[31] which in a patient allows acquisition of images for 5 slices (eg, long-axis slices) per heartbeat, for heart rates up to 65 beats per minute.[34] It was implemented on a clinical MR scanner with fast gradient rise times (1.5 T VISION, Siemens Medical Systems, Erlangen, Germany). Specifications were a gradient rise-time of 24 $\mu s \cdot mT^{-1} \cdot m^{-1}$ and a maximum gradient amplitude of 25 mT·ms^{-1}. This allows snapshot FLASH imaging with an image acquisition time as short as 160 ms per slice, a 128 × 60 (readout points × phase encoding steps) matrix size, and a rectangular field of view (repetition time for phase encode steps TR = 2.5 ms; echo time TE = 1.2 ms; flip angle α = 15°–18°; slice thickness of 10 mm). The MR first-pass images were acquired either for double-oblique short-axis views or long-axis views of the heart, or a combination thereof.

A saturation recovery magnetization preparation is used to provide insensitivity to heart rate changes.[31] It is is started with a nonslice selective 90^F radiofrequency pulse that nulls the longitudinal magnetization, and is followed by a gradient crusher pulse to dephase the transverse magnetization. The FLASH read-out with linear k-space ordering occurs during saturation recovery. Both the magnetization preparation and the acquisition of k-space data during saturation recovery are preferably repeated sequentially for each slice. The main advantage of a sequential versus interleaved readout for each image plane, is the reduction of blurring from cardiac motion, as the image read-out time for each image plane is reduced. Images for a given slice position are acquired for the same cardiac phase, but images for different slice positions fall into different phases of the cardiac cycle. This does not represent a problem for a consistent assessment of blood flow.

Protocols for Magnetic Resonance First-Pass Studies

With ultra-rapid imaging sequences optimization of the signal-to-noise ratio becomes of critical importance. A receive-only phase array coil should preferably be used for cardiac first-pass imaging studies. The whole-body coil serves to transmit radiofrequency pulses with a homogeneous B_1 field over the region of interest. The patient is generally imaged in a supine position and breath-hold[18] or non-breath-hold[19,34] protocols have been used for perfusion imaging. Breath-holding does not improve the image quality as the first-pass images are mostly acquired in a single-shot mode within a heartbeat. Breath-holding is nevertheless of advantage for postprocessing of the images, as the position of a region of interest remains constant. With non-breath-holding, the motion of the diaphragm requires that the position of regions of interest be adjusted from frame-to-frame to keep them fixed relative to landmarks of the heart. Alternatively the effects of respiratory motion can be reduced through postprocessing, either by image registration[35] or time domain Fourier filtering.[19] It is also not absolutely necessary to cardiac-gate the first-pass imaging sequence, except for added complications due to differences in diastolic and systolic myocardial blood volume and more cumbersome image postprocessing.

For patients, a venous catheter line advanced through the cubital vein to, or close to the superior vena cava and use of a power injector will result in a compact bolus. Figure 1 shows first pass signal curves for rest and hyperemia (140 μ/kg/min adenosine intravenous) obtained in a patient with this injection protocol. Figure 2 shows first-pass signal

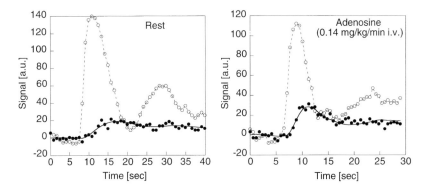

FIGURE 1. First-pass signal time curves for resting (3 image planes; HR = 75 beats per minute and hyperemic conditions (2 image planes; HR = 106 beats per minute) in a patient. The figures show the signal time course in the LV blood pool (dotted line with circles) and for one myocardial region of interest in the anterior wall (solid circles). The contrast agent was administered peripherally through an cubital vein catheter with a power injector (Medrad Inc., Pittsburgh, PA) at a rate of 10 mL/s, followed by a 15-mL saline flush at the same rate. The solid lines are from a least squares to a Fermi function distribution of tracer residence times.[34,43,44]

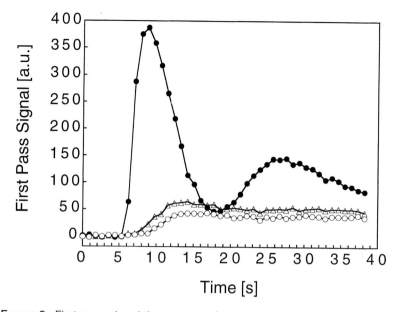

FIGURE 2. First-pass signal time courses for one slice position in a three-slice set of first-pass images acquired in a closed-chest porcine model. The signal time courses correspond to regions of interest in the LV blood pool (solid circles), the posterior papillary muscle (triangles) and the anterior papillary muscle (circles).

time courses from a three-slice set of first-pass images acquired in a closed-chest porcine model where the contrast agent (CA) was centrally injected. The signal time courses correspond to regions of interest in the LV blood pool (solid circles), the posterior papillary muscle (triangles) and the anterior papillary muscle (circles). Measurements with radioisotope labeled microspheres indicated that the tissue blood flows were 1.51 and 1.08 mL/min/g, respectively.

How Can One Quantify Perfusion?

Most approaches to quantify myocardial perfusion start with the generation of regional signal versus time curves. This is done either manually or automated for the generation of parametric images. Various parameters have been proposed as semiquantitative measures of myocardial perfusion, such as the maximum signal intensity,[36] the maximum rate of signal enhancement during contrast agent wash-in (up-slope),[11,37,38] the time-to-peak,[28] and the mean residence time.[8,39] The relative merit of these parameters has been established to varying degrees through comparison with gold standards for blood flow measurements such as the microsphere technique.[8] In part, the choice of perfusion parameter is determined by the observed contrast agent kinetics for normal myocardium. For example, for Gd-DTPA[40] the maximum up-slope during contrast agent wash-in is least affected by changes in capillary permeability compared with other parameters such as the mean residence time or the maximum signal intensity.[41] The maximum up-slope therefore provides a more direct measure of blood flow changes than the maximum signal intensity.

Modeling

A more fundamental issue with semiquantitative parameters such as the up-slope is the difficulty of quantifying changes in myocardial blood flow between baseline and stress conditions, as required for the determination of the myocardial blood flow reserve. In this latter case, the changes in hemodynamic conditions and cardiac output require comparison of the tissue signal curve parameters after correcting for differences in the blood pool input functions. In mathematical terms this can only be accomplished by calculation of the tissue residue impulse response through deconvolution of the measured tissue signal time course with the blood pool input function. In most myocardial perfusion studies,[20] including nuclear imaging studies,[22] it was found that the time course of tracer concentration in the left ventricular blood pool is an appropriate and feasible choice for an arterial input function.[30] We follow this convention here when mention is made of the input function.

For a linear and stationary system the inflow and outflow concentration versus time curves, $c_{in}(t)$ and $c_{out}(t)$, are related through convolution of $c_{in}(t)$ with the transfer function, $h(t)$[42]:

$$c_{out}(t) = \int_0^t c_{in}(\tau) \cdot h(\tau - t) \cdot d\tau = c_{in}(t) \otimes h(t) \qquad (1)$$

The transfer function, $h(t)$, gives the probability that a tracer molecule has left the region of interest (ROI) at time t. By definition at $t=0$ no tracer molecule has yet left the ROI and therefore $h(0)=0$. A characteristic of most tomographic imaging methods is the inability to measure the concentration at the entrance of the ROI, in part because the ROI does not have a single, well-defined vascular input. As an approximation, the signal time course is measured upstream of the ROI, and in practice this generally means in the left ventricle.

MR first-pass imaging allows the detection of the mass of contrast material, $m(t)$, residing in a tissue ROI, instead of measurement of the

ROI outflow curve, as in a classic indicator dilution experiment.[43] From the priniciple of mass balance it follows that the mass of contrast material in the ROI at any time, $m(t)$, is simply the difference between what has entered and flown out of the ROI[43]:

$$m(t) = F\int_0^t [c_{in}(s) - c_{out}(s)] \cdot ds = F\int_0^t c_{IN}(s) \otimes [1 - h(s)] \cdot ds \quad (2)$$

$$= c_{IN}(t) \otimes R(t). = c_{IN}(t) \otimes R_F(t) = F \cdot c_{IN}(t) \otimes R(t)$$

Here F denotes the rate of flow. The residue impulse function, $R(t)$, represents the fraction of the bolus that has not left the ROI at time t. It is a slowly decreasing function of time and because $1-h(0)=1$ we have $R_F(0)=F$.[43] This means that the initial amplitude of the impulse response function is a measure of the flow F. A Fermi function was previously found to approximate well the form of the residue impulse response function, $R(t)$, observed in first-pass experiments.[44] It provides a parametrized representation of the tissue impulse response function and this constrained deconvolution can be used in myocardial perfusion imaging as a numerically robust model for the distribution of vascular residence times. The first pass portion of the observed tissue signal time courses can be fit to the above model with a Marquardt-Levenberg nonlinear least squares fitting algorithm.

The Kety-Schmidt model has also been applied as a parametric deconvolution technique to determine the unidirectional flux constant which is the product of flow and extraction fraction.[15,45] Flow and extraction fraction cannot be distinguished in this model, unless the extraction fraction is known *a priori*, or can be determined independently, which is an invasive and cumbersome proposition.[15] The Kety-Schmidt model is therefore most suitable for modeling the kinetics of freely diffusible tracers such as ^{17}O labeled water for PET studies, because the extraction can then be set to unity.[22] The extraction fraction for Gd-DTPA has been determined in canines with radioisotope labeled Gd-DTPA and the peak extraction fraction was found to decrease from 0.6 to 0.35 with flow increasing from 0.44 mL/min/g to 1.37 mL/min/g.[15] The Kety-Schmidt model was used in the analysis of MR measurements during slow infusion of an extracellular CA.[45] An increase of the unidirectional influx constant was observed to occur with the administration of dipyridamole despite the decrease of extraction fraction expected at higher flows.[46]

Myocardial Perfusion Reserve and Collateral Flow

The coronary flow reserve (CFR), defined as the ratio of hyperemic blood flow to resting blood flow, is generally thought to be a good

TABLE 1

Clinical Applications of Magnetic Resonance Perfusion Studies

Diagnostic Information	Perfusion MR Techniques
Infarct size and extent	1) Multislice first pass imaging 2) T_1, T_2-sensitive techniques for tissue characterization
Detection of subendocardial perfusion defect; Transmural blood flow	1) First pass imaging with high spatial and temporal resolution
Myocardial perfusion reserve; Delineation of area at risk	1) First pass measurements under basal and hyperemic conditions
Assessment of collateral blood supply	1) First pass imaging 2) Myocardial perfusion reserve assessment
Assessment of myocardial viability	1) Combined MR wall motion and perfusion studies 2) Equilibrium contrast agent studies 3) ^{31}P MR spectroscopy

indicator of the functional significance of a coronary artery lesion.[23,25] However, compensation of a coronary stenosis by the induction of collateral circulation suggests, that the degree to which a coronary lesion causes myocardial ischemia, could be better assessed through determination of the regional myocardial perfusion reserve. As an analog to the CFR, the myocardial perfusion reserve is defined as the ratio of regional myocardial blood flows under hyperemic and resting conditions.[21,47] To correct for the hemodynamic changes inherent to the determination of the perfusion reserve, one should deconvolve the myocardial signal time course with the signal time course observed in the left ventricular blood pool, as already discussed earlier. It has been shown that the myocardial blood flow reserve can be obtained from two first pass measurements under resting conditions and during maximal hyperemia by calculating the ratio of the amplitudes of the impulse response for rest and maximal hyperemia.[34]

Figure 3 shows a comparison of the LAD coronary flow reserve, measured with an intracoronary Doppler probe, and the MR estimate of the myocardial perfusion reserve in the LAD perfusion bed. Patients with the syndrome of chest pain and nonsignificant coronary artery

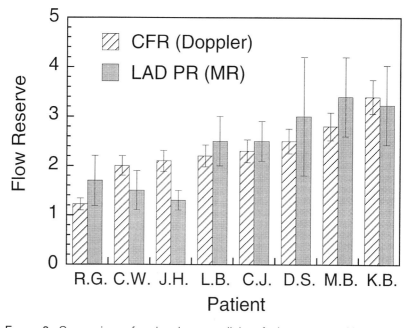

FIGURE 3. Comparison of regional myocardial perfusion reserve with coronary flow reserve in patients with angina and nonsignificant coronary artery lesions. The perfusion reserve was estimated for the territory of the LAD, and the coronary flow reserve in the LAD was measured with an intracoronary Doppler probe.

lesions (syndrome X) were selected for this study. A linear correlation was observed between the LAD CFR and the regional flow reserve in the territory of the LAD ($r = 0.80$). The CFR under maximal vasodilation with adenosine averaged 2.29/ ±0.5 that is significantly lower than for patients with normal coronary arteries, or less than 50% diameter stenosis, where CFR was previously found to be 3.5 or higher.[48] Based on considerations of mass balance, the CFR and myocardial perfusion reserve should be the same, in patients with microvascular disease but normal arteriograms. The MR results for the myocardial perfusion reserve in response to adenosine agree well with previous findings of an abnormal response to vasoconstrictor stimuli at the prearteriolar level of the coronary vasculature.[49] These MR studies showed for the first time that the myocardial perfusion reserve correlates with Doppler flow measurements in patients with syndrome X.[34,50]

The Kety-Schmidt model was also applied to the determination of the myocardial flow reserve, and the ratio of unidirectional flux constants for hyperemic and basal flows fell into a range of 2 to 3 in normals.[51] This is, however, less than the myocardial perfusion reserve measured in normals with PET through absolute flow quantification[52] and may reflect the fact that the extraction fraction is thought to decrease with increasing flow.[15]

Validation with the Gold Standard

With pharmacologically induced vasodilation (eg, with adenosine) the coronary pressure falls and the CFR is exhausted first in the territory of a stenosed coronary artery.[24] Consequently, the regional heterogeneity in myocardial blood flow tends to be more pronounced under stress conditions.[47] Such regional differences in perfusion can be quantified with a relative perfusion index, defined as a ratio of myocardial perfusion in the territory of the stenosed coronary artery, and perfusion in a remote, normal region.[47] Ratios of parameters such as the maximum signal intensity,[36,53] the maximum upslope during CA wash-in,[11] or the residue impulse response height[41] have been proposed to quantify the relative variation of myocardial perfusion between different myocardial regions.

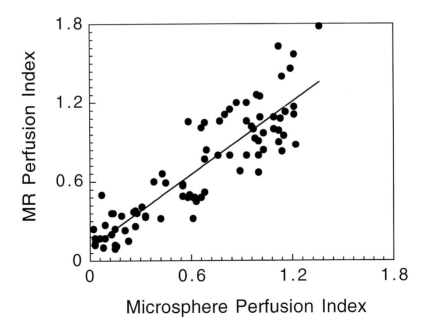

FIGURE 4. Comparison of the relative MR perfusion indices lateral/anterior and (anterior papillary muscle)/septal with corresponding ratios of blood flow, measured with radiolabeled microspheres. The MR perfusion index was calculated as the ratio of the maximum amplitude of the tissue impulse response for the regions of interest entering in the ratio.

Figure 4 shows (n = 8) a comparison between such an MR perfusion index defined as the ratio of the respective heights of the residue impulse response for two myocardial regions (eg. lateral/anterior), and the corresponding ratio of microsphere flows. Ligation of the first two marginal branches of the left circumflex coronary artery (LCx) caused a moderate to severe perfusion deficit in the lateral segments, and blood flow in the anterior papillary muscle usually suffered only a mild to moderate reduction.

Two relative perfusion indices were determined, giving the ratios of the average of the maximum impulse response amplitude in the lateral (LAT) and anterior (ANT) regions of interest, and the anterior papillary muscle (APM) and septal (SEPT) regions, respectively. The correlation (slope 0.93 ± 0.05; r = 0.88) between the relative myocardial perfusion indices (ratios LAT/ANT and APM/SEPT; n = 84) obtained from MR experiments and microsphere flow measurements respectively are shown in Figure 4. Significant changes in the blood flow index on the order of 0.3, measured with radiolabeled microspheres, were paralleled by similarly significant changes (P < .05) in the MR perfusion index.[41]

Absolute Quantification of Myocardial Blood Flow

Simulations with a multipath, spatially distributed mathematical model of blood tissue exchange,[42] have shown that the leakage of Gd-DTPA into the interstitial space is small during the wash-in of Gd-DTPA if the contrast agent is rapidly injected as a bolus.[35] To account for the effects of contrast agent leakage into the interstitial space requires a multicompartment model. A simple embodiment[54] comprises a vascular compartment of volume v_p (mL/g of tissue), through which contrast agent is carried at a flow rate f_p (in units of mL/s per g of tissue). A second compartment represents the interstitial space of volume v_i (mL/g of tissue). The leakage of contrast agent from the vascular into the interstitial space is determined by the permeability surface area product PS. The concentrations of CA in the vascular and interstitial spaces, $C_p(t)$ and $C_i(t)$, obey a system of two coupled ordinary differential equations that can be solved numerically.

Figure 5 shows a comparison between the values of absolute blood flow in mL/min/g obtained with radiolabeled microspheres, and from multislice MR first-pass measurements. The MR data were averaged for three immediately adjacent slice locations and the microsphere data for three corresponding autopsy rings. The averaging reduces errors from mismatching of the MR slice positions with the autopsy ring positions. The error bars give the standard deviations of those averages. The two-compartment model parameters were adjusted through nonlinear least squares fitting, except for v_i for the interstitial compartment vol-

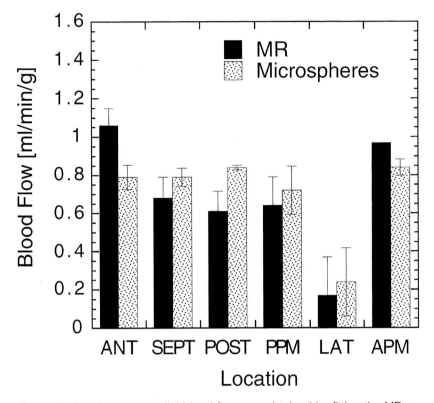

FIGURE 5. Absolute myocardial blood flow was obtained by fitting the MR regional signal time courses to a two-compartment model. Images for three adjacent slices were acquired in the first-pass experiment at a rate of three images per heartbeat. The resulting estimates of absolute flow were averaged for three slice positions and compared with the blood flow determined with radiolabeled microspheres.

ume that was held fixed at 0.18 mL/g for the sake of being able to identify unique best-fit values for *PS*. Pooling the data for six canines results in a linear correlation of the MR flow estimate versus the microsphere blood flow data with a slope of 0.95 ± 0.06 and an intercept value of 0.1 ± 0.07 mL/min/g ($r = 0.81$). These preliminary results demonstrate that the determination of absolute myocardial blood flow from first-pass measurements with an extracellular contrast agent is indeed feasible.

Through the seminal work of Bassingthwaighte and colleagues[42] more realistic, multipath, spatially distributed models have become available to analyze the kinetics of MR contrast agents in the heart.[14] Applying these more realistic, but necessarily also more complex models to the analysis of MR first-pass time courses is still in an exploratory stage and beyond the scope of this chapter.[30]

Magnetic Resonance Perfusion Assessment in Coronary Artery Disease

The MR first-pass technique in concert with the extracellular MR contrast agent Gd-DTPA has been used to assess myocardial perfusion in patients with ischemic heart disease at rest[4,5] and during pharmacological stress.[11,55] Wilke et al[5,20] examined patients with stable, mild, or moderate angina who had undergone selective coronary angiography for evaluation of chest pain. Coronary angiography and scintigraphy were performed within 48 hours. No patient had associated heart diseases. The selection criteria were as follows: (a) no acute myocardial infarction; (b) no myocardial ischemia or angina at rest; (c) unequivocal evidence of coronary artery disease; (d) presence of angina and/or ST segment changes at stress; (e) normal left ventricular volumes and systolic function at rest as proved by levocardiography and two-dimensional echocardiography. Serial ultrafast imaging was performed under resting conditions and subsequently. An infusion of dipyridamole was started through an intravenous catheter in the right antecubital vein without moving the patient. A low-dose Gd-DTPA bolus (0.06 mL/kg - 0.02 mmol/kg, Magnevist, Schering AG, Berlin) was administered after maximal vasodilatation. Dipyridamole was administered through the IV line over a four minute period at a constant rate of 0.02 mg/kg/min.

The first-pass images obtained in a patient with subtotal LCx occlusion and collateral supply from the LAD at rest are shown in Figure 6. A perfusion defect became clearly visible during dipyridamole stress (steal phenomenon), but was mostly confined to the subendocardial

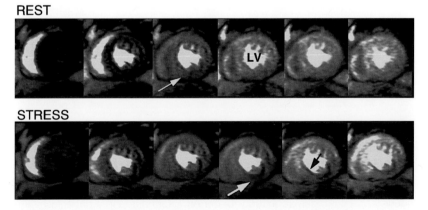

FIGURE 6. First-pass images for rest and dipyridamole stress obtained in a patient with subtotal LCx occlusion and collateral supply at rest from the LAD.

layer. These images serve as an example for the ability to detect with MR first-pass imaging hypoperfusion in the subendocardial layer, where the blood flow deficit will be most severe as a result of a proximal coronary stenosis.[56]

Coronary Revascularization and Reperfusion

Figure 7 shows first images acquired at a rate of 1 image per heartbeat for all three slices in a patient with angioplasty performed 2 hours postacute myocardial infarction. The patient had an occlusion of the LCx and the x-ray angiograms before and after angioplasty are shown in Figure 8. Left ventricular end-diastolic pressure (30 mm Hg) increased and ejection fraction postangioplasty was reduced. The first-pass images reveal a zone of mild hypoperfusion in the lateral wall, demonstrating that the restoration of coronary artery patency did not result in fully successful microvascular reperfusion. An MR cine wall motion study before the first-pass measurements showed that the observation of hypoperfusion in the lateral wall coincided with reduced regional and global left ventricular function. Incomplete reperfusion after angioplasty can give rise to the no-reflow phenomenon, also suggested in MR studies of the contrast agent equilibrium distribution.[57] However this case demonstrates the ability to visualize with MR first-pass imaging discrete perfusion alterations associated with postischemic, hibernating and stunned myocardium.

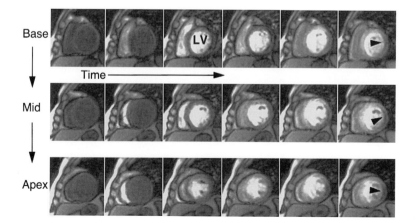

FIGURE 7. First images acquired with the AICE technique in a patient postangioplasty 2 hours after acute myocardial infarction.

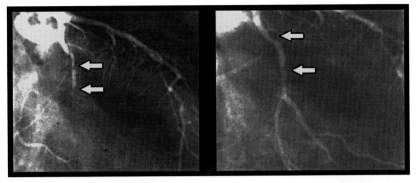

pre PCTA   post PCTA

FIGURE 8. X-ray angiograms pre- and postangioplasty 2 hours after myocardial infarction. The angiogram suggests that the patency of the LCx was successfully restored with a remaining 25% stenosis.

Infarct Size and Extent

Postmortem, histochemical staining of myocardial tissue samples is one of the gold standards for determination of infarct size. With the MR first-pass technique it is possible to quantify the extent of the infarct and assess at the same time any restored myocardial blood flow in the ischemic segment. Figure 9 shows a comparison between the infarct zone visible in 2,3,5-triphenyltetrazolium chloride (TTC) stained slices of the heart and zones of severe hypoperfusion visible in the MR first-pass images. The images illustrate the fact that MR first-pass imaging can indeed determine infarct size, if a multislice first-pass imaging technique is used for full coverage of the heart. The potential of assessing the infarct size by imaging the equilibrium distribution of Gd-DTPA was previously studied in animal models.[13,57,58] These hypo- or hyperenhancement patterns emerging over a time period of 5 to 30 minutes reflect a combination of changes in capillary permeability, distribution volume, and blood flow. It was found that the hypoenhanced area seen after reperfusion was larger than the necrotic region.[59]

Noninvasive Transmural Contraction Perfusion Matching

It has been recognized that the combined study of first-pass perfusion and regional myocardial deformation with MR tagging carries

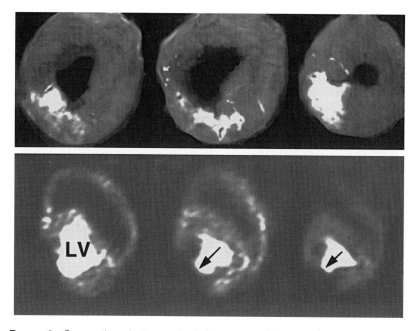

FIGURE 9. Comparison between the infarct zone visible in 2,3,5-triphenyltetra-zolium chloride (TTC)-stained slices of the heart (upper row) and MR first-pass images (lower row) showing zone of hypoperfusion in lateral wall segment.

considerable promise for the assessment of contraction perfusion matching in one integrated examination.[38] In a recent experiment, images with spatial modulation of magnetization (SPAMM) for tissue were obtained in a closed-chest canine model for a control state, during moderate stenosis, and moderate stenosis combined with pharmacological stress.[38] The SPAMM images were analyzed with the custom-written analysis package, SPAMMVU.[6] The myocardial principal strains, displacements and rotations were quantitatively assessed in the subepicardial and subendocardial layers of the normal perfused and hypoperfused segments. Figure 10 shows the displacement (T) for endocardial and epicardial regions in the anterior wall normalized by the average displacement in the posterior wall. Similarly, the myocardial blood flow (MBF) data from microsphere measurements are shown for the corresponding endocardial and epicardial tissue samples.

Conclusions

Quantitative MR first-pass imaging provides an unbiased, observer independent assessment of myocardial perfusion. Such a quanti-

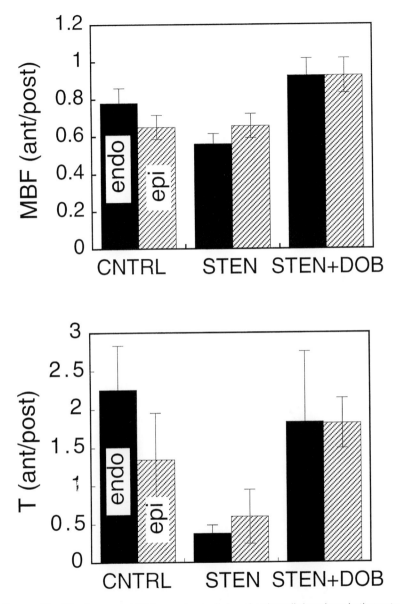

FIGURE 10. Displacement (T) for endocardial and epicardial regions in the anterior wall normalized by average displacement in the posterior wall. Similarly the myocardial blood flow (MBF) data from microsphere measurements are shown for the corresponding endocardial and epicardial tissue samples.

tative assessment will ultimately lead to a better understanding of the pathophysiology of myocardial ischemia post-treatment and during the follow-up period. True MR first-pass imaging, preferably with multislice coverage of the heart, has sufficient sensitivity for the detection and quantification of mild to severe perfusion deficits. This allows a quantitative assessment of the area at risk, the degree of collateral blood supply, as well as determination of infarct size as predictor for outcome. First-pass perfusion studies are an important complement to MR wall motion studies, and possibly MR phase contrast coronary flow measurements. MR contraction-perfusion matching[38] will allow for a more in-depth noninvasive evaluation of stunned or hibernating myocardium in men. Because perfusion limitations usually begin in the subendocardium as coronary flow is gradually reduced, first-pass imaging with the prerequisite spatial and temporal resolution would allow much earlier detection of mild coronary stenosis than any other diagnostic imaging modality. Clinical outcome trials in a larger patient population and comparative studies to nuclear medicine are needed for the further acceptance of MR myocardial perfusion imaging in the cardiological community, and for the management of patients with ischemic heart disease.

Acknowledgments

The authors are indebted to Dr. K. Kroll and Dr. J. B. Bassingthwaighte (University of Washington, Seattle) for generously sharing their experience and insight.

References

1. White RD, Holt WW, Cheitlin MD, et al. Estimation of the functional and anatomic extent of myocardial infarction using magnetic resonance imaging. *Am Heart J.* 1988;115:740–748.
2. Baer FM, Voth E, Theissen P, et al. Gradient-echo magnetic resonance imaging during incremental dobutamine infusion for the localization of coronary artery stenoses. *Eur Heart J.* 1994;15:218–225.
3. Atkinson DJ, Burstein D, Edelman RR. First-pass cardiac perfusion: Evaluation with ultrafast MR imaging. *Radiology.* 1990;(3 pt 1):757–762.
4. Manning WJ, Atkinson DJ, Grossman W, et al. First-pass nuclear magnetic resonance imaging studies using gadolinium-DTPA in patients with coronary artery disease. *J Am Coll Cardiol.* 1991;18:959–965.
5. Wilke N, Maching T, Engels G. Dynamic perfusion studies by ultrafast MR imaging: Initial clinical results from cardiology. *Electromedica.* 1990;58:102–108.
6. Axel L, Goncalves RC, Bloomgarden D. Regional heart wall motion: Two-

dimensional analysis and functional imaging with MR Imaging. *Radiology.* 1992;183:745–750.

 7. Zerhouni EA, Parish DM, Rogers WJ, et al. Human heart: tagging with MR imaging—A method for noninvasive assessment of myocardial motion. *Radiology.* 1988;169:59–63.

 8. Wilke N, Simm C, Zhang J, et al. Contrast-enhanced first pass myocardial perfusion imaging: Correlation between myocardial blood flow in dogs at rest and during hyperemia. *Magn Reson Med.* 1993;29:485–497.

 9. Wendland MF, Saeed M, Yu KK, et al. Inversion recovery EPI of bolus transit in rat myocardium using intravascular and extravascular gadolinium-based MR contrast media: Dose effects on peak signal enhancement. *Magn Reson Med.* 1994;32:319–329.

10. Edelman RR, Li W. Contrast-enhanced echo-planar MR imaging of myocardial perfusion: preliminary study in humans. *Radiology.* 1994;190:771–777.

11. Eichenberger AC, Schuiki E, Kochli VD, et al. Ischemic heart disease: Assessment with gadolinium-enhanced ultrafast MR imaging and dipyridamole stress. *J Magn Reson Imaging.* 1994;4:425–431.

12. Saeed M, Wendland MF, Tomei E, et al. Demarcation of myocardial ischemia: Magnetic susceptibility effect of contrast medium in MR imaging. *Radiology.* 1989;173:763–767.

13. Lima JA, Judd RM, Bazille A, et al. Regional heterogeneity of human myocardial infarcts demonstrated by contrast-enhanced MRI. Potential mechanisms. *Circulation.* 1995;92:1117–1125.

14. Wilke N, Kroll K, Merkle H, et al. Regional myocardial blood volume and flow: First pass MR imaging with polylysine-gadolinium-DTPA. *J Magn Reson Imaging.* 1995;5:227–237.

15. Tong CY, Prato FS, Wisenberg F, et al. Measurement of the extraction efficiency and distribution volume for Gd-DTPA in normal and diseased canine myocardium. *Magn Reson Med.* 1993;30:337–346.

16. Saeed M, Wendland MF, Masui T, Higgins CB. Reperfused myocardial infarctions on T1- and susceptibility-enhanced MRI: Evidence for loss of compartmentalization of contrast media. *Magn Reson Med.* 1994;31:31–39.

17. Wilke N, Koronaeos A, Feistel H, et al. Magnetic resonance first pass myocardial perfusion imaging at stress compared to Tc-99m SPECT. Presented at Joint XIIth World Congress of Cardiology & European Society of Cardiology, Berlin, 1994.

18. Keijer JT, vanRossum AC, vanEenige MJ, et al. First-pass contrast enhanced MRI of myocardial perfusion in single vessel coronary artery disease: A quantitative comparison with 201thallium-SPECT at rest and during pharmacological stress (abstract). ISMRM, 4th Scientific Meeting, New York, NY, 1996;vol. 1, p. 180.

19. Walsh EG, Doyle M, Lawson MA, et al. Multislice first-pass myocardial perfusion imaging on conventional clinical scanner. *Magn Reson Med.* 1995; 34:39–47.

20. Wilke N, Jerosch-Herold M, Stillman AE, et al. Concepts of myocardial perfusion imaging in magnetic resonance imaging. *Magn Reson Q.* 1994;10: 249–286.

21. Beanlands RS, Muzik O, Melon P, et al. Noninvasive quantification of regional myocardial flow reserve in patients with coronary atherosclerosis using nitrogen-13 ammonia positron emission tomography. Determination of extent of altered vascular reactivity. *J Am Coll Cardiol.* 1995;26:1465–1475.

22. Araujo LI, Lammertsma AA, Rhodes CG, et al. Noninvasive quantification

of regional myocardial blood flow in coronary artery disease with ^{15}O-labeled carbon dioxide inhalation and positron emission tomography. *Circulation.* 1991;83:875–885.

23. Wilson RF, Marcus ML, White CW. Prediction of the physiologic significance of coronary arterial lesions by quantitative lesion geometry in patients with limited coronary artery disease. *Circulation.* 1987;75:723–732.

24. Klocke FJ. Measurements of coronary flow reserve: defining pathophysiology versus making decisions about patient care. *Circulation.* 1987;76:1183–1189.

25. Gould KL, Lipscomb K. Effects of coronary stenosis on coronary flow reserve and resistance. *Am J Cardiol.* 1974;34:48–55.

26. Clarke GD, Eckels R, Chaney C, et al. Measurement of absolute epicardial coronary artery flow and flow reserve with breath-hold cine phase-contrast magnetic resonance imaging. *Circulation.* 1995;91:2627–2634.

27. Sakuma H, Blake LM, Amidon TM, et al. Coronary flow reserve: Noninvasive measurement in humans with breath-hold velocity encoded cine MR imaging. *Radiology.* 1996;198:745–750.

28. Pearlman JD, Hibberd MG, Chuang ML, et al. Magnetic resonance mapping demonstrates benefits of VEGF-induced myocardial angiogenesis. *Nature Med.* 1995;1:1085–1089.

29. Mirhoseini M, Shelgikar S, Cayton MM. New concepts in revascularization of the myocardium. *Ann Thorac Surg.* 1988;45:415–420.

30. Kroll K, Wilke N, Jerosch-Herold M, et al. Accuracy of modeling of regional myocardial flows from residue functions of an intravascular indicator. *Am J Physiol. (Heart Circ Physiol).* 1996;40:H1643–H1655.

31. Tsekos N, Zhang Y, Merkle H, et al. Fast anatomical imaging of the heart and assessment of myocardial perfusion with arrythmia insensitive magnetization preparation. *Magn Reson Med.* 1995;34:530–536.

32. Haase A, Matthaei D, Bartkowski R, et al. Inversion recovery snapshot FLASH MR imaging. *J. Comp Assist Tomogr.* 1989;13:1036–1040.

33. Doyle M, Walsh EG, Blackwell GG, Pohost GM. Block regional interpolation scheme for k-space (BRISK): a rapid cardiac imaging technique. *Magn Reson Med.* 1995;33:163–170.

34. Wilke N, Jerosch-Herold M, Wang Y, et al. Myocardial perfusion reserve: Assessment with multisection, quantitative, first-pass MR imaging. *Radiology.* 1997;204:373–384.

35. Jerosch-Herold M, Wilke N, Stillman AE, et al. Functional myocardial perfusion maps from MR first pass images. Society of Magnetic Resonance, 3rd Annual Meeting, Nice, 1995;459.

36. Wendland MF, Saeed M, Masui T, et al. Echoplanar MR imaging of normal and ischemic myocardium with gadodiamide injection. *Radiology.* 1993;186:535–542.

37. Matheijssen NAA, Rugge FPv, Louwerenburg HW, et al. Wall. Comparison of ultrafast dipyridamole magnetic resonance imaging with dipyridamole SestaMIBI SPECT for detection of perfusion abnormalities in patients with one-vessel coronary artery disease. *Magn Reson Med.* 1996;35:221–228.

38. Kraitchman DL, Wilke N, Hexeberg E, et al. Myocardial perfusion and function in dogs with moderate coronary stenosis. *Magn Reson Med.* 1996;35:771–780.

39. Keijer JT, Rossum ACv, Eenige MJv, et al. Semiquantitation of regional myocardial blood flow in normal human subjects by first-pass magnetic resonance imaging. *Am Heart J.* 1995;130:893–901.

40. Weinmann HJ, Brasch RC, Press WR, Wesbey GE. Characteristics of Gadolinium-DTPA complex, a potential NMR contrast agent. *AJR.* 1984;142: 619–624.
41. Jerosch-Herold M, Wilke N, Wang Y, Stillman AE. Quantification of relative myocardial blood flow changes with true first pass MR imaging and extracellular contrast agents. ISMR, Fourth Scientific Meeting, New York, 1996; 677.
42. Bassingthwaighte JB, Goresky CA. Modeling in the analysis of solute and water exchange in the microvasculature. In: Renkin EM, Michel CC, eds. *Handbook of Physiology—The Cardiovascular System.* Bethesda, MD: American Physiology Society; 1984;549–626.
43. Clough AV, Al-Tinawi A, Linehan JH, Dawson C. Regional transit time estimation from image residue curves. *Ann Biomed Eng.* 1994;22:128–143.
44. Axel L. Tissue mean transit time from dynamic computed tomography by a simple deconvolution technique. *Invest Radiol.* 1983;18:94–99.
45. Larsson HBW, Fritz-Hansen T, Rostrup E, et al. Myocardial perfusion imaging using MRI. *Magn Reson Med.* 1996;35:716–726.
46. Fritz-Hansen T, Larsson HBW, Rostrup E, et al. Quantification of myocardial perfusion at rest and during dipyridamole infusion in humans. Society of Magnetic Resonance in Medicine, 3rd scientific meeting. Nice, France, 1995;21.
47. Gould KL, Kirkeeide RL, Buchi M. Coronary flow reserve as a physiologic measure of stenosis severity. *J Am Coll Cardiol.* 1990;15:459–474.
48. Wilson RF, Wyche K, Christensen BV, et al. Effects of adenosine on human coronary arterial circulation. *Circulation.* 1990;82:1595–1606.
49. Epstein SE, Cannon R III. Site of increased resistance to coronary flow in patients with angina pectoris and normal epicardial coronary arteries. *J Am Coll Cardiol.* 1986;8:459–461.
50. Jerosch-Herold M, Wilke N, Wang Y, Stillman AE. Comparison of MR-derived regional perfusion reserve with coronary flow reserve in patients with syndrome X. Radiological Society of North America, 82nd Scientific Assembly and Annual Meeting, Chicago, 1996.
51. Fritz-Hansen T, Rostrup E, Larsson HBW. Comparison of qualitative and quantitative methods for evaluation of the myocardial perfusion reserve. International Society of Magnetic Resonance in Medicine, 4th scientific meeting, New York, 1996;685.
52. Geltman EM, Henes CG, Senneff MJ, et al. Increased myocardial perfusion at rest and diminished perfusion reserve in patients with angina and angiographically normal coronary arteries. *J Am Coll Cardiol.* 1990;16:586–595.
53. Saeed M, Wendland MF, Lauerma K, et al. First-pass contrast-enhanced inversion recovery and driven equilibrium fast GRE imaging studies: Detection of acute myocardial ischemia. *J Magn Reson Imaging.* 1995;5:515–523.
54. Sangren WC, Sheppard CW. Mathematical derivation of the exchange of a labeled substance between a liquid flowing in a vessel and an external compartment. *Bull Math Biophys.* 1953;15:387–394.
55. Schaefer S, Tyen Rv, Saloner O. Evaluation of myocardial perfusion abnormalities with gadolinium-enhanced snapshot MR imaging in humans. *Radiology.* 1992;185:795–801.
56. Bache RJ, Schwartz JS. Effect of perfusion pressure distal to a coronary stenosis on transmural myocardial blood flow. *Circulation.* 1982;65:928–935.
57. Judd RM, Lugo-Olivieri CH, Arai M, et al. Physiological basis of myocardial contrast enhancement in fast magnetic resonance images of 2-day-old reperfused canine infarcts. *Circulation.* 1995;92:1902–1910.

58. Lauerma K, Saeed M, Wendland MF, et al. The use of contrast-enhanced magnetic resonance imaging to define ischemic injury after reperfusion. Comparison in normal and hypertrophied hearts. *Invest Radiol.* 1994;29: 527–535.
59. Yuasa K, Sugimura K, Kawamitsu H, et al. Quantification of occlusive and reperfused myocardial infarct size with Gd-DTPA-enhanced MR imaging. *Eur J Radiol.* 1993;17:150–154.

## Chapter 13

Magnetic Resonance Contrast Media in Ischemic Heart Disease

Charles B. Higgins, MD, Maythem Saeed, DVM, PhD, and Michael Wendland, PhD

A number of studies in animal models[1-7] and patients[8-15] have demonstrated that magnetic resonance (MR) contrast media are important for current and future magnetic resonance imaging (MRI) for the evaluation of ischemic heart disease. The utility of MR contrast media have increased in recent years and will likely continue to do so because of the introduction of fast gradient-echo (GRE) and echoplanar (EPI) imaging techniques that can be made sensitive to the effects of the media and can monitor their first passage through the central blood pool and myocardium.

The specific potential applications of MR contrast media in ischemic heart disease include the following:

(1) earlier and improved demarcation between infarcted and normal myocardium;

(2) quantification of the size of myocardial infarctions;

(3) differentiation between occlusive and reperfused myocardial infarctions;

(4) determination of myocardial nonviability (or viability) after ischemic injury;

(5) characterization of ischemically stunned myocardium;

(6) evaluation of myocardial perfusion including the identifi-

From: Higgins CB, Ingwall JS, Pohost GM, (eds). *Current and Future Applications of Magnetic Resonance in Cardiovascular Disease.* Armonk, NY: Futura Publishing Company, Inc.; © 1998.

cation of hemodynamically significant coronary arterial stenoses;

(7) improvement of coronary MR angiography.

This chapter reviews these various applications of contrast enhanced MRI for the evaluation of ischemic heart disease.

Magnetic Resonance Contrast Media

MR contrast media can be classified according to their effect on signal intensity of tissues in relationship to the major MR mechanism of this effect.[3,7,16] Both positive and negative contrast media for MRI have been tested in the heart (Figures 1 and 2). T1-enhancing agents increase myocardial signal intensity with T1-sensitive imaging sequences. Efficient enhancement of T1 relaxation requires molecular contact between the contrast agent and water molecules, whereby the water molecules are briefly coordinated to the paramagnetic metal. Agents that rapidly diffuse throughout the interstitium are more potent than those confined to the intravascular space.

T2* or susceptibility agents cause signal loss with T2-sensitive imaging sequences. Spin dephasing is caused by microscopic field gradients in the tissue close to regions or compartments that contain contrast agent. The potency of the contrast agent is a function of its magnetic susceptibility and its distribution within the tissue.[17] T2* agents have been shown to provide substantial signal loss in the myocardium.[18-21]

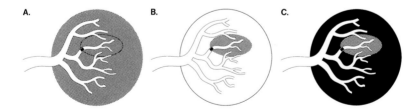

FIGURE 1. Diagrams displaying the methods for demarcating the ischemic zone of the myocardium caused by a coronary occlusion. In the early hours after acute occlusion, there is no contrast between normal and ischemic myocardium (**A**). After administration of T1-enhancing contrast medium (**B**) the signal is increased in the normal myocardium and the ischemic region is demarcated as a zone of low signal (cold spot). After administration of a magnetic susceptibility contrast medium (**C**), the signal is decreased or eliminated in the normal myocardium and the ischemic region is demarcated as a zone of high signal (hot spot).

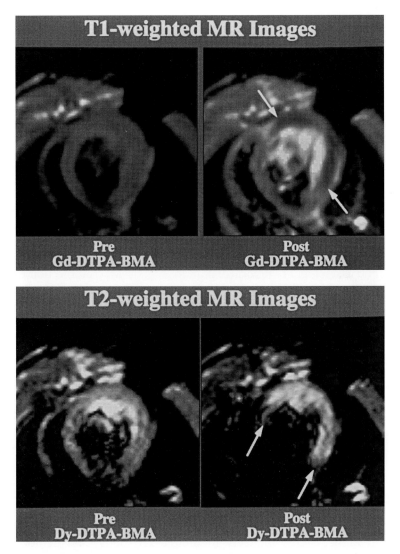

FIGURE 2. **A:** ECG-gated T1-weighted spin echo images of a rat with acute occlusion of the anterior coronary artery before (**left**) and after (**right**) injection of gadolinium DTPA-BMA (Gadodiamide injection, Nycomed, Oslo). After contrast medium the ischemic zone is demarcated as a low signal region (cold spot). **B:** ECG-gated T2-weighted spin-echo images of the same rat before (**left**) and after (**right**) injection of dysprosium DTPA-BMA (Sprodiamide injection, Nycomed, Oslo). After contrast medium the ischemic zone is demarcated as a high signal region (hot spot).

MR contrast media may also be classified according to their early distribution in tissues. Contrast media may be distributed to the extracellular, to both intracellular and extracellular spaces, or predominantly confined for a prolonged period to the intravascular space. All x-ray (iodinated) and MR contrast media currently approved for human use are extracellular agents. There are intravascular MR agents currently being experimentally evaluated in animals.[22–25]

Low molecular weight agents are excluded from the intracellular compartment but are free to equilibrate throughout the interstitium. These agents distribute rapidly to the extravascular space and undergo early renal excretion. Distribution of both T1 and T2* agents to the intravascular space can be achieved by conjugating the paramagnetic ligand to macromolecules such as albumin or polylysine (molecular weight, >50,000 d), which prevents glomerular filtration or leakage through the capillary wall. Gadolinium diethylenetriaminepentaacetic acid (DTPA)-albumin and polylysine have been used for characterization and assessment of myocardial injuries.[22,24,25] Macromolecular contrast media such as gadolinium dendrimers and ferrite particles have been used for enhancing magnetic resonance angiography (MRA) and may prove very useful for improving coronary MRA.

Demarcation of Acute Myocardial Infarction

In normal myocardium, water is distributed almost homogeneously and moves relatively freely across the capillary wall and cellular membrane. The extraction fraction of water is close to unity and is not sensitive to flow changes.[26] Edema with an increase in protein in the interstitium of infarcted myocardium has been reported[27]; this observation may be due to an increase in capillary permeability, loss of cellular integrity, and compression of the lymphatic system.[28] Edema associated with myocardial infarction prolongs tissue relaxation times, resulting in higher signal intensity in infarcted regions than in normal myocardium on unenhanced T2-weighted spin-echo images.[29] In reperfused infarcted myocardium, disruption of the cellular membrane during the process of cell death provides an expanded volume for distribution of contrast medium.[6,7,21] In this case, a T1-enhancing agent may diffuse even into the intracellular space and cause much greater signal enhancement than that in normal myocardium.[19,30] Magnetic susceptibility contrast media and high doses of gadolinium chelates cause a diametric appearance of occlusive myocardial infarctions in animal models; the infarction displays high signal intensity due to reduction of signal in the normal myocardium caused by the action of this type of contrast agent.[19–21,31] Dysprosium DTPA-BMA (sprodiamide injection) or a relatively high dose of Gd-DTPA-BMA (gadodiamide injection) induce a marked decrease in signal intensity of normal myocardium and no change or less change in signal of the infarcted region on T2-weighted spin-echo images of rats with occlusive acute myocardial infarctions.

The dual utility of a single contrast medium for T1- and T2-enhancement in creating differential contrast between normal and acutely infarcted myocardium has also been explored with use of spin-echo and echoplanar imaging.[16,31,32] Postcontrast T1-sensitive images, spin-echo with short TR and TE and inversion recovery (IR) echoplanar images, clearly delineated the infarcted region as an area of low signal intensity. However, on T2-sensitive images, spin-echo with long TR and TE and driven-equilibrium echoplanar images the infarcted region appeared as an area of high signal intensity. These effects were obtained with two different doses of Gd-DTPA-BMA, in normal and ischemic hearts. The low dose caused increased signal of normal myocardium while the high dose caused decreased signal of normal myocardium.

Measurement of the size of infarction and the area in jeopardy can potentially provide valuable information for guiding therapeutic interventions aimed at limiting the size of the infarction. MRI has been effective for sizing regions of acute and subacute infarction.[33] The accuracy of quantification of acutely reperfused infarctions with Gd-DTPA-BMA-enhanced MRI has been exhibited by comparison with histochemical morphometry.[21] Yu et al[34] found a close correlation between the area in jeopardy on Dy-DTPA-BMA-enhanced T2-weighted images ($51\% \pm 3\%$) and the area in jeopardy measure at thallium-201 autoradiography ($46\% \pm 3\%$). They concluded that Dy-DTPA-BMA-enhanced T2-weighted imaging can potentially be used to accurately quantify the area in jeopardy after acute coronary occlusion. de Roos et al[35] used Gd-DTPA-enhanced imaging to estimate the size of occlusive and reperfused infarcts in 21 patients. They found that the infarct size was significantly reduced in patients with reperfusion relative to patients without reperfusion.

Differentiation Between Occlusive and Reperfused Myocardial Infarctions

Current management of many myocardial infarctions uses thrombolytic drugs and/or catheter interventions in order to reopen acutely occluded coronary arteries. The success of this therapy depends on reperfusion at the tissue (capillary) level rather than merely affecting patency of conductance vessels. Inadequate reperfusion at the capillary level can be caused by persistent occlusion of a coronary artery; severe myocardial edema causing collapse of small intramyocardial vessels; or destruction of small vessels (intramural hemorrhage). Using albumen encapsulated microbubbles as an ultrasonic contrast media injected into reopened coronary arteries, thrombolysis failed to reperfuse ischemically injured myocardium in about 25% of patients.[36] Contrast-enhanced MRI strategies have been explored as a noninvasive method for both documenting reperfusion at the tissue level and defining the presence and extent of irreversible cellular injury.

In animal models, occlusive infarcts have shown significantly greater enhancement of the peripheral zone (peri-infarction region) than the normal myocardium or the center of the infarct,[25,30] whereas reperfused infarcts have shown almost homogeneous enhancement after the administration of T1-enhancing agents using T1-weighted spin-echo imaging.[25,30,37,38] Contrast-enhanced dynamic MRI has also been used to discriminate between occlusive and reperfused infarcts. Echoplanar imaging has been tested for this purpose in the rat model of occlusive and reperfused infarction (Figure 3).[39] In animals subjected

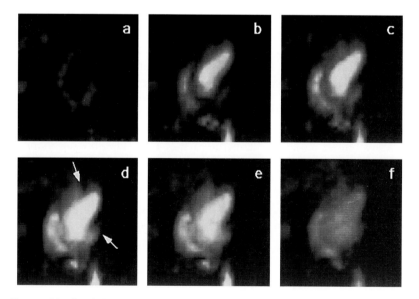

FIGURE 3A. Real-time inversion recovery echoplanar MR images of occlusive myocardial infarction during the transit of 0.025 mmol/kg gadolinium-BOPTA/Dimeglumine. Images were obtained (**a**) before and at (**b**) 4 seconds, (**c**) 6 seconds, (**d**) 10 seconds, and (**e**) 20 seconds and (**f**) 86 seconds after administration of contrast agent. The infarcted region was detected as a zone of low signal intensity (arrows) compared with normal myocardium and chamber blood. Note that unlike reperfused infarction, contrast agent is excluded from the occlusive infarction during the entire observation period.

Signal Intensity
(% of fully relaxed)

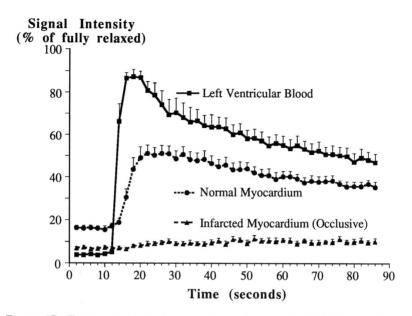

Time (seconds)

FIGURE 3B. Temporal signal changes during the transit of 0.025 mmol/kg on inversion-recovery echoplanar images in nine animals subjected to 2-hour coronary occlusion. Sharp enhancement was observed in normal myocardium and left ventricular chamber blood, but not in the infarcted zone.

to occlusive infarction, inversion recovery echoplanar images exhibited no change in signal intensity in the infarcted region during the first passage of Gd-BOPTA dimeglumine, whereas uninjured myocardium showed rapid enhancement. Reperfused infarcted myocardium showed delayed enhancement and a subsequent gradual increase in signal intensity. By 2 minutes after injection, the signal intensity of reperfused infarctions had increased to a larger value than that of normal myocardium at the peak of the effect of the bolus.

Recent studies have indicated that deoxyhemoglobin has the potential to significantly influence myocardial signal intensity by altering the T2* relaxation rate.[40,41] This intrinsic contrast mechanism has been used to identify areas of reperfused myocardial infarction. In these experiments, significant signal loss was shown in normal myocardium compared with no change in signal of the reperfused infarction during a 60-second period of apnea, thereby demarcating the reperfused injured myocardial region. The hyperintense region depicted during apnea was similar to that noted on follow-up Dy-DTPA-BMA-enhanced echoplanar images. The lack of signal loss in the reperfused infarct during apnea suggests that the injured vascular bed is incapable of altering regional myocardial blood volume in response to a hypoxic challenge.

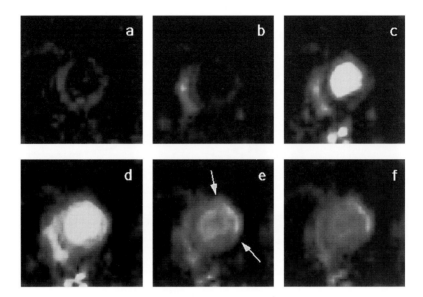

FIGURE 3C. Real-time inversion recovery echoplanar MR images of reperfused irreversibly injured myocardium during the first pass of 0.025 mmol/kg gadolinium-BOPTA/Dimeglumine. Images were acquired (**a**) before and at (**b**) 2 seconds, (**c**) 4 seconds, (**d**) 8 seconds, (**e**) 44 seconds, and (**f**) 86 seconds after administration of contrast agent. Contrast agent initially enters the right ventricle blood in (b), left myocardium in (d). Clearance of contrast agent from reperfused infarcted myocardium is delayed compared with normal myocardium and provided visualization of the injury (arrows) as a zone of relative high signal intensity (hot-spot) in (e) and (f).

Despite the success in differentiating between occlusive and reperfused infarctions in different animal models, in a study of patients, these two types of infarcts could not be consistently discriminated with use of spin-echo imaging.[42] This finding may be related to the long acquisition time, which results in images displaying the steady-state phase of contrast medium distribution. This type of image is influenced by the presence of collateral flow and rapid diffusion of the contrast agent into the center of the infarct, even in occlusive infarcts.

Heterogeneous signal intensity on contrast-enhanced images acquired during the near equilibrium phase of distribution of intravenous injected MR contrast media may reflect intramyocardial hemorrhage and/or functional status of intramyocardial vessels. In rats subjected to increasing severity of myocardial ischemic injury, using low molecular weight contrast media, foci of intramyocardial hemorrhage showed less or no hyperintensity while the remainder of the infarct was hyperintensive.[43] In another similar set of experiments, large infarctions were hyperintense throughout with low molecular weight gadolinium chelates,

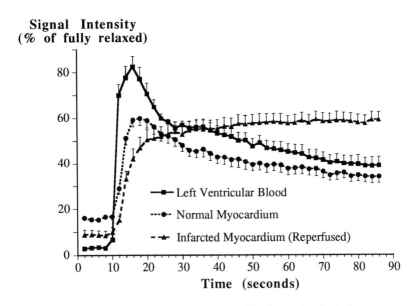

FIGURE 3D. Signal intensity changes observed in nine animals during passage of 0.025 mmol/kg gadolinium-BOPTA/Dimeglumine on inversion recovery echoplanar NMR images. The T1-weighted inversion recovery data were obtained once every 2 seconds. Note that enhancement of signal intensity in the normal myocardium generally preceded that in the reperfused infarcted region, while clearance of contrast agent from the infarcted regions was delayed.

but showed a central zone of lower intensity with high molecular weight (blood pool) gadolinium contrast medium (gadolinium DTPA-albumin).[44] It is theorized that low molecular weight media may reach the central zone by diffusion, whereas blood pool media requires convection or blood flow, this observation suggests loss of intramyocardial vascular function. Loss of intramyocardial vascular function means loss of nutrient vessels due to intramyocardial vascular collapse from severe edema, clogging by neutrophils and other debris, or vessel disintegration (bursting). The latter complication would be expected in association with myocardial hemorrhage.

In addition to evaluating successful reperfusion, contrast-enhanced MRI has been used to discriminate between reversible and irreversible myocardial ischemic injury. This topic is discussed in the next section.

Characterization of Ischemic Myocardial Injuries: Myocardial Viability

Two approaches to characterizing viable versus nonviable myocardium have been pursued using either T1-enhancing contrast media alone or using T1-enhancing and magnetic susceptibility agents together. A number of studies in experimental models have shown that T1-enhancing agents (gadolinium and manganese chelates) increase signal of reversibly injured (ischemically injured but viable) myocardium to a degree similar to normal myocardium.[37,38,,45,46] Likewise, magnetic susceptibility agents (T2* enhancing) reduce signal similarly in ischemically affected viable myocardium and normal myocardium.[1,20]

T1-enhancing media, however produce considerably greater enhancement of irreversibly injured compared with normal myocardium on images acquired at the equilibrium distribution phase.[37,38,45] This observation implies that a relatively greater quantity of contrast medium has distributed into the injured myocardial region. Sequential measurements of the change in T1 relaxivity produced by a gadolinium chelate in normal and injured myocardium compared with the blood pool during the equilibrium distribution phase provides an estimation of the distribution space of the contrast agent.[47] These experiments in rats with reperfused irreversible injury (infarction) estimated a distribution volume equivalent to the intracellular and extracellular space for infarcted myocardium (Figure 4). It is proposed that calculation of the distribution space for T1-enhancing agents in a region of interest encompassing a jeopardized myocardial region could provide a measure of the percentage of necrotic cells in this volume.

After the administration of T2* enhancing agents, the decrease in signal intensity in normal myocardium is caused by dephasing of water molecules, which diffuse through local magnetic field gradients induced by heterogeneous distribution of susceptibility-enhancing agents. Because loss of membrane selectivity is an indicator of cell death, alterations in the potency of susceptibility-dependent signal loss can be related to cell viability. In normal myocardium, cell membranes act as a barrier and limit the distribution of the contrast agent into the intracellular space and thereby cause signal reduction.[17] If the contrast agent distributes homogeneously throughout the cells and interstitium, the local field strength increases slightly without change in field homogenicity and spin dephasing will be much less affected.[19,21] In reperfused infarcted regions, the T2*-enhancing agent initially distributes within the intravascular and interstitial compartments and then rapidly diffuses throughout the intracellular compartments. Equilibration of the T2* contrast agent into the intracellular compartment results in a loss of its effect. This effect is evident on T2*-sensitive images.[19,21]

A rat study in situ showed that Dy-DTPA-BMA caused less signal loss in reperfused infarcted myocardium than normal myocardium on T2-weighted spin-echo images.[21] The results of another study[19] in excised hearts confirmed this finding; Gd-DTPA-BMA and Dy-DTPA-

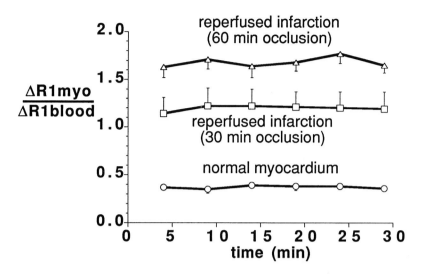

FIGURE 4. Change in ratio of ΔR1 values for myocardium to blood after administration of 0.1 mmol/kg GdDTPA. Note that for both reperfused infarcted myocardium and normal myocardium the ratio value remains constant during the initial 30 minutes after contrast, indicating that equilibrium phase distribution has been achieved during the measurement. Then the fractional distribution volume of the contrast agent can be determined from the product of the δR1 ratio value and the fractional distribution volume for the blood pool (plasma volume ~ 0.6). Accordingly, normal myocardium has fractional distribution volume of 0.22, while that for reperfused infarction prepared by 30- and 60-minute coronary artery occlusions were 0.72 and 1.02, respectively (n = 8).

BMA were adminstered in tandem to rats subjected to irreversible myocardial injury and reperfusion, and spin-echo and GRE imaging were performed. Gd-DTPA-BMA was used to document the presence of flow in the reperfused region and the delivery of contrast agents, whereas Dy-DTPA-BMA was used to assess myocardial viability (Figure 5). While Gd-DTPA-BMA caused a greater increase in signal of the reperfused infarcted region, Dy-DTPA-BMA did not cause the expected decrease in signal of the infarcted region. Chemical analysis confirmed a higher concentration of Dy-DTPA in the infarcted region compared with normal myocardium. The results of these studies indicate that Dy-DTPA-BMA can be used to determine cellular membrane integrity and Gd-DTPA-BMA can be used as a marker of successful reperfusion.

Thus, proof of the concept of using MR strategies for determining myocardial viability and necrosis after ischemic injury now exists. It remains another matter to determine if this approach is sufficiently simple and reliable for clinical application.

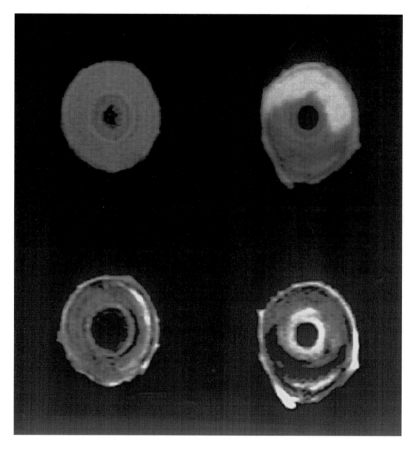

FIGURE 5. Ex vivo rat hearts from animals subjected to 2 hours of occlusion of the anterior coronary artery followed by 1 hour of occlusion prior to sacrifice. Images in **top row** were acquired using T1-weighted spin-echo sequences before (**left**) and after (**right**) injection of both gadolinium DTPA-BMA (Gadodiamide injection, Nycomed, Oslo) and dysprosium DTPA-BMA (Sprodiamide injection, Nycomed, Oslo). Images in **bottom row** were acquired using T2-weighted spin-echo sequences before (**left**) and after (**right**) injection of the two contrast media. The greater enhancement of the infarcted region by the gadolinium chelate indicates reperfusion and increased extracellular space of the infarct. The dysprosium chelate has the same distribution as the gadolinium chelate, but the potency of this agent is greatly reduced in the infarcted region. This is considered to be due to loss of compartmentalization of the agent due to loss of cellular membrane integrity of infarcted myocardium.

Characteristics of Ischemically Stunned Myocardium

Differentiation of stunned, ischemic but viable, from infarcted myocardium has become an important clinical issue in the current era of thrombolytic therapy. Stunned myocardium refers to a reversible postischemic mechanical dysfunction that occurs after reperfusion despite the absence of irreversible damage.[48,49] Noninvasive diagnostic modalities that have the potential to identify myocardial stunning may provide important prognostic information.

MRI has the capability to simultaneously evaluate regional perfusion and contractile function.[50,51] After brief episodes of ischemia and reperfusion, regional myocardial function may be depressed for prolonged periods of time in the absence of sustained abnormalities in perfusion constituting the state of stunned myocardium. Under these circumstances, fast GRE imaging can be used as a noninvasive method to characterize the presence and extent of regional contraction and perfusion abnormalities characteristic of stunned myocardium.

In a recent study, the extent of wall thickening abnormalities, as detected by fast cine MRI, was correlated with the extent of the regional perfusion inhomogeneity, as determined by fast dynamic contrast-enhanced MRI during acute coronary artery occlusion and early reperfusion in a canine model.[52] This study showed that contrast-enhanced inversion recovery fast GRE imaging demonstrates the redistribution of regional blood volume/flow during occlusion and reperfusion. The same ischemic region was defined as a region of low and then high signal intensity during coronary occlusion and reperfusion, respectively. The bright reperfused region on contrast enhanced images was detectable for at least 10 minutes and was dependent on reflow hyperemia. In addition, fast cine MRI documented the presence and quantified the extent of the regional contraction abnormalities in postischemic myocardium. In an area corresponding to the perfusion deficit, fast cine MRI demonstrating systolic wall thinning during occlusion and reduced wall thickening during reperfusion, consistent with the definition of myocardial stunning. Initial but transient recovery in regional wall thickening was associated with increase in regional blood volume/flow as reflected by greater MR contrast enhancement of reperfused myocardium. By 15 to 30 minutes after reperfusion, there was progressive decline in wall thickening in the reperfused region in spite of complete recovery of regional blood flow. Thus, simultaneous monitoring of myocardial perfusion and function, using fast MRI, can be used to characterize regional function and perfusion or blood volume of stunned myocardium.

Evaluation of Myocardial Perfusion: Identification of Hemodynamically Significant Coronary Arterial Stenoses

In the early stage of myocardial ischemia after coronary occlusion, normal and ischemic myocardium show no differential contrast without the aid of MR contrast media. After the administration of Gd-DTPA-BMA[14,42] or Dy-DTPA-BMA,[26] the signal intensity of the ischemic region remains unchanged, and the signal of normally perfused myocardium increases with gadolinium enhancement and decreases with dysprosium administration. The lesser influence of the MR contrast media in the ischemic region at steady-state distribution or during the first passage of the contrast agent at conventional spin-echo or fast

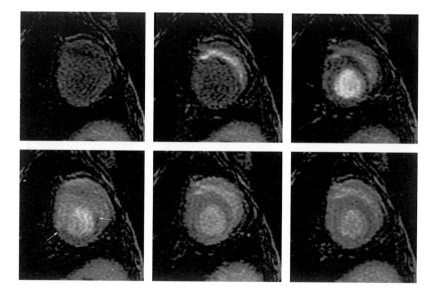

FIGURE 6A. Inversion recovery fast gradient recalled echo images (TR/TE/T1-7.0/2.9/700) during transit of 0.03 gadodiamide through the heart following the infusion of 0.1 mg/kg/min dipyridamole. Selected images are shown in the following order: **top row**; precontrast baseline image **(left)**, after the leading edge of the bolus of gadodiamide entered the right ventricular chamber **(center image)** and then into the left ventricular chamber **(right image)**. **Bottom row**; left image shows the entry of gadodiamide into normally perfused myocardium, but not into the hypoperfused region; center and right images show the redistribution and washout of the contrast medium in the hypoperfused and normal myocardium, respectively. The area at risk (posterior wall of the left ventricle) is shown as a region of low signal intensity compared with normal myocardium.

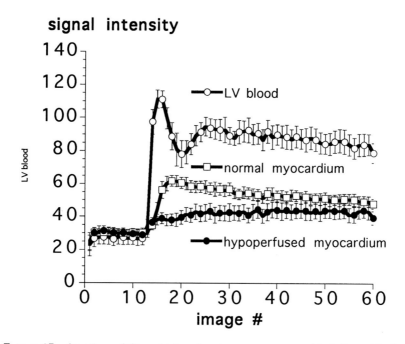

FIGURE 6B. *(continued)* Signal intensity changes measured in left ventricular blood, normal and hypoperfused myocardium of eight dogs during the transit of gadodiamide. In the vasodilated state, the area subserved by the critically stenotic coronary artery was observed as a region of decreased intensity at the peak of the bolus.

imaging, respectively, is caused by exclusion of the contrast medium from the territory of the occluded vessel. The duration of delineation is influenced by the density of the collateral circulation, diffusion of the contrast medium, and the size of the ischemic region.[42,46] In rats, which have poor collateral circulation, gadolinium-enhanced images acquired early after administration (3–15 minutes) exhibit the greatest difference in signal intensity between normal and acutely ischemic myocardium. Later, the contrast agent redistributes into the ischemic region,[24] and contrast between normal and injured myocardium is lost. However, definition of the ischemic myocardium is much more difficult in patients because of better collateral circulation. For this reason, in patients, small ischemic regions are difficult to identify with conventional imaging sequences.[39,40] This problem is less important during the first pass of contrast agent; thus, dynamic studies with fast imaging techniques should allow more accurate depiction of jeopardized myocardium.

Echoplanar and fast GRE imaging have been used to detect regional ischemia in experimental models. In the rat model of ischemia examined with both IR and GRE echoplanar imaging, signal intensity in the territory of the occluded vessel did not change, and the ischemic region was identified as a zone of either low or high signal intensity depending on the dose of the contrast medium and the pulse sequence used.[1,4,5,32] Similar results were obtained in dogs subjected to regional ischemia by means of acute occlusion of the left anterior descending coronary artery, with the use of IR-prepared GRE and fast driven-equilibrium-prepared GRE sequences. While this technique provides definition of the ischemic zone within a single section, it does not provide good coverage of the entire area of injury. Coverage can be improved at the expense of temporal resolution on dynamic images by acquiring images in multiple sections during passage of the bolus.

The region of potential myocardial ischemia served by a critical stenosis of the left anterior descending artery has been demonstrated

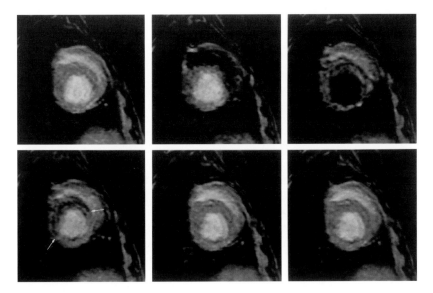

FIGURE 7A. Driven equilibrium fast gradient-recalled echo images (TR/TE/DE delay = 10.2/4.2/60) during transit of 0.4 sprodiamide through the heart. MR images were obtained from the same dog shown in Figure 6, after the infusion of 0.1 mg/kg/min dipyridamole. Selected images were shown in the following order: **top row**; precontrast baseline image (**left**) and after the leading edge of the bolus of sprodiamide entered the right ventricular chamber (**center image**) and then into the left ventricular chamber (**right image**). **Bottom row**; left image shows the hypoperfused region of high signal intensity compared to normally perfused region (arrows); center and right images show the rapid washout of sprodiamide from normally perfused myocardium and the absence of contrast between the two regions.

signal intensity

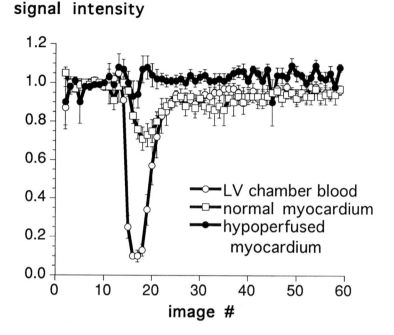

FIGURE 7B. Signal intensity changes measured in left ventricular blood, normal and hypoperfused myocardium of eight dogs during the transit of sprodiamide. Note in the vasodilated state that the hypoperfused myocardium subserved by the critically stenotic coronary artery was demonstrated as a region of high signal intensity compared with normally perfused myocardium.

using both T1 enhancing (Gd-DTPA BMA, gadodiamide) and T2* (Dy-DTPA-BMA, sprodiamide) by comparing images in the basal and vasodilated (dipyridamole) states.[2,53,54] In general, the ischemic region is better demarcated on the first pass of gadodiamide on inversion recovery prepared fast GRE images compared with sprodiamide on driven equilibrium prepared fast GRE images,[54] (Figures 6 and 7).

At the current time two noninvasive imaging techniques are in competition for the clinical detection of significant coronary arterial stenosis, stress nuclear perfusion imaging and stress echocardiographic evaluation of regional myocardial function. Both regional perfusion and contractile function can be assessed with fast GRE or echoplanar imaging.[50,55] Recent studies in our laboratory have used this dual approach for characterizing stunned myocardium[52] and for identifying nonocclusive coronary arterial stenosis. The latter study has shown that the extent of the regional contractile dysfunction is greater than the perfusion deficit demarcated by a gadolinium chelate in the vasodilated (dipyridamole) state. Moreover, contractile dysfunction could sometimes be detected in the basal state in the absence of a recognizable perfusion deficit.

Improvement of Coronary Magnetic Resonance Angiography

Early reports on the feasibility and clinical applications of coronary MRA provided enthusiasm for this as a noninvasive alternative to selective coronary angiography in selected patient populations.[56,57] Another report indicated a diagnostic accuracy of around 50%[58] as compared with greater than 90% in an earlier report.[56] These inconsistent results reveal the limitations of the most popular approach to coronary MRA, breath hold fat saturated two-dimensional acquisitions. Recently, excellent coronary MRA have been achieved using respiratory compensated (navigator echoes) three-dimensional acquisitions.[59,60] The quality and reproducibility of MRA of the chest and abdomen have been greatly improved using a fast three-dimensional time-of-flight method with slow constant infusion of a double or triple dose of gadolinium chelate during most of the acquisition period.[61,62] Because of the time requirement, this approach to respiratory compensated or gated three-dimensional time-of-flight MRA of the coronary arteries is not feasible. Moreover, during the long acquisition period low molecular weight contrast media equilibrates in the extracellular space, causing depression of T1 of myocardium as well as the blood pool so that contrast between vessel and extravascular tissue due to flow effects is diminished. Consequently, high molecular weight (intravascular) MR contrast media seem to be necessary for optimizing respiratory compensated or respiratory gated three-dimensional time-of-flight coronary MRA.

Recently, we have used a blood pool MR contrast medium (Gd-DTPA-albumin) in an attempt to provide a high-contrast three-dimensional data set for reconstruction of the coronary arteries. This technique uses respiratory gating, electrocardiographic referencing, and three-dimensional fast GRE acquisition after the administration of the Gd-DTPA albumin.

Ischemic heart disease is the most prevalent cause of mortality and morbidity in many countries of the world. Consequently, the importance of MR in cardiovascular disease depends on its recognition as an important noninvasive imaging technique for this disease. It seems evident that the attainment of reliable coronary MRA is crucial to the emergence of MR in the evaluation of ischemic heart disease. With the attainment of this capability, MR could realize the so often vocalized hope of a one-stop imaging technique for ischemic heart disease. It would serve as a single noninvasive test for defining coronary morphology, coronary function (flow in basal and vasodilated states), myocardial contractile function and perfusion, and myocardial viability.

References

1. Wendland MF, Saeed M, Masui T, et al. First pass of an MR susceptibility contrast agent through normal and ischemic heart: Gradient-recalled echoplanar imaging. *J Magn Reson Imaging.* 1993;3:755–760.
2. Wilke N, Simm C, Zhang J, et al. Contrast-enhanced first pass myocardial perfusion imaging: Correlation between myocardial blood flow in dogs at rest and during hyperemia. *Magn Reson Med.* 1993;29:485–497.
3. Saeed M, Wendland MF, Higgins CB. Contrast media for MR imaging of the heart. *J Magn Reson Imaging.* 1994;4:269–279.
4. Yu KK, Saeed M, Wendland MF, et al. Real-time dynamics of an extravascular magnetic resonance contrast medium in acutely infarcted myocardium using inversion recovery and gradient-recalled echo-planar imaging. *Invest Radiol.* 1992;27:927–934.
5. Wendland MF, Saeed M, Masui T, et al. Echo-planar MR imaging of normal and ischemic myocardium with gadodiamide injection. *Radiology.* 1993;186: 535–542.
6. Higgins CB, Saeed M, Wendland MF, et al. Contrast media for cardiothoracic MR imaging. *J Magn Reson Imaging.* 1993;3:265–276.
7. Higgins CB, Saeed M, Wendland MF. Contrast enhancement for the myocardium. *Magn Reson Med.* 1991;22:347–353.
8. Manning WJ, Atkinson DJ, Grossman W, et al. First-pass nuclear magnetic resonance imaging studies using gadolinium-DTPA in patients with coronary artery disease. *J Am Coll Cardiol.* 1991;18:959–965.
9. Schaefer S, van Tyen R, Saloner D. Evaluation of myocardial perfusion abnormalities with gadolinium-enhanced snapshot MR imaging in humans: work in progress. *Radiology.* 1992;185:795–801.
10. van Rugge FP, Borell JJ, van der Wall EE, et al. Cardiac first-pass and myocardial perfusion in normal subjects assessed by sub-second Gd DTPA enhanced MR imaging. *J Comput Assist Tomogr.* 1991;15:959–965.
11. Eichgstaedt WH, Felix F, Dougherty RC. Magnetic resonance imaging at different stages of myocardial infarction using contrast agent gadolinium DTPA. *Clin Cardiol.* 1986;9:527–535.
12. Dulce MC, Duerinckx AJ, Hartiala J, et al. MR imaging of the myocardium using nonionic contrast medium: Signal-intensity changes in patients with subacute myocardial infarction. *AJR.* 1993;160:963–970.
13. Nishimura T, Kobayashi H, O'Hara Y, et al. Serial assessment of myocardial infarction by using gated MR imaging and Gd-DTPA. *AJR.* 1989;153: 715–720.
14. van der Wall EE, van Dijkman PR, de Roos A, et al. Diagnostic significance of gadolinium-DTPA (diethylenetriamine pentaacetic acid) enhanced magnetic resonance imaging in thrombolytic treatment for acute myocardial infarction: its potential in assessing reperfusion. *Br Heart J.* 1990;63:12–17.
15. de Roos A, Mathejissen NA, Doornbos J, et al. Myocardial infarct size after reperfusion therapy: Assessment with Gd-DTPA-enhanced MR imaging. *Radiology.* 1990;176:517–521.

16. Saeed M, Wendland MF, Masui T, et al. Dual mechanisms for change in myocardial intensity by means of a single MR contrast medium: Dependence on concentration and pulse sequence. *Radiology.* 1993;186:175–182.

17. Thuborn K, Waterton J, Mathews P, Radda G. Oxygenation dependence of the transverse relaxation time of water protons in whole blood at high field. *Biochim Biophys Acta.* 1982;717:265–270.

18. Rozenman Y, Zou XM, Kantor HI. Cardiovascular MR imaging with iron oxide particles: Utility of a superparamagnetic contrast agent and the role of diffusion in signal loss. *Radiology.* 1990;175:655–659.

19. Geschwind JF, Saeed M, Wendland MF, et al. Evidence for loss of compartmentalization in reperfused infarcted myocardium on contrast-enhanced MR imaging. Presented at the 94th Annual Meeting of the American Roentgen Ray Society, New Orleans, LA, April 24–29, 1994.

20. Saeed M, Wendland MF, Tomei E, et al. Demarcation of myocardial ischemia: Magnetic susceptibility effect of contrast medium in MR imaging. *Radiology.* 1989;173:763–767.

21. Saeed M, Wendland MF, Masui T, Higgins CB. Myocardial infarction on T1- and susceptibility-enhanced MRI: Evidence for loss of compartmentalization of contrast media. *Magn Reson Med.* 1994;31:31–39.

22. Schmiedl U, Sievers RE, Brasch RC, et al. Acute myocardial ischemia and reperfusion: MR imaging with albumin-Gd DTPA. *Radiology.* 1989;170: 351–356.

23. Schmiedl U, Brasch RC, Ogan MD, Moseley ME. Albumin labeled with Gd DTPA: An intravascular contrast-enhancing agent for magnetic resonance blood pool and perfusion imaging. *Acta Radiol.* 1990;374(suppl):99–102.

24. Wolfe CL, Moseley ME, Wikstrom MG, et al. Assessment of myocardial salvage after ischemia and reperfusion using magnetic resonance imaging and spectroscopy. *Circulation.* 1989;80:969–982.

25. Saeed M, Wendland MF, Masui T, et al. Myocardial infarction: assessment with an intravascular MR contrast medium: Work in progress. *Radiology.* 1991;180:153–160.

26. Bol A, Melin JA, Vanoverschelde JL, et al. Direct comparison of [13–N] ammonia and [15–O] water estimates of perfusion with quantification of regional myocardial blood flow by microspheres. *Circulation.* 1993;87: 512–525.

27. Cavagna FM, Marzola P, Dapra M, et al. Binding of Gd-BOPTA/dimeg to proteins extravasated into interstitial space enhances conspicuity of reperfused infarcts. *Invest Radiol.* 1994;29(suppl 2): S50–S53.

28. Willerson H, Watson J, Hutton I, et al. Reduced myocardial reflow and increased coronary vascular resistance following prolonged myocardial ischemia in the dog. *Circ Res.* 1975;36:771–781.

29. Higgins CB, Herfkens R, Lipton MJ, et al. Nuclear magnetic resonance imaging of acute myocardial infarction in dogs: Alterations in magnetic resonance relaxation times. *Am J Cardiol.* 1983;53:184–188.

30. Saeed M, Wendland MF, Takehara Y, Masui T, Higgins CB. Reperfusion and irreversible myocardial injury: Identification with a nonionic MR imaging contrast medium. *Radiology.* 1992;182:675–683.

31. Saeed M, Wendland MF, Yu KK, et al. Dual effects of gadodiamide injection in depiction of the region of myocardial ischemia. *J Magn Reson Imaging.* 1993;3:21–29.

32. Wendland MF, Saeed M, Higgins CB. Strategies for differential enhancement of myocardial ischemia using echo-planar imaging. *Invest Radiol.* 1991; 26:S236–S238.

33. Caputo GR, Sechtem U, Tscholakoff D, Higgins CB. Measurement of myocardial infarction size at early and late time intervals using MR imaging. *AJR.* 1987;149:237–243.
34. Yu KK, Saeed M, Wendland MF, et al. Comparison of T1-enhancing and magnetic susceptibility magnetic resonance contrast agents for demarcation of the jeopardy area in experimental myocardial infarction. *Invest Radiol.* 1993;28:1015–1023.
35. de Roos A, Kundel HL, Joseph PM, et al. Variability of myocardial signal on magnetic resonance images. *Invest Radiol.* 1990;25:1024–1028.
36. Ito H, Toomoki T, Sakai N, et al. Lack of myocardial reperfusion immediately after successful thrombolysis. *Circulation.* 1992;85:1699–1705.
37. Saeed M, Wagner S, Wendland MF, et al. Occlusive and reperfused myocardial infarcts: Differentiation with Mn-DPDP-enhanced MR imaging. *Radiology.* 1989;172:59–64.
38. Saeed M, Wendland MF, Takehara Y, Higgins CB. Reversible and irreversible injury in the reperfused myocardium: Differentiation with contrast material-enhanced MR imaging. *Radiology.* 1990;175:633–637.
39. Saeed M, Wendland MF, Yu KK, et al. Identification of myocardial reperfusion using echo planar MR imaging: Discrimination between occlusive and reperfused infarctions. *Circulation.* 1994;90:1492–1501.
40. Wendland MF, Saeed M, Lauerma K, de Crespigny A, Moseley ME, Higgins CB. Endogenous susceptibility contrast in myocardium during apnea measured using gradient recalled echo planar imaging. *Magn Reson Med.* 1993;29:273–276.
41. Atalay MK, Forder JR, Chacko VP, Kawamoto S, Zerhouni EA. Oxygenation in the rabbit myocardium: Assessment with susceptibility-dependent MR imaging. *Radiology.* 1993;189:759–764.
42. de Roos A, van Rossum AC, van der Wall E, et al. Reperfused and nonreperfused myocardial infarction: Diagnostic potential of Gd-DTPA-enhanced MR imaging. *Radiology.* 1989;172:717–720.
43. Canet E, Wendland MF, Saeed M, et al. Validation of contrast enhanced MRI to detect "no reflow" zones in reperfused myocardial infarction: Lack of specificity of thioflavine S to define the no reflow zone. In: Proceedings of the International Society of Magnetic Resonance in Medicine, New York, 1996, p. 1983.
44. Shwitters J, Saeed M, Wendland MF, et al. Characterization of injured myocardium using gadolinium based MR contrast media. In: Proceedings of the International Society of Magnetic Resonance in Medicine. New York, 1996, p. 688.
45. Masui T, Saeed M, Wendland MF, Higgins CB. Occlusive and reperfused myocardial infarcts: MR differentiation with nonionic Gd-DTPA BMA. *Radiology.* 1991;181:77–83.
46. Lim TH, Lee DH, Kim YH, et al. Occlusive and reperfused myocardial infarction: Detection by using MR imaging with gadolinium polylysine enhancement. *Radiology.* 1993;189:765–768.
47. Wendland MF, Saeed M, Lauerma K, et al. Alterations in T1 in normal and reperfused infarcted myocardium following Gd BOPTA or Gd DTPA on inversion recovery EPI. *Magn Reson Med.* 1997;37:448–456.
48. Braunwald E, Kloner RA. The stunned myocardium: Prolonged, post-ischemic ventricular dysfunction. *Circulation.* 1982;66:1146–1149.
49. Bolli R. Mechanism of myocardial stunning. *Circulation.* 1990;82:731–738.
50. Steffens JC, Sakuma H, Bourne MW, Higgins CB. MR imaging in ischemic heart disease. *Am Heart J.* 1996;132:156–173.

51. Pflugfelder PW, Sechtem UP, White RD, Higgins CB. Quantification of regional myocardial function by rapid (cine) magnetic resonance imaging. *AJR*. 1988;150:523–530.
52. Szolar DH, Saeed M, Wendland MF, et al. MR imaging characterization of post ischemic myocardial dysfunction ("stunned myocardium"): relationship between functional and perfusion abnormalities. JMRI 1996 (in press).
53. Saeed M, Wendland MF, Sakuma H, Geschwind J-F, Derugin N, Cavagna FM, Higgins CB. Coronary artery stenosis: Detection with contrast-enhanced MR imaging in dogs. *Radiology*. 1995;196:79–84.
54. Saeed M, Wendland MF, Szolar D, et al. Quantification of extent of area at risk with fast contrast enhanced MRI in experimental coronary artery stenosis. *Am Heart J*. 1996;132:921–932.
55. Higgins CB, Saeed M, Wendland M, et al. Evaluation of myocardial function and perfusion in ischemic heart disease. *MAGMA*. 1994;128(2):326–332.
56. Manning WJ, Li W, Edelman RR. A preliminary report comparing MR angiography with conventional angiography. *N Engl J Med*. 1994;328:828–832.
57. Pennell DJ, Keegan J, Firmin DN, et al. Magnetic resonance imaging of the coronary arteries: Technique and preliminary results. *Br Heart J*. 1993;70:315–326.
58. Deurinckx AJ, Urman MK. Two-dimensional coronary MRA analysis of initial clinical results. *Radiology*. 1994;193:732–738.
59. Wang Y, Rossman PJ, Grimm RC, et al. Navigator echo based real time respiratory gating and triggering of respiratory effects in 3D coronary MRA. *Radiology*. 1996;198:55–60.
60. Haacke EM, Li D, Kaushikkar S. Cardiac MR imaging: Principles and techniques. *Topic Magn Reson Imaging*. 1995;7:200–217.
61. Prince MR. Gadolinium-enhanced MR aortography. *Radiology*. 1994;191:155–164.
62. Prince MR, Narasingham DC, Stanley JC, et al. Breath hold gadolinium-enhanced MRA of the abdominal aorta and its major branches. *Radiology*. 1995;197:785–792.

Chapter 14

Assessment of Regional and Transmural Myocardial Function Using Tagging Techniques

Leon Axel, PhD, MD

Magnetic resonance imaging (MRI) provides a powerful tool for the study of cardiac function. It is noninvasive and does not require the use of ionizing radiation. The generally excellent contrast between the heart wall and the blood within the cardiac chamber provides good delineation of the myocardial borders without the need for the injection of a contrast agent. MRI is tomographic in nature, with a free choice of orientation of the imaging planes and with true three-dimensional registration between different images. Thus, the three-dimensional structure of the heart can be reconstructed accurately. In addition to the measures of regional function that can be derived from such three-dimensional tomographic imaging, MRI has intrinsic sensitivity to motion that can be exploited for further analysis of regional wall function. The motion effects of MRI that can be used for the study of heart function are primarily the phase shifts acquired by moving excited spins, which can be used to derive local myocardial velocities, and the ability to create regional patterns of perturbation of the magnetization, which can serve as MRI visible tags to demonstrate regional motion and deformation. In this chapter, we will be primarily concerned with the analysis of such tagged MRI studies of the heart wall. Finally, MRI provides the potential capability of studying many other aspects of the heart, such as regional perfusion. As these other aspects of the state of the heart can be acquired at the same imaging session as regional function studies, this will permit accurate spatial registration of regional mea-

Research supported by NIH grant HL43014.

From: Higgins CB, Ingwall JS, Pohost GM, (eds). *Current and Future Applications of Magnetic Resonance in Cardiovascular Disease.* Armonk, NY: Futura Publishing Company, Inc.; © 1998.

sures of both mechanical function and these other parameters, such as perfusion. This should permit improved analysis of such conditions as stunning and hibernation.

Using conventional MRI, we can calculate the cardiac chamber volume as a function of cardiac phase by integrating the cavity area in sequential stacked image slices and then computing the equivalent enclosed volume based on the spacing between the slices. This can be used to calculate conventional measures of global cardiac function such as stroke volume and ejection fraction. Visual assessment of a dynamic cine loop display of consecutive phases of the cardiac cycle is also helpful for qualitative assessment of both overall cardiac function and regional wall motion. Methods similar to those used to analyze echocardiographic images can also be used to assess local wall motion and thickening more quantitatively from serial magnetic resonance (MR) images of a given slice. However, in common with the echocardiographic methods, there are several problems associated with such quantitative analyses of regional motion from conventional MRI. First, what reference frame should be used to assess local wall motion? If the motion is referred to the magnet coordinate system, any overall motion of the heart will be reflected in an apparent regional variation of the local motion. If the reference frame is chosen to be centered on a point that moves with the heart, such as the centroid of the ventricular cavity, the motion of this reference point may still be affected by local variations in cardiac function. As the heart generally moves through space in a somewhat complex manner, in general, there will be a component of motion through the plane of the image. As the heart is a tapered conical structure, its motion through a fixed imaging plane can result in an artifactual apparent motion of the portion of the wall imaged (as the intersection of the imaging plane and the heart). Similarly, variations in the angle of intersection between the heart wall and the imaging plane can result in apparent changes in the imaged thickness of the heart wall. Finally, the paucity of trackable landmarks in the heart, and the essential lack of them within the heart wall, means that any components of motion other than those perpendicular to the heart wall are essentially invisible, including any transmural variation in regional wall motion.

The use of the additional motion information provided by the intrinsic motion sensitivity of MRI permits us to overcome many of these limitations of conventional MRI studies of regional cardiac function. In particular, magnetization tagging studies, using techniques such as spatial modulation of magnetization (SPAMM),[1] provides a robust and direct method of assessing displacement of the tag locations within the imaged heart wall. Using SPAMM, we can create a regular grid of tags

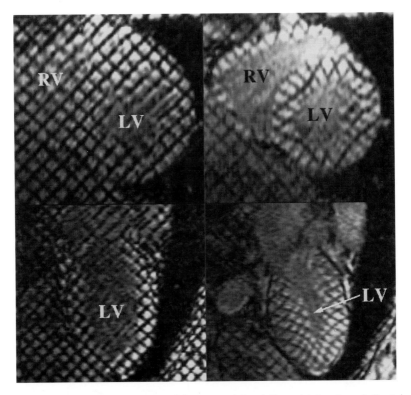

FIGURE 1. Midventricular tagged images of the left ventricle at end-diastole (**left**) and end systole (**right**). Both endocardial and epicardial contours as well as SPAMM stripe intersection points can be seen.

(Figure 1). As the motion of these tags in the image directly reflects the motion of the underlying heart wall, analysis of the motion and deformation of this grid permits us to analyze the corresponding underlying wall motion. The limitation on resolution of these tag patterns is essentially determined by the corresponding limits of resolution of the imaging process itself. Tag lines that are finer than the corresponding resolution elements of the image will have a decreased apparent image contrast. Tag lines that are too closely spaced may be blurred together. It also may be more difficult to track individual tag lines from one image frame to the next if the spacing is too small for the imaging resolution and the time interval between consecutive frames. As the tagging is performed as essentially a preconditioning pulse sequence, analogous to the inversion pulses used for inversion in inversion-recovery imaging, they can be readily combined with any desired MRI techniques. In particular, they can be used in conjunction with breathhold imaging techniques to reduce the degrading effects of respiratory motion on the tagged images. One limitation of the magnetization tagging method is that the tags fade with time, due to relaxation of the local magnetization perturbation. However, for appropriate choices of tagging methods and imaging techniques, the tags can be followed for a large fraction of the cardiac cycle.

In order to validate the reliability of magnetization tags as markers for the motion of the underlying tissue, phantom studies have been performed using deformable objects whose motion can be controlled.[2] In particular, the observed motion of the magnetization tags can be compared both with direct optical observation of physical markers on a deforming phantom and with theoretical predictions of the distribution of motion within the object. Such studies have shown excellent correlation of the magnetization tag motion with the independently determined motion of the phantoms.

Analysis of Tagged Cardiac Images

Magnetization tags are generally created by perturbing the magnetization in planes perpendicular to the imaging plane, so that the intersection of the tagged planes and the imaging plane is seen as a corresponding set of dark stripes. Even if there is motion through the imaging plane between the times of tagging and subsequent imaging, the initial location of points within a given stripe being tracked will still be known in the direction orthogonal to the stripe. This is important, as it permits us to provide a set of one-dimensional constraints on the motion of the heart wall, even with the general three-dimensional motion of the heart relative to the imaging system. By combining such motion information from orthogonal sets of tags and from orthogonal sets of tagged images, a full three-dimensional picture of the motion of the heart wall can be reconstructed. This, in turn, can be used to calculate different measures of local function, and the results can be used to create functional image displays of the regional function.

A clear qualitative assessment of regional function can be quickly gained by visual analysis of a dynamic display of tagged cardiac images. Those areas with poor cardiac function show corresponding diminished displacement and distortion of the local tag pattern during the cardiac cycle. However, for a quantitative assessment of cardiac function, we must extract the corresponding position information for the tagged locations from the images, for further numerical processing. This can be done either manually or with more automated methods

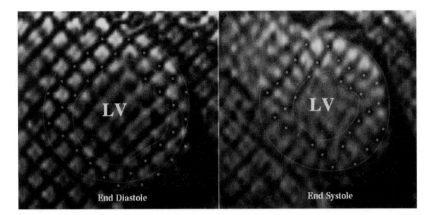

FIGURE 2. Midventricular short-axis (**top**) and long-axis (**bottom**) tagged images of the left ventricle at end diastole (**left**) and end systole (**right**). SPAMM stripe deformation can clearly be seen between end diastole and end systole.

(Figure 2). While manual methods for tracking tag positions are straightforward, they are also tedious and time consuming. More automated methods can be more rapidly performed, but generally require some supervision to avoid interference from image artifacts or other imperfections.

Automated Approaches to Tagged Image Analysis

In extracting tag position information from images, we can look for the intersections of tag grids, using a matched-filter approach of detecting those portions of the image that most resemble a stored or computed representation of a "standard" grid intersection,[3] or we can track the tag lines themselves. As one way to track the tag lines, we could track the whole grid pattern, assuming we can predict its local intensity variation, with optical flow methods.[4] One approach our group has focused on is the use of "snakes" or "active contours,"[5-7] in which the tracked line is modeled as if it were a physical spline, with controllable stiffness and rigidity, acted on by image forces, such as the image intensity or strength of edges. An attractive feature of the snakes approach is that it can also incorporate the use of user-supplied forces, eg, through the screen cursor, to provide user interaction. This permits easy guidance of the tag tracking process, as the user can easily push the line being extracted away from undesired image features and onto the tag to be tracked. This snakes approach can be similarly incorporated into the extraction of tag grid intersections.[8]

The development of automated or semiautomated approaches to tag position analysis is important, as it can speed up the analysis to more clinically usable times than is possible with manual tracking. As many tag positions must be tracked through multiple cardiac cycle phases, this can otherwise be a major task. The use of more automated methods also has the potential to reduce variability in the extracted position information.

Motion Variables

The use of conventional MRI has permitted measurement of the radial component of the motion of the inner or outer surfaces of the heart wall, eg, relative to the centroid of the ventricular cavity in the image. However, with tagged MRI, we can now follow the motion of material points within the heart wall. This makes possible many more ways to analyze the local motion of the myocardium. Once we have derived a model of the distribution of the material point motions within the wall from the tag displacements (as discussed further below), we can calculate different variables to characterize the motion in each local region. It is convenient to consider the local motion as composed of a rigid body component, encompassing displacement and rigid body rotation, and deformation (or strain); the calculation of these variables from the raw motion data is relatively straightforward.

The displacement of a given region is easy to understand. It is a vector quantity (with magnitude and direction), and tells us how far and in what direction the region has moved, after removing the effects of rotation and deformation. It is similar to the kinds of information obtained from conventional imaging, but we are not confined only to the radial component and we have the potential to look at the transmural variation in motion. When used with three-dimensional motion data analysis, it can also account for through-plane motion.

The rigid body rotation of a region is also relatively easy to understand, although it cannot be determined with conventional imaging methods. For two-dimensional imaging, it will be a signed scalar quantity, reflecting the direction and amount of local rotation. For three-dimensional motion analysis, there is additional information on the orientation of the local axis of rotation.

The local strain is a less familiar concept, and is a tensor quantity, which is somewhat more complex than a vector. Essentially, the value of the strain reflects the fractional change in length of a hypothetical line segment in the tissue, due to the motion. In general, this will be dependent on the orientation of the line segment, as the tissue at a given location may be lengthening in one direction, eg, radially, at the same time as it is contracting in another, eg, circumferentially. The distribution of the strain values in different directions at a given location will describe an ellipsoid (or an ellipse in a two-dimensional image of motion). The directions of the axes of this ellipsoid are called the principal directions or eigenvectors of the strain tensor, and the lengths of the axes are the "principal values" or eigenvalues. Considering the strain along the eigenvectors has the nice property that the deformation only causes a change in length; in other directions, the associated shear will also result in some rotation.

A major advantage of decomposing the motion into rigid body and strain components is that the resulting strain values are independent of the choice of external reference frame, and reflect only the local change in the state of the tissue. Thus, we can avoid the problems associated with the choice of reference frame found with analysis of conventional wall motion imaging. While the eigenvectors and eigenvalues provide a convenient way to characterize the strain, we can alternatively calculate the corresponding strain values in any desired direction, eg, in local radial, longitudinal and circumferential directions; we will also then need to calculate the corresponding shear values.

To calculate the regional strain and other motion variables from two-dimensional images of a tagging grid, we can follow two approaches. First, we can use the tracked positions of the intersections of the tagging grid to divide the wall into a set of triangles delineated by adjacent triplets of intersection points. If we assume that the deformation is homogeneous within these triangles, sequential positions of the vertices of the triangles will fully determine the rigid body motion and strain within the triangular regions.[9] Alternatively, we can use the sequential positions of the tagging grid to estimate the motion within the wall as a smoothly varying function of position, using finite element techniques. We can then calculate the corresponding (inhomogeneous) distribution of the motion variables.

This two-dimensional analysis of motion can be useful for identifying and characterizing wall motion abnormalities. However, as the heart actually moves in a complex three-dimensional pattern, we would like to analyze the corresponding motion variables for this full three-dimensional motion. We can do so by combining the motion data from two orthogonal sets of tagged images to create a three-dimensional model of the local wall motion, again using finite element techniques (Figure 3).[7,10] We can do this as long as the two orthogonal sets of tagged images are acquired in good spatial registration with each other. While most subjects are able to remain immobile for the time required to acquire these image sets, there may be some motion between the two acquisitions. However, as long as each of the two data sets is in

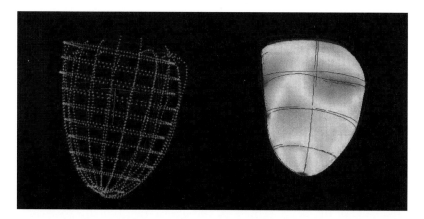

FIGURE 3. Three-dimensional wire model of the left ventricle (FEM). The crosses represent contour data points; the lines represent the element borders (**left**). Three-dimensional strain map of the same model (**right**). The variations in shading (when in color) represent different amounts of strain across the heart.

good registration internally, the two sets of motion data can be moved together to bring the whole set into registration.

For application to analysis of the motion of the right ventricle (RV), we must modify these methods to account for the normally much thinner RV free wall. However, using one-dimensional tagging grids to track the motion of the free wall, and adapting the finite element methods, we can reconstruct the motion of the midwall of the RV free wall and calculate the corresponding motion variables in the local plane of the wall.

Display

The motion of the heart, and the associated motion variables, are intrinsically difficult to display, as they describe a thick-walled structure that is evolving in time. The use of pseudocolor displays of the local values of scalar quantities, such as the magnitude of the displacement or the eigenvalues, can be used to create functional images of the motion between two time points in the cardiac cycle by mapping the colors onto the corresponding two-dimensional images or a three-dimensional surface such as the midwall of the heart. The higher order motion quantities, such as the displacement vectors or the strain tensors, can be displayed with regional superimposed arrow or trihedral symbols. Having an interactive computer display available is valuable both for dynamic displays of the time evolution of the motion and for better displaying three-dimensional structures.

An alternative approach to analysis and display of regional motion is to represent the motion as a set of relatively intuitive parametric functions such as twist or radial contraction, that can be used to fit the observed motion data derived from the tagged images. The local values of these parametric functions can then be used to generate a set of functional images, again using a pseudocolor representation of the corresponding parameter values on a desired surface.

The normal regional variation in the values of the motion variables must be taken into account in considering the significance of the value at a given location. As the experience with these motion measurement techniques grows, so that the normal values and ranges of these variables get better defined, this information will be able to be incorporated into the display so that abnormal areas can be highlighted.

As the ability of MRI to produce regional maps of other myocardial function measures, such as perfusion, is developed further, we will need to consider how best to produce combined displays. While pairs of functional images can simply be presented side by side, displays of combined measures may be valuable for highlighting areas such as perfusion/function mismatches.

Conclusion

The use of tagged MRI to study the heart offers a new and potentially powerful way to evaluate regional and transmural variation in cardiac function. While the methods to perform this analysis and to display the results are still under development, it is likely that we will obtain useful new information about cardiac function from them, particularly in conjunction with other MRI-derived measures of the heart such as perfusion.

References

1. Axel L, Dougherty L. Heart wall motion: Improved method of spatial modulation of magnetization for MR imaging. *Radiology.* 1988;172:349–350.
2. Young A, Axel L, Dougherty L, et al. Validation of tagging with MR imaging to estimate material deformation. *Radiology.* 1993;188:101–108.
3. Fisher D. Automated Tracking of Cardiac Wall Motion Using Magnetic Resonance *Markers*. Iowa City: University of Iowa; 1990. Ph. D. dissertation.
4. Prince JL, McVeigh ER. Motion estimation form tagged MR image sequences. *IEEE Trans Med Imaging.* 1992;11:238–249.
5. Kass M, Witkin A, Terzopoulos D. Snakes: Active contour models. *Int J Comput Vision.* 1987;1:321–331.
6. Kumar S, Goldgof D. Automatic tracking of SPAMM grid and the estima-

tion of deformation parameters from cardiac MR images. *IEEE Trans Med Imaging* 1994;13:122–132.

7. Young AA, Kraitchman DL, Dougherty L, et al. Tracking and finite element analysis of stripe deformation in magnetic resonance tagging. *IEEE Trans Med Imaging* 1995;14:413–421.

8. Kraitchman DL, Young AA, Chang C-N, et al. Semi-automatic tracking of myocardial motion in MR tagged images. *IEEE Trans Med Imaging* 1995; 14:422–433.

9. Axel L, Gonçalves R, Bloomgarden D. Regional heart wall motion: Two-dimensional analysis and functional imaging with MR tagging. *Radiology.* 1992;183:745–750.

10. Young AA, Axel L. Three-dimensional motion and deformation in the heart wall: Estimation from spatial modulation of magnetization—A model-based approach. *Radiology.* 1992;185:241–247.

## Chapter 15

Assessment of Myocardial Viability By Magnetic Resonance Techniques

Udo Sechtem, MD, Frank M. Baer, MD,
Peter Theissen, MD, Eberhard Voth, MD,
and Harald Schicha, MD

Introduction

Magnetic resonance imaging (MRI) is probably the best technique to visualize the anatomy and function of the left ventricular myocardium. One of the early reports on visualization of ischemically damaged left ventricles noted that patients with chronic myocardial infarcts showed severely thinned myocardium in the infarct region.[1] Severe thinning of the myocardium is a typical feature of transmural scar without significant amounts of residual viable cells as observed at necropsy.[2] Thus, in analogy to the findings at necropsy, the observation of severely thinned and akinetic myocardium by MRI might permit the identification of long-term myocardial scar and exclude the presence of viable myocardium in the respective region.

Viable myocardium is characterized by severe dysfunction at baseline that recovers with time (stunned myocardium) or after revascularization (hibernating myocardium). Whether the ischemically injured myocardium is potentially able to recover or not can be predicted by using low-dose dobutamine infusions and observing the contractile reserve of the myocardial region of interest.[3] The advent of rapid magnetic resonance pulse sequences permits functional evaluation of the left ventricle within 30 minutes that is comparable to the time needed

From: Higgins CB, Ingwall JS, Pohost GM, (eds). *Current and Future Applications of Magnetic Resonance in Cardiovascular Disease.* Armonk, NY: Futura Publishing Company, Inc.; © 1998.

for an echocardiographic dobutamine study. Improved contraction after dobutamine stimulation corresponds to viable myocardium and the combination of functional and anatomic information makes MRI a very attractive technique for studying myocardial viability.

Magnetic resonance techniques are, however, not limited to depicting myocardium anatomy and function. Other information pertaining to myocardial viability includes the signal intensity of acutely ischemically injured myocardium, the signal intensity and time course after the application of intravenous contrast agents, the application of myocardial tagging to study three-dimensional myocardial motion, and the direct observation of high-energy phosphates within the injured myocardium by using magnetic resonance spectroscopy (MRS). This chapter focuses on features of viable and scarred myocardium as characterized by magnetic resonance techniques and compares the information provided by magnetic resonance techniques with that provided by scintigraphic techniques that are currently the standard of reference for the identification of viable myocardium.

Stunning and Hibernation

The concept of myocardial viability arose from the observation that severely dysfunctional myocardium had the potential to recover either spontaneously or after revascularization. The dysfunctional state of the myocardium that can be produced by a brief occlusion of a coronary artery and the subsequent restoration of blood flow is termed stunning. After restoration of blood flow, stunned myocardium recovers spontaneously, but the time course of recovery depends on the extent of the perfusion abnormality during the preceding phase of ischemia and dysfunction may be present for several weeks although coronary blood flow is normal.[4]

In contrast to stunning, hibernation refers to a condition characterized by a prolonged dysfunction of the myocardium due to prolonged periods of ischemia or chronically reduced perfusion in severe coronary artery disease.[5] Clinically, this condition can be found in patients with occluded coronary arteries with or without a history of myocardial infarction. Residual perfusion may be maintained through collaterals, preventing complete irreversible structural damage to the myocardial region perfused by the occluded artery. Identification of myocardial hibernation is a challenge to the clinician because revascularization of these regions may result in complete restitution of regional contractile function.[6] The pathophysiology of hibernation has not yet entirely clarified due to the inability to develop an animal model of hibernation in which a state of low perfusion and absent contraction could be preserved for a longer period of time.

Magnetic Resonance Identification of Viable Myocardium in Acute Myocardial Infarcts

Signal Intensity Measurements

An early attempt to identify the presence and the extent of myocardial necrosis early after the ischemic event was using the increased signal intensity of freshly infarcted myocardium for defining the infarct zone. However, the increase in signal intensity is due to myocardial edema that can also be observed within interspersed surviving myocardium (Figure 1). Therefore, early after the infarct, the planimetered area of high signal intensity overestimates the area of necrosis. However, 3 weeks after the infarct, true infarct size shows a good correlation the area of increase signal intensity presumably because the edema surrounding infarct zone has regressed.[7] Ryan and coworkers[8] demonstrated that magnetic resonance signal intensity measurements can indeed be used to distinguish between viable and infarcted myocardium.[8] Stunned and infarcted myocardial regions were produced in dogs by reversibly occluding a coronary artery for various time intervals. In contrast to infarcted myocardium, stunned myocardium did not show increases in signal intensity despite regional systolic dysfunction. The same phenomenon may be expected to also occur in humans but there have been no reports concerning signal intensity measurements in patients with stunned myocardium.

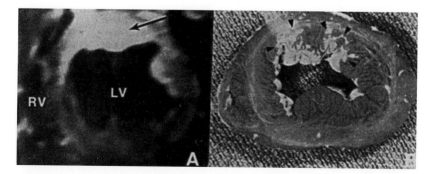

FIGURE 1. Short-axis spin-echo image (echo time 60 ms) of ex vivo dog heart **(A)** and corresponding triphenyltetrazolium chloride-stained specimen **(B)**. The heart was subjected to 3 hours of coronary artery occlusion. The infarct is small, patchy, and predominantly subendocardial (black arrowheads). The region of increased signal intensity on the MR image (large arrow) is more transmural and clearly overestimates true infarct size. LV indicates left ventricle; RV, right ventricle. (Reprinted with permission from Reference 8.)

Contrast Agents

Gadolinium and manganese-based compounds have been used as contrast agents in animal models to differentiate between reversible and irreversible injury (stunning and necrosis) on the basis of signal enhancement.[9,10] Reversibly injured myocardium, which is reperfused early, enhances in similar way as normal myocardium. In contrast, irreversibly injured myocardium shows more signal enhancement than either normal or irreversibly injured myocardium. In contrast to T1 enhancing contrast agents such as gadolinium and manganese, T2* enhancing agents such as dysprosium-based agents cause a decrease in signal intensity in normal myocardium by dephasing water molecules, which diffuse through local magnetic field gradients induced by an inhomogeneous distribution of the contrast agent. The access of the contrast agent to the intracellular space is limited by myocyte cell membranes acting as a barrier. Consequently, necrosis of myocardial cells, which results in destruction of cell membranes, should result in less spin dephasing and less signal loss. This effect has been confirmed in an animal model of reperfused myocardial infarcts, where less signal loss was observed in reperfused myocardial infarcts than in normal myocardium after administration of dysprosium-DTPA-bis(methylamide).[11]

In humans, there is relatively little information on the use of contrast agents to identify acute myocardial injury. After intravenous injection of gadolinium-DTPA, infarcted myocardium shows more signal enhancement than normal myocardium and the signal intensity of infarcted relative to normal myocardium increases from 1.06 ± 0.16 before to a maximum of 1.39 ± 0.13 after gadolinium-DTPA ($P<.001$).[12] Although the administration of gadolinium-DTPA improves visualization of the infarct region in humans, quantitation of infarct size, and differentiation between reversible injury and myocardial necrosis in humans has not yet been reported.

It is very attractive to use localized ^{31}P-MRS in acute myocardial infarcts because the changes of metabolism within myocardial cells from ischemia to infarction can be directly observed.[13] Early after the onset of ischemia, the contents of phosphocreatine and adenosine triphosphate (ATP) decrease, whereas the inorganic phosphate peak increases. By applying coils directed to the surface of the heart it is possible to demonstrate in vivo that phosphocreatine recovers after brief coronary occlusion and reperfusion[14,15] indicating that stunned myocardium can be identified and distinguished from myocardial scar by MRS. Complete myocardial scar is characterized by the absence of high-energy phosphates, but this phenomenon can only be demonstrated without interference by surrounding viable myocardium if surface coils are small enough to only sample the small central area of complete necrosis. However, in humans the volume of interest is still relatively large as compared to myocardial wall thickness thus limiting the clinical use of MRS at the present time.

Wall Thickening Measurements

After an acute ischemic event, structural changes occur within the infarct zone and infarct healing with scar formation is completed in approximately 3 to 4 months.[16] Although thinning of the infarct region may occur early, especially in large anterior myocardial infarcts, both viable and acutely necrotic myocardium may have the same gross appearance both in terms of anatomy and complete absence of resting function early after the acute event. Therefore, observing anatomy and function of the left ventricle by MRI may not be helpful to detect viability. However, even a small amount of wall thickening in a region of interest indicates the presence of residual contracting cells in that area thus confirming the presence of viability. Measurements of left ventricular wall thickening by using MRI are probably more accurate than by echocardiographic imaging and even small amounts of wall thickening will be reliably detected. However, as with all cross-sectional and projectional imaging techniques, the complex motion of the heart in relation to the body axes makes it impossible to observe exactly the same portion of myocardium during systole and diastole in the same image. These problems can now be overcome using MR tagging techniques[17] and tracing of identical portions of the myocardium is thus possible. Using these techniques, wall thickening measurements by MRI have been shown to be as accurate as with using the current gold standard, ultrasonic crystals sewn to the heart.[18]

If no wall thickening at all is present or the amount of wall thickening is so small as to leave serious doubt about the potential for recovery of regional ventricular function, inotropic stimulation by various pharmacological agents, which result in improved contractile function of viable but not of necrotic myocardium, can be used with MRI to assess residual viability in patients with recent infarct after thrombolysis.[19] This concept has been evaluated in a closed-chest dog model of 90 minutes left anterior descending (LAD) coronary artery occlusion followed by 48 hours of reperfusion. Stunned but viable myocardium demonstrated enhanced contraction during dobutamine infusion and could thus be distinguished from myocardial scar.[20] Consequently, MRI is an attractive imaging modality for the depiction of acute infarcts and determine residual viability and may become useful, both scientifically and clinically, to follow the time course of infarct healing and ventricular remodeling.

Viability in Chronic Myocardial Infarcts

Infarct healing is completed 12 to 16 weeks after the acute event and at that time the maximum of regional wall thinning occurs in transmural infarcts. Necropsy studies confirmed that healed transmural myocardial infarcts exhibit a wall thickness of usually <6 mm.[21] Therefore, identification of substantial wall thinning with absent systolic wall thickening is evidence of complete scar formation in a region. However, one must be very cautious to assume that the entire region perfused by an occluded coronary artery will be completely scarred because life may be present in the border zone and border zone ischemia alone may cause substantial symptoms in a patient. Therefore, in a patient with single-vessel disease and anginal symptoms, restoration of blood flow by re-establishing patency of the occluded artery would be justified despite evidence of necrosis in the center of the infarct zone. Although such therapy will usually relieve symptoms, the central zone of necrosis will not recover function.

Myocardial Wall Thickness

The hypothesis that thinned and akinetic myocardium represents chronic scar has been tested by comparing MRI findings with findings by positron emission tomography (PET) and single-photon emission computer tomography (SPECT) findings in identical myocardial regions.[22,23] Comparison of MRI with scintigraphic techniques is attractive because identical regions can be matched, which is difficult for comparisons between projectional imaging techniques such as angiography and cross-sectional techniques such as MRI.

Regional wall thickness measurements from short-axis MR tomograms were compared in 35 patients with chronic infarcts and regional akinesia on left ventricular angiograms to short-axis PET tomograms after injection of [18]fluorodeoxyglucose (FDG).[22] The study confirmed that regions with an end-diastolic wall thickness of <5.5 mm, which was the mean regional left ventricular wall thickness on gradient-echo MRI images minus 2.5 standard deviations obtained from a group of normal volunteers,[24] showed FDG uptake of less 50% (Figure 2). Viability of the infarct region was diagnosed by positron emission tomography with [18]fluorodeoxyglucose (FDG-PET) in 23 of 35 patients and gradings based on FDG uptake and myocardial morphology as assessed by MRI were identical in 29 of 35 patients. Of the 234 akinetic segments with preserved end-diastolic wall thickness, 214 were viable resulting in a positive predictive accuracy of this MR finding for PET defined viability of 91%. Sensitivity of wall thickness reduction was

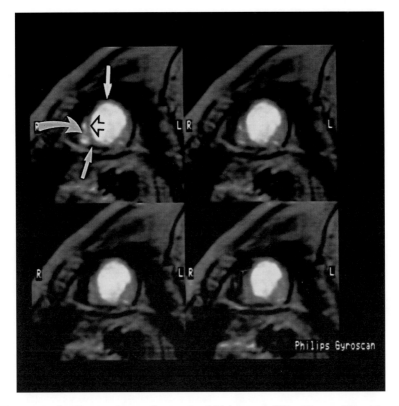

FIGURE 2. **A:** Short-axis gradient-echo MR images (TR = 28 ms, TE = 12 ms) of the left ventricle near the apex in a patient with a 3-year-old anteroseptal myocardial infarct. **Upper left:** End-diastolic image showing severe wall thinning of the anterior wall (white arrow top) and the interventricular septum (black arrow). The curved arrow points to the right ventricle. The inferior wall (partially obscured by shift artifact, see white arrow bottom) and the lateral wall have normal wall thickness. **Upper right:** Early systolic image. **Lower left:** Midsystolic image. **Lower right:** End-systolic image. There is normal wall thickening in the inferior and lateral walls, whereas the anterior wall and the intraventricular septum fail to show any thickening.

72% and specificity was 89%. There was a significant difference in FDG uptake between segments with preserved diastolic wall thickness and those with substantial myocardial thinning (Figure 3). Importantly, relative FDG uptake did not differ between segments with systolic wall thickening at rest or akinesia at rest, as long as wall thickness was preserved. Thus, end-diastolic regional left ventricular wall thickness in akinetic regions gives substantial information about the presence or absence of viable myocardium in that region.

The abovementioned study did not report on the results of revascu-

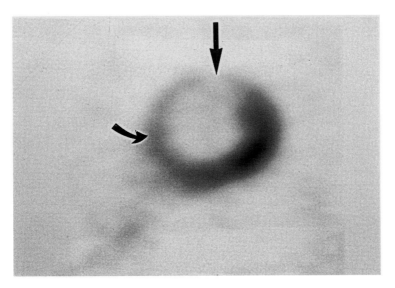

FIGURE 2. *(continued)* **B:**[18F]fluorodeoxyglucose PET image at the same position as the gradient-echo MR images confirms absence of viable myocardium anteriorly (arrow) and septally (curved arrow)

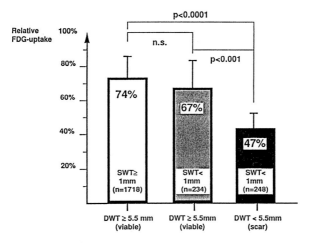

FIGURE 3. Mean segmental FDG-uptake related to diastolic wall thickness and systolic wall thickening at rest as assessed by MRI. DWT indicates end-diastolic wall thickness; FDG, [18F]-fluorodeoxyglucose; SWT, systolic wall thickening at rest

larization, which must be regarded as the gold standard for the clinical definition of myocardial viability. However, left ventricular wall thickness has been confirmed as an accurate predictor of myocardial viability in a small number of revascularized patients.[25] Cine MRI with myocardial tagging during dobutamine infusion was used to quantify regional contractile reserve and recovery of myocardial function after revascularization. Total imaging time was less than 20 minutes. Of the 43 segments without normal wall motion at baseline, no segment with a resting end-systolic wall thickness of <7 mm demonstrated contractile reserve or improvement after revascularization. Of the 28 segments that improved after revascularization, contractile reserve was present in 25, but in only 1 of 15 segments that did not improve after revascularization. There was an excellent correlation between end-systolic wall thickness at peak dobutamine infusion and after revascularization with a correlation coefficient of $r = 0.95$. Moreover, the observation of significantly reduced regional wall thickness <5 mm in transmural infarcts was recently confirmed by an echocardiographic study.[26]

The relation between wall thickness and viability has been disputed by other researchers,[27] who found FDG uptake largely independent of regional end-diastolic wall thickness. This astonishing finding can be explained in two ways. First, both patients with recent and with chronic infarcts could have been included in the study as this inclusion criterion was not specified. This would explain why regions with normal wall thickness were found to have no FDG uptake. Second, myocardial wall thickness could have been overestimated in this particular study because a spin-echo technique with a short echo time of 20 ms was used. Considering the available evidence, left ventricular wall thickness must be regarded as an important parameter of myocardial viability and severe wall thinning in regions without contractile function at rest exhibiting such severe wall thinning are highly likely to represent transmural scar.

Myocardial Thickening During Dobutamine Infusion

MRI is, however, not limited to observing myocardial wall thickness and systolic wall thickening but can also be used to provide information about the myocardial response to stimulation with positive inotropic agents. In the study by Baer and coworkers, the presence or absence of a dobutamine induced contractile reserve correctly predicted the presence or absence of more than 50% relative FDG uptake in 31 of the 35 patients (Figure 4). Of 251 initially akinetic myocardial regions, which had wall thickening of >1 mm after dobutamine stimulation, 242 or 96% had FDG uptake of more than 50% on PET images.

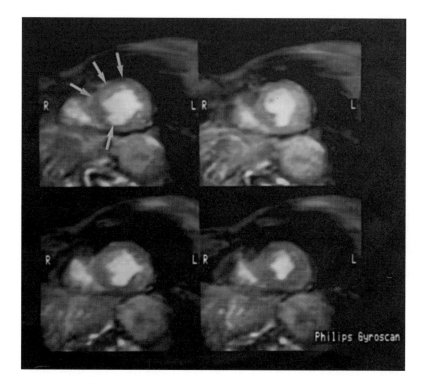

FIGURE 4. **A:** Short-axis gradient-echo MR images (TR = 28 ms, TE = 12 ms) during dobutamine infusion (10 μg/kg/min) in a patient with chronic anteroseptal myocardial infarction. **Upper left:** End-diastolic image. There is some wall thinning in the anteroseptal region (three white arrows) and less pronounced in the inferior wall (single white arrow). **Upper right:** The end-systolic image demonstrates akinesia of the anteroseptal region, the inferior region shows minimal wall thickening. **Lower left:** End-diastolic image during dobutamine: **Lower right:** At end systole, there is perfectly normal wall thickening of the inferior wall and obvious dobutamine-induced wall thickening of the anteroseptal region.

The combination of the morphological parameter end-diastolic wall thickness and the functional parameter dobutamine induced systolic wall thickening gave the best result for sensitivity (88%) and positive predictive accuracy (92%).

Magnetic Resonance Spectroscopy

The most exciting way to measure viability is by using MRS. Quantitation of MR spectra offers the possibility to determine the amount

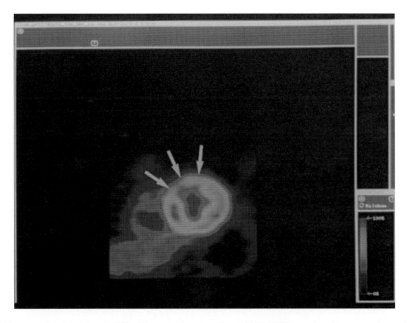

FIGURE 4. *(continued)* **B:** The corresponding FDG-PET image shows reduced uptake in the anteroseptal region (arrows), but relative uptake is larger than 50%. Therefore, this region is also viable by PET criteria. The inferior wall shows normal FDG uptake.

of viable myocardium present in the region of interest. A recent article by Yabe and coworkers[28] evaluated whether quantitative MRS was useful to distinguish between patients with LAD-stenosis with and without signs of viability as evidenced on thallium scans. Two groups of patients were distinguished: one group had reversible thallium defects whereas the other group had irreversible defects on the basis of an abnormal exercise-redistribution study. MR spectra were localized by one-dimensional chemical shift imaging with slice selection in the sagittal direction. Spectra were acquired with ECG gating at end systole. Slice thickness was between 60 and 80 mm in the sagittal direction and 20 mm in the coronal direction. Thus, the volume of interest was relatively large. Eleven normal patients were studied as controls. Quantification of spectra was done as compared to a vial of hexamethylphosphoric triamide (HMPT). Representative spectra from the three groups are shown in Figure 5. Phosphocreatine (PCr) content was significantly lower in the group without thallium redistribution (which may indicate absence of viability) and in the group with reversible defects (indicating residual viability) as compared to the group of normal persons. The ATP concentration, however, was significantly lower than in normals

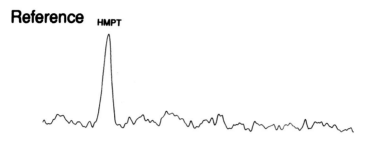

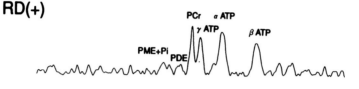

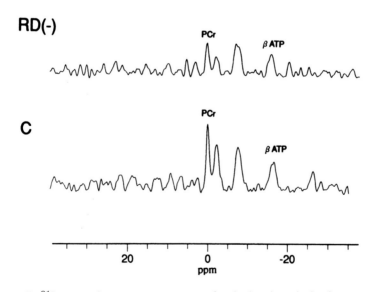

FIGURE 5. ^{31}P magnetic resonance spectra of typical patients in the three groups examined by Yabe et al.[28] The patient in the group with prior myocardial infraction and extensive anterior wall^{201} Tl defects at rest without redistribution [(RD(−)] had a lower myocardial PCr content compared with patients in the group with LAD stenosis but reversible thallium defects in the anterial wall [RD(+)] and the control group consisting of normal volunteers. In addition, the patient in the RD (+) group had a lower PCr content than the patient in the control group. However, ATP content decreased only in the patient in the RD (−) group. C indicates healthy control group; HMPT, hexamethylphosphoric triamide; PCr, phosphocreatine; PME, phosphor monoesters; Pi, inorganic phosphate; PDE, phosphor diesters. (Reprinted with permission from Reference 28.)

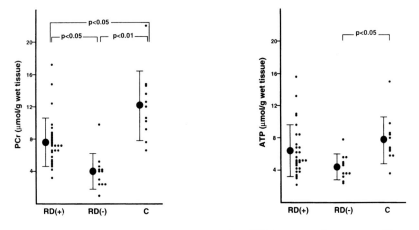

FIGURE 6. Group values for phosphocreatine (PCr) content in groups with reversible [201]T1 defects [RD (+)], fixed [201]T1 defects [RD (−)], control (C). ANOVA reveiled significant differences among the three groups (C, 12.14±4.25 > RD (+), 7.64±3.00 > RD (−), 3.94±2.21 μmol/g wet tissue). On the right, the ATP content in the three groups is shown. Subjects in the RD (−) group had significantly lower myocardial ATP content than those in the control group (*P*<.05). However, no significant differences existed between the RD (+) and control group [RD (+), 6.35±3.17; RD (−), 4.35±1.52; and C 7.72±2.97 μmol/g wet tissue]. (Reprinted with permission from Reference 28.)

only in the no redistribution group (Figure 6). Although much overlap was found between groups, this study demonstrated that quantitative MRS measurements are possible in patients after myocardial infarction and that MRS can be used in the clinical setting to gain information about the presence of myocardial viability. Does this confirm that magnetic resonance spectroscopy is the ideal tool to identify viable myocardium in the clinical setting? Unfortunately, the size of the region of interest is still in the order of 30 to 90 cm^3. Therefore, the volumes of interest usually incorporate mixtures of scar, normal and ischemically injured viable myocardium. Further development of localization techniques is necessary to obtain spectroscopic information from smaller volumes of interest. Only then will MRS fulfill its promise of providing the most direct information on myocardial viability.

Conclusions

MRI is a highly accurate method of obtaining information on residual myocardial viability after myocardial infarction. Indirect signs of viability are a lack of signal increase in an acutely ischemic region on spin-echo images, any sign of wall thickening at rest (which may not be detectable by techniques less accurate than MRI), wall thickening after stimulation by dobutamine and preserved wall thickness. However, in contrast to PET, MRI is not able to directly demonstrate preserved myocardial metabolism in the region of interest. Nevertheless, comparative studies with FDG-PET indicate the potential of MRI to correctly identify regions with residual viability and clearly distinguish them from regions with predominant chronic scar. More data are needed in patients undergoing revascularization on how accurate MRI is able to predict functional recovery of akinetic areas after revascularization.

MRI of the entire left ventricle can now be performed in 20 to 30 minutes using breath-hold segmented k-space segmented techniques. Image quality is as good as for standard cine MRI. Rapid acquisition of high-quality images make MRI an attractive means of evaluating myocardial viability in patients in whom revascularization of the infarct region is a clinical issue.

Assessment of viability by fast gradient-echo MR techniques has several advantages over other imaging techniques. Compared with echocardiography, MRI often has superior image quality, which is important for deriving quantitative data, and MRI gives a truly three-dimensional series of images covering the entire left ventricle. Compared with scintigraphic techniques, MR is faster to perform and does not expose the patient to ionizing radiation. Ultimately, the clinical usefulness of MRI for assessing viability can only be defined by comparing fast gradient-echo MRI directly with the other imaging modalities in patient groups undergoing revascularization.

MRS is less likely than MRI to become used clinically for diagnosing myocardial viability. Nevertheless, MRS provides unique physiological information and may enhance the understanding of metabolic changes occurring in acute ischemia.

References

1. Higgins CB, Lanzer P, Stark D, et al. Imaging by nuclear magnetic resonance in patients with chronic ischemic heart disease. *Circulation.* 1984;69: 523–531.
2. Schlichter J, Hellerstein HK, Katz LN. Aneurysm of the heart. A correlative study of 102 proven cases. *Medicine.* 1954;33:43–86.
3. Pierard LA, De Landsheere CM, Berthe C, et al. Identification of viable myocardium by echocardiography during dobutamine infusion in patients with myocardial infarction after thrombolytic therapy: Comparison with positron emission tomography. *J Am Coll Cardiol.* 1990;15:1021–1031.
4. Bolli R, Zhu WX, Thornby JI, et al. Time course and determinants of recov-

ery of function after reversible ischemia in conscious dogs. *Am J Physiol.* 1988;254:102–114.

5. Rahimtoola SH. The hibernating myocardium. *Am Heart J.* 1989;117: 211–221.
6. Bodenheimer MM, Banka VS, Hermann GA, et al. Reversible asynergy. Histopathologic and electrographic correlations in patients with coronary artery disease. *Circulation.* 1976;53:792–796.
7. Wisenberg G, Prato FS, Carroll SE, et al. Serial nuclear magnetic resonance imaging of acute myocardial infarction with and without reperfusion. *Am Heart J.* 1988;115:510–518.
8. Ryan T, Tarver RD, Duerk JL, et al. Distinguishing viable from infarcted myocardium after experimental ischemia and reperfusion by using nuclear magnetic resonance imaging. *J Am Coll Cardiol.* 1990;15:1355–1364.
9. McNamara MT, Tscholakoff D, Revel D, et al. Differentiation of reversible and irreversible myocardial injury by MR imaging with and without gadolinium-DTPA. *Radiology.* 1986;158:765–769.
10. Saeed M, Wendland MF, Takehara Y, Higgins CB. Reversible and irreversible injury in the reperfused myocardium: Differentiation with contrast material-enhanced MR imaging. *Radiology.* 1990;175:633–637.
11. Saeed M, Wendland MF, Masui T, Higgins CB. Reperfused myocardial infarctions on T1- and susceptibility-enhanced MRI: Evidence for loss of compartmentalization of contrast media. *Magn Reson Med.* 1994;31:31–39.
12. Van Rossum AC, Visser FC, Van Eenige MJ, et al. Value of gadolinium-diethylene-triamine pentaacetic acid dynamics in magnetic resonance imaging of acute myocardial infarction with occluded and reperfused coronary arteries after thrombolysis. *Am J Cardiol.* 1990;65:845–851.
13. Bottomley PA, Smith LS, Brazzamano S, et al. The fate of inorganic phosphate and pH in regional myocardial ischemia and infarction: a noninvasive ^{31}P NMR study. *Magn Reson Med.* 1987;5:129–142.
14. Guth BD, Martin JF, Heusch G, Ross JJ. Regional myocardial blood flow, function and metabolism using phosphorus-31 nuclear magnetic resonance spectroscopy during ischemia and reperfusion in dogs. *J Am Coll Cardiol.* 1987;10:673–681.
15. Camacho SA, Lanzer P, Toy BJ, et al. In vivo alterations of high-energy phosphates and intracellular pH during reversible ischemia in pigs: A 31P magnetic resonance spectroscopy study. *Am Heart J.* 1988;116:701–718.
16. Mallory GK, White PD, Salcedo-Galger J. The speed of healing of myocardial infarction: A study of the pathologic anatomy in 72 cases. *Am Heart J.* 1939;18:647–671.
17. Zerhouni EA. Myocardial tagging by magnetic resonance imaging. *Coron Artery Dis.* 1993;4:334–339.
18. Lima JA, Jeremy R, Guier W, et al. Accurate systolic wall thickening by nuclear magnetic resonance imaging with tissue tagging: Correlation with sonomicrometers in normal and ischemic myocardium. *J Am Coll Cardiol.* 1993;21:1741–1751.
19. Nienaber CA, Rochau T, Chatterjee T, Nicolas V. Dobutamin-Magnetresonanztomographie und 201-Thallium-SPECT: Nachweis von vitalem Myokard in der Postinfarktphase (abstract). *Z Kardiol.* 1993;82 (Suppl 1):17.
20. Croisille P, Judd RM, Lima JAC, et al. Combined dobutamine stress 3-D tagged and contrast enhanced MRI differentiate viable from non-viable myocardium after acute infarction and reperfusion. *Circulation.* 1995;92 (Suppl. I):I–508.

21. Dubnow MH, Burchell HB, Titus JL. Postinfarction left ventricular aneurysm. A clinicomorphologic and electrocardiographic study of 80 cases. *Am Heart J.* 1965;70:753–760.
22. Baer FM, Voth E, Schneider CA, et al. Comparison of low-dose dobutamine-gradient-echo magnetic resonance imaging and positron emission tomography with [18F]fluorodeoxyglucose in patients with chronic coronary artery disease. A functional and morphological approach to the detection of residual myocardial viability. *Circulation.* 1995;91:1006–1015.
23. Baer FM, Smolarz K, Jungehulsing M, et al. Chronic myocardial infarction: Assessment of morphology, function, and perfusion by gradient echo magnetic resonance imaging and 99mTc-methoxyisobutyl-isonitrile SPECT. *Am Heart J.* 1992;123:636–645.
24. Baer FM, Smolarz K, Jungehülsing M, et al. Magnetresonanztomographische Darstellung transmuraler Myokardinfarkte im Vergleich zur 99Tc-methoxyisobutyl-isonitrile-SPECT. *Z Kardiol.* 1992;81:423–431.
25. Sayad DE, Willett DWL, Hundley G, et al. Dobutamine magnetic resonance imaging with myocardial tagging predicts quantitative and qualitative improvement in regional function after revascularization. *Circulation.* 1995;92 (Suppl I):I–507.
26. Athanassopoulos G, Koutelou M, Maginas A, et al. Wall thickness in akinetic segments at rest correlates with dobutamine stress echocardiography and T1-201 SPECT re-injection for the detection of myocardial viability. *Circulation.* 1994;90 (Suppl I):I–117.
27. Perrone-Filardi P, Bacharach SL, Dilsizian V, et al. Metabolic evidence of viable myocardium in regions with reduced wall thickness and absent wall thickening in patients with chronic ischemic left ventricular dysfunction. *J Am Coll Cardiol.* 1992;20:161–168.
28. Yabe T, Mitsunami K, Inubushi T, Kinoshita M. Quantitative measurements of cardiac phosphorus metabolites in coronary artery disease by ^{31}P magnetic resonance spectroscopy. *Circulation.* 1995;92:15–23.

Chapter 16

Positron Emission Tomography for the Quantification of Myocardial Blood Flow and Viability

Heinrich R. Schelbert, MD

Introduction

Myocardial viability as a state of reversibly impaired regional contractile function may result from ischemia, hibernation, and stunning. Ischemia represents an acute imbalance between supply and demand that progresses to necrosis and scar tissue formation. If, however, flow is restored before irreversible damage occurs, function will ultimately recover fully although it may remain initially impaired, a state referred to as "stunning." In contrast, myocardial hibernation might be considered a more chronic downregulation of contractile function in response to persistently diminished blood flow and thus supply, so that a new precarious balance between supply and demand at a lower level of function is achieved. Yet, maintenance of such new steady state might not be fully possible as for example in the human myocardium with diseased coronary arteries where demand or supply or both may change in response to neurohumoral alterations or to physical activity.

Operated for the U.S. Department of Energy by the University of California under Contract #DE-AC03-76-SF00012. This work was supported in part by the Director of the Office of Energy Research, Office of Health and Environmental Research, Washington D.C., by Research Grants #HL 29845 and #HL 33177, National Institutes of Health, Bethesda, MD and by an Investigative Group Award by the Greater Los Angeles Affiliate of the American Heart Association, Los Angeles, CA.

From: Higgins CB, Ingwall JS, Pohost GM, (eds). *Current and Future Applications of Magnetic Resonance in Cardiovascular Disease.* Armonk, NY: Futura Publishing Company, Inc.; © 1998.

Lastly, it is also possible that "repetitive stunning" may lead to chronic impairment in regional contractile function.

This chapter briefly describes the tools available with positron emission tomography (PET) for the detection and characterization of myocardial viability as the common denominator for various states of reversible myocardial contractile dysfunction. It discusses observations with PET that offer insights into the underlying pathophysiology and reviews clinical investigations that have underscored the value of PET measurements of blood flow and metabolism for managing patients with ischemic cardiomyopathy.

Measurements of Blood Flow and Metabolism

Essential ingredients for the evaluation of abnormal myocardial states and, in particular, of myocardial viability are the assessment and quantification of blood flow and substrate metabolism. For PET, several radiotracers and approaches are available for determining the relative distribution of myocardial blood flow as well as for estimating absolute rates of regional flow. The most widely available and accepted PET tracers of blood flow include Oxygen-15 (O-15) labeled water, rubidium-82, and N-13-labeled ammonia.[1-3] Myocardium accumulates and retains rubidium-82 and N-13 ammonia in proportion to regional myocardial blood flow so that the resulting myocardial tissue concentrations as visualized on static PET images depict the relative distribution of blood flow. Oxygen-15-labeled water, in contrast, equilibrates rapidly between blood and myocardium; as blood tracer concentrations decline, O-15 water clears from the myocardium so that the static images of the myocardial O-15 concentrations are frequently of limited diagnostic quality. Yet, this radiotracer as well as N-13 ammonia affords measurements of regional myocardial blood flow.[4-7] Such measurements are predicted on rapid serial image acquisition beginning at the time of tracer administration and continuing for several minutes. After assigning regions of interest to the left ventricular blood pool and myocardium, the arterial tracer input function and the myocardial tissue response to it can be derived. Fitting of these time activity curves with a one-compartment (for O-15 water) and a two-compartment (for N-13 ammonia) tracer kinetic model yields regional rates of myocardial blood flow in absolute units ($ml \cdot min^{-1} \cdot g^{-1}$). The accuracy of such measurements has been validated against independent flow measurements by the arterial reference sampling technique with radiolabeled microspheres.[4,8-10] The noninvasive flow estimates were found to correlate directly and linearly with microsphere flow estimates over flow ranges from near 0 to as much as 5 to 6 $ml \cdot min^{-1} \cdot g^{-1}$. In the human myocardium, both approaches, the O-15 water and the N-13 ammonia technique were found to be equally accurate in tracking myocardial blood flow.[11]

Regional rates of myocardial exogenous glucose utilization can be measured with F-18 2-fluoro 2-deoxyglucose.[12,13] This agent exchanges across the capillary and sarcolemmel membranes in proportion to glucose and then competes with glucose for hexokinase to become phosphorylated to F-18 2-fluoro 2-deoxyglucose-6-phosphate. Unlike native glucose, the phosphorylated tracer then becomes effectively trapped in the myocardium so that static images of the regional F-18 concentrations as acquired with PET or, more recently, with single-photon emission computed tomographs (SPECT) equipped with high-energy collimators[14] depict the relative distribution of regional exogenous glucose utilization rates. Again, absolute rates of exogenous glucose utilization in μmol·min^{-1}·g^{-1} can be derived from serially acquired PET images. The arterial tracer input function together with the myocardial tissue response to it are fitted then with a three-compartment tracer kinetic model.[13,15,16]

Blood Flow and Metabolism in Chronic Coronary Artery Disease

Typically, acute myocardial ischemia is associated with regionally reduced blood flow that is readily demonstrated with positron emitting tracers of blood flow. Yet, this may be associated with a marked increase in glycolytic flux that then can be demonstrated with F-18 2-fluoro 2-deoxyglucose. If blood flow is restored in time, myocardial blood flow will return to normal although F-18 2-fluoro 2-deoxyglucose uptake may be reduced, normal, or even enhanced[17,18] and wall motion remains initially impaired. In contrast, by definition blood flow will be decreased in "hibernating myocardium" and F-18 2-fluoro 2-deoxyglucose uptake may be reduced slightly, normal, or elevated. Importantly, F-18 2-fluoro 2-deoxyglucose uptake exceeds blood flow as a reflection of increased glucose extraction.[19,20] Lastly, relatively recent studies report normal or mildly reduced flows and normal or enhanced F-18 2-fluoro 2-deoxyglucose uptake in collateral dependent though dysfunctional myocardium.[21] Associated with this pattern is a markedly impaired myocardial flow reserve. The latter might argue in favor of "repetitive stunning" where increases in local demand as for example in response to physical work or mental stress cannot be met by adequate increases in blood flow and supply. In this situation, repeated episodes of demand-induced ischemia may produce repetitive stunning as another mechanism of chronic impairment of regional myocardial wall motion. Table 1 lists the different patterns. The different possible patho-

TABLE 1

Patterns of Myocardial Blood Flow and F-18 2-fluoro 2-deoxyglucose Uptake

	MBF	F-18 2-fluoro 2-deoxyglucose uptake
Ischemia	Reduced	Enhanced
Stunning	Normal	Normal or enhanced
Hibernation	Reduced	Greater than MBF
Repetitive stunning	Normal	Normal or enhanced
Necrosis/scar	Reduced	Reduced in proportion to MBF

MBF indicates Myocardial blood flow.

Resting Perfusion

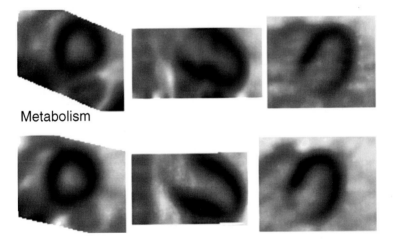

Metabolism

A   *p04065*

FIGURE 1. Examples of blood flow metabolism patterns as observed in patients with chronic coronary artery disease. For each patient, a vertical and long axis together with a short axis cut is shown. **A:** In this patient with mild hypokinesis of the anterior wall, myocardial blood flow as seen on the N-13 ammonia images and exogenous glucose utilization as seen on the F-18 2-deoxyglucose images are normal. This is consistent with pattern A.

Resting Perfusion

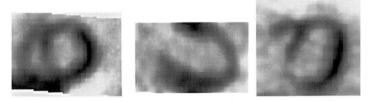

Metabolism

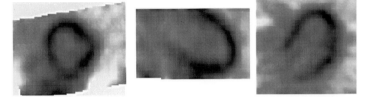

B   *p50707*

Resting Perfusion

Metabolism

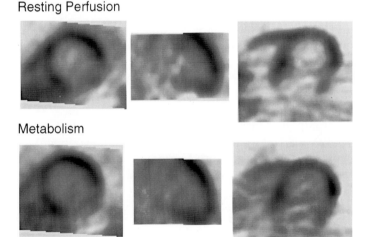

C   *p50375*

FIGURE 1. *(continued)* **B:** This patient revealed akinesis of the anterior wall. As seen on the N-13 ammonia images, blood flow is moderately decreased. Yet, F-18 2-deoxyglucose concentrations are normal or slightly enhanced. This is consistent with Pattern B. **C:** Again, this patient revealed akinesis of the lateral and inferolateral walls which as seen on the N-13 ammonia images is associated with a severe reduction in myocardial blood flow. Unlike the patient shown in B, glucose utilization is reduced in proportion to blood flow. This pattern is consistent with a blood flow metabolism match or Pattern C.

TABLE 2

Flow Measurements in Dysfunctional Myocardium

	MBF-rest mL·min^{-1}·g^{-1}	% of normal	MBF-Dipyr mL·min^{-1}·g^{-1}	MFR	% Normal
	Normally or Minimally Reduced Blood Flow				
Vanoverschelde, 1993	0.77 ± 0.25	81%	1.12 ± 0.44	1.27	42%
Marzullo, 1995	0.69 ± 0.14	69%	1.64 ± 0.70	2.5 ± 1.6	90%
	Modest to Severe Blood Flow Reductions				
Czernin, 1992	0.60 ± 0.25	60%	0.80 ± 0.30	1.25 ± 0.30	48%
Marzullo, 1995	0.42 ± 0.12	42%	1.07 ± 0.50	2.6 ± 1.30	94%

MBF indicates myocardial blood flow at rest or after dipyridamole induced (Dipyr) hyperemia. The percent of normal indicate the comparison of resting blood flows and of the myocardial flow reserve (MFR) to the corresponding values in normal remote myocardium.

physiological scenarios may be consistent with the various blood flow metabolic patterns as depicted on PET and as reported originally.[19,20] Defined by the operational terms, pattern A consists of normal blood flow and glucose use rates in dysfunctional myocardial regions. Pattern B includes reductions in blood flow yet relative or absolute increases in glucose use rates. In contrast, pattern C consists of a segmental reduction in the glucose use rate that parallels the reduction in regional myocardial blood flow (Figure 1).

Both patterns A and B predict with a rather high degree of accuracy a postrevascularization improvement in regional contractile dysfunction.[20,22–29] Conversely, pattern C predicts a failure of functional improvement following revascularization (Table 2).

Quantitative Studies of Blood Flow and Glucose Use

Several investigations have quantified regional myocardial blood flow (mostly with N-13 ammonia) and rates of glucose use in dysfunctional myocardium. They offer some insights into the underlying mechanisms accounting for the initially observed blood flow metabolism patterns. In patients with left anterior coronary artery disease, two studies have reported either normal or minimally reduced blood flow.[21,30] In both studies, wall motion was impaired. Yet, there were differences in observed myocardial flow reserve (Table 3). Marzullo and colleagues[30] found normally or near normally preserved flow reserve. In contrast, Vanoverschelde and coinvestigators[21] noted a marked attenu-

TABLE 3

PET Metabolic Imaging For Recovery of Left Ventricular Function After Revascularization

Patients	Number of segments	Procedure	Segments with improved WM		Reference
			With FDG uptake	No FDG uptake	
17	67	CABG	35/41 (85%)	2/26 (8%)	Tillisch 1986
22	46	CABG	18/23 (78%)*	5/23 (22%)	Tamaki 1989
11	56	CABG	40/50 (80%)*	0/6 (0%)	Tamaki 1991
16	85	PTCA, CABG	25/37 (68%)*	10/48 (21%)	Marwick 1992
14	54	CABG	37/39 (95%)*	3/15 (20%)	Lucignani 1992
21	23	CABG	16/19 (84%)	1/4 (25%)	Carrel 1992
34	116	CABG, PTCA	38/73 (52%)	8/43 (19%)	Gropler 1992, 1993
48	90	PTCA, CABG	23/87 (85%)	10/63 (16%)	Knuuti 1994
37	110	PTCA, CABG	24/59 (41%)**	7/51 (14%)**	vom Dahl 1994
43	130	CABG, PTCA	45/59 (76%)*	6/71 (8%)	Tamaki 1995
12#	12	PTCA, CABG	12/12 (100%)	—	Vanoverschelde 1993
20#	20	CABG	8/12 (67%)	2/8 (25%)	Maes 1994
Total 295	809		321/451 (71%)	54/358 (15%)	

* Metabolic imaging performed in the fasting state. ** Segments with moderate hypokinesis or worse function.
\# Histopathological correlation performed. NR indicates not reported; WM, wall motion.

ation of the flow reserve to only 1.27 in collateral dependent and dysfunctional myocardium. In contradistinction, the flow reserve averaged 3.05 and thus was essentially normal in collateral dependent yet normally functioning myocardium in other patients. It is the latter observation that might point to repetitive stunning as the pathophysiology underlying the PET flow metabolism pattern A. Increases in demand prompted by physical activity or mental stress cannot be met by an appropriate supply in the presence of a restricted flow reserve. Repetitive episodes of demand induced ischemia alternate with reperfusion and stunning ultimately resulting in a chronic impairment of contractile function.

Other investigations have noted more severe flow reduction in blood flow-metabolism mismatch. Such reduction varied considerably between patients. The mean reduction in each investigation ranged from 40% to 58% below flow in remote control myocardium.[30,31] Again, there were differences in the magnitude of the residual flow reserve. In the study by Czernin et al[31] dipyridamole produced variable responses, although on average hyperemic flows did not differ significantly from those at baseline (Table 3). On the other hand, Marzullo et al[30] reported a significant, 48% flow increase in response to dipyridamole that was, however, strikingly reduced relative to that in normal myocardium. Whereas a fixed reduction in blood flow (eg, with loss of flow reserve) in the presence of enhanced glucose use favors hibernation as the possible underlying mechanism, the preservation of a significant though attenuated flow reserve tips the balance toward stunning as the pathophysiological process underlying the blood flow metabolism pattern A. It is also possible that both processes may coexist with significant amounts of scar tissue. Consistent with stunning are other observations of one investigation where low-dose dobutamine raised regional blood flow from 0.46 ± 0.12 to 0.63 ± 0.18 ml·min^{-1}·g^{-1} in mismatch regions.[32] This 44% flow increase was markedly less than the 71% increase (from 0.75 ± 0.20 to 1.28 ± 0.31 ml·min^{-1}·g^{-1}) in remote myocardium and was associated with a selective increase in the exogenous glucose use rate from 0.46 ± 0.12 to 0.63 ± 1.2 μmol·min^{-1}·g^{-1}. In remote myocardium, dobutamine lowered the glucose use rate by 31%, probably as a consequence of higher circulating free fatty acid levels. Again, the dobutamine-induced enhancement of blood flow-metabolism mismatch might be consistent with acute myocardial ischemia followed by renewed stunning. It thus might also argue in favor of repetitive stunning at least to some extent in chronically hypoperfused segments or in favor of a superimposition of stunning on hibernation.

Although rates of glucose use have also been quantified for the various blood flow metabolism patterns on PET, these are highly variable and dependent on the study conditions, especially the dietary state with variations in the circulating substrate and hormone levels. The magnitude of the flow reductions and the degree of cell injury are other important factors. Nevertheless, as glucose use rates are by definition elevated relative to blood flow, the steady-state extraction fractions of glucose as the quotient of glucose uptake and blood flow are by definition elevated.

Regional Blood Flow as a Marker of Viability

Given the rather well-preserved flows in pattern A and the variable flow reductions noted for patterns B and C, the question arises whether measurements of blood flow alone or of regional flow reserve can distinguish between viable and nonviable myocardium. One study of 26 patients with prior myocardial infarction compared regional blood flow with the presence of residual metabolic activity as demonstrated with F-18 2-fluoro 2-deoxyglucose.[33] Blood flow in remote myocardium averaged 0.81 ± 0.31 mL·min^{-1}·g^{-1}. There was no statistically significant correlation between the magnitude of the blood flow-metabolism mismatch as determined by the difference between relative F-18 2-fluoro 2-deoxyglucose and N-13 ammonia concentrations. However, none of the myocardial regions with flows less than 0.25 mL·min^{-1}·g^{-1} (relative flow reductions by more than 65%) exhibited metabolic evidence of myocardial viability. Another study in 14 patients with prior myocardial infarction[30] reported comparable reduction in blood flow at rest in mismatch and match regions (0.42 ± 0.12 and 0.39 ± 0.27 mL·min^{-1}·g^{-1} versus 1.0 ± 0.2 mL·min^{-1}·g^{-1} in normally functioning remote myocardium). However, myocardial flow reserve significantly differed between both types of regions. It averaged 2.6 ± 1.3 in mismatch, but only 1.3 ± 0.5 in match regions. The authors conclude that viable myocardium can be identified using preserved myocardial flow reserve. Lastly, another study of 43 chronic coronary artery disease patients concluded that severe flow reduction as well as the absence of stress-induced flow defects accurately identified irreversibly compromised contractile function.[34] However, less severe flow reduction was only 48% accurate in predicting a postrevascularization improvement in contractile function. The presence of a stress induced flow defect enhanced the predictive accuracy to 63% yet was still lower than the 76% predictive accuracy for a blood flow-metabolism mismatch.

Morphological Substrates of Blood Flow Metabolism Patterns

Several investigations have reported striking morphological changes in myocardium with either blood flow-metabolism match or mismatch patterns.[21,35,36] These morphological changes were observed on biopsy specimens harvested from dysfunctional myocardium during coronary artery bypass surgery. The findings included scar tissue and degenerated myocytes as well as interstitial changes. Of particular interest were the degenerated cells that characteristically exhibited a more central loss of myofibrils, excessive glycogen accumulation most prominent in the proximity of the nucleus, multiple small though normally appearing mitochondria and a reduction or loss of sarcomeres (Figure 2). Immunochemical techniques revealed alterations of the cytoskeleton as evidenced by an enhanced expression of α-actinin and titin. Both Depré and Maes and coworkers[35,36] reported the presence of fibrotic tissue in normally contracting segments but more so in mismatch and match myocardium. On average, fibrotic tissue accounted for about 35% of the tissue mass in match and for about 11% in mismatch seg-

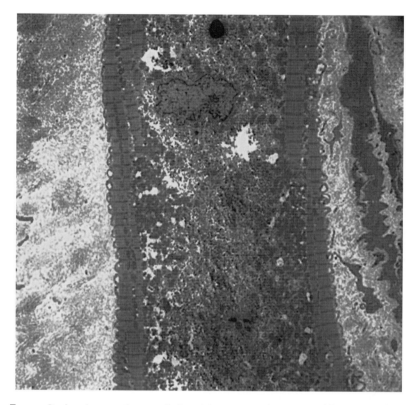

FIGURE 2. An abnormal myocyte in a biopsy sample removed from a dysfunctional anterior myocardial wall during coronary artery bypass grafting. Note the central loss of myofibrils associated with deposition of glycogen. (Courtesy of Dr. Marcel Borgers, Janssen Research Foundation, Heerse, Belgium).

ments.[35] Conversely, the tissue mass exhibited histologically normal myocardium in about 41% of match and about 74% of mismatch segments. Both, match and mismatch regions contain similar fractions of "degenerated cells", amounting to about 25% in the study by Maes and coworkers.[35] However, Depré et al[36] reported significantly higher fractions of scar tissue in functionally nonreversible than in reversible myocardium whereas reversible compromised myocardium contained significantly more dedifferentiated cells than reversibly injured myocardium (Figure 3). In fact, in this study, the fraction of scar tissue in the biopsy samples were correlated inversely with blood flow (Figure 4). Although the reason for these discrepancies between the two studies remain unclear, interstudy differences, for example, as in the myocardial site for harvesting the biopsy samples (eg, center of the dysfunctional region versus fixed anatomic site) might serve as one explanation.

Post Revascularization

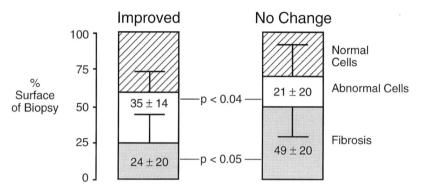

FIGURE 3. Fractional distribution of fibrotic tissue, normal myocytes and "degenerated" cells. Myocardial biopsy specimens removed from the dysfunctional wall during coronary artery bypass grafting. The left column represents the average distributions for those segments that improved contractile function following revascularization with the column on the right the mean values for segments without change in contractile function after revascularization. (Reproduced with permission from Reference 36.)

These morphological findings raise several questions. First, does such degeneration of cells represent a dedifferentiation, especially if some of the features resemble those found in neonatal cells as for example the increased glycogen content. If so, does restoration of blood flow lead to a redifferentiation with rebuilding of the contractile machinery with an arrangement of contractile fibers in a meaningful fashion so that contractile function improves. The correlation between the rate of functional recovery and the tissue fraction of degenerated cells appears to support such a possibility. Second, does the degeneration result from the absence of contractile work as observed in isolated myocytes or, conversely, does the loss of the contractile machinery produce the impairment of contractile function? Third, if degenerated cells cannot redifferentiate, does reconstitution of myocardial blood flow result in hypertrophy of adjacent normal myocytes that then might account for the postrevascularization improvement in contractile function?

According to more recent, still unpublished findings, there appears to also be a group of mismatches without any or only very minimal morphological changes.[37] This then raises another question, namely whether the morphological changes may be chronic and stable or, conversely, progressive with necrosis and scar tissue formation as end points.

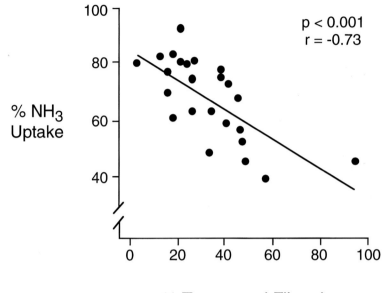

FIGURE 4. Comparison of relative myocardial blood flow with a fraction of scar tissue formation as determined from biopsy samples removed from the anterior dysfunctional wall during bypass grafting. (Reproduced with permission from Reference 36.)

Equally important is the question whether these degenerated cells account for the enhanced glucose use especially in view of the excessive accumulation of glycogen. Maes et al[35] rejected this possibility because the tissue fraction of degenerated cells failed to correlate with the F-18 2-fluoro 2-deoxyglucose uptake. Yet, Depré and colleagues[36] implied that this may in fact be the case because of a direct, statistically significant correlation between the fraction of degenerated cells and F-18 tissue concentration (Figure 5). Nevertheless, the observed absence of morphological changes in mismatch segments as observed by others argues against such a hypothesis. Assuming that dysfunctional myocardium contains cells with a broad spectrum of different degrees of compromise and injury, it may well be that functionally compromised although morphologically intact myocytes coexisting with morphologically altered cells account for the most part for the enhanced glucose use.

In this respect, the recently observed increased expression of the insulin independent glucose transporter GLUT 1 in acutely ischemic[38] and more recently in biopsy samples from reversibly dysfunctional

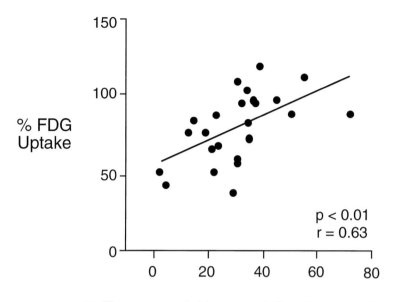

FIGURE 5. Correlation between the fraction of degenerated cells in each biopsy sample obtained during surgery and the relative F-18 2-deoxyglucose uptake. (Reproduced with permission from Reference 36.)

myocardium in coronary artery disease patients[39] is of interest. This may account for the attenuated response of F-18 2-fluoro 2-deoxyglucose uptake in such segments in response to changes in plasma insulin and glucose levels.[40] Yet, whether the augmentation of GLUT 4 relative to the insulin sensitive glucose transporter GLUT 1 is in fact the cause of the enhanced glucose uptake or the response to other still unknown mechanisms remains uncertain at present.

Detection of Myocardial Viability by Positron Emission Tomography

The various blood flow metabolism patterns as observed on PET in patients with coronary artery disease contain considerable predictive and prognostic value. The initial study by Tillisch and colleagues[20] observed all three flow metabolism patterns in dysfunctional myocardial regions of coronary artery disease patients scheduled for surgical revascularization. Blood flow metabolism matches were 92% accurate in predicting that regional wall motion would not improve following revascularization. Conversely, segmental blood flow metabolism mismatches (pattern B) predicted a postrevascularization improvement in regional wall motion with an 81% accuracy. Further, 88% of all dysfunctional segments with normal blood flow and metabolism (pattern A) had improved wall motion after revascularization. In a subsequent study from our own laboratory[41] the extent of the blood flow metabolism mismatch was found to predict the postangioplasty improvement in segmental wall motion.

Numerous investigators have now confirmed the predictive value of the blood flow metabolism patterns for the revascularization outcome in regional contractile function (Table 3). Differences in study protocols need to be emphasized. Whereas some investigations strictly compared the relative distribution of blood flow by PET with that by F-18 2-fluoro 2-deoxyglucose,[20,22–24,26] others evaluated the relative distribution of blood flow by Tc-99m sestaMIBI by SPECT and F-18 2-fluoro 2-deoxyglucose uptake by PET,[25] but others relied on regional F-18 2-fluoro 2-deoxyglucose uptake alone.[28] Also, some investigators examined their patients in the fasting state when F-18 2-fluoro 2-deoxyglucose uptake is predominantly enhanced in reversibly dysfunctional regions but low or absent in normal myocardium.[22] Yet, most investigators augment glucose use in normal myocardium by either a prestudy glucose administration or, during the study, by insulin or glucose infusion (euglycemic-hyperinsulinemic clamp).[24,25,42] Despite these differences in study protocols, the various studies report comparable predictive accuracies.

As a *sine qua non*, viability depends on some residual blood flow. Inhibitory metabolites such as lactate or hydrogen ions must be removed and substrate delivered. Because of this, attempts have been made to assess the presence or absence of viable myocardium by the severity of the regional reduction in blood flow alone.[34] Yet, as both, Maes and Depré and their coworkers[35,36] found there is a considerable overlap in the flow reductions between viable and nonviable myocardium so that blood flow alone appears rather unreliable for distinguishing between reversible and irreversible dysfunction. This is especially true for intermediate flow reductions, but severely reduced flow rather accurately signifies the absence and rather well-preserved flow in the presence of viability in dysfunctional myocardium. Admixture of scar tissue and normal myocardium or of normal and reversibly dysfunctional myocardium most likely account for the inability of flow alone to discriminate between reversibly and irreversibly impaired myocardial regions.

Use of F-18 2-Fluoro 2-Deoxyglucose as the Sole Marker of Viability

Partial volume related regional reductions in observed rather than true tracer tissue concentrations raise additional concerns for assessing myocardial viability from F-18 2-fluoro 2-deoxyglucose images alone. This effect, common to all imaging procedures, causes images to represent the true tracer activity concentrations only if the object size approaches or exceeds the spatial image resolution by a factor of two.[43] Most state-of-the-art PET offers an effective spatial resolution of 6 to 10 mm full-width at half-maximum (FWHM) after image filtering. Applied to the left ventricular myocardium with a normal average wall thickness of 10 to 12 mm, a regional loss of systolic thickening results in a decrease in the average wall thickness and thus in an artifactual decline in the regionally observed tracer tissue concentrations which might be as much as 40% to 50% as demonstrated in animal experiments.[44] True wall thinning might further accentuate this effect. The correlations between regional wall thickness as determined by gated magnetic resonance imaging (MRI) and myocardial F-18 2-fluoro 2-deoxyglucose concentrations, as imaged by PET and as described in several reports, are therefore expected, at least to some extent, and must be interpreted with some caution.[45,46] Comparison of the F-18 2-fluoro 2-deoxyglucose concentrations to regional flow tracer concentration, however, eliminates such potential partial volume related artifacts as both measurements are subject to the same effect and therefore cancels out. Yet, this does not fully apply to comparisons of the F-18 2-fluoro 2-deoxyglucose uptake on PET images to regional flow tracer concentrations as, for example, imaged with Tc-99m sestamibi and SPECT[25] because of the different spatial resolutions of both imaging devices.

Remodeled Left Ventricular Myocardium

Both, Maes' and Depré's[35,36] observations derive from patients with relatively well-preserved global left ventricular function and were limited to the myocardium subtended by the left anterior descending coronary artery. Obviously, this particular myocardial region was chosen as it is most suitable for removal of biopsy specimens during surgical revascularization. Furthermore, it seems reasonable to extrapolate these regional findings to other myocardial territories such as the lateral or the inferior wall of the left ventricle. Yet, as revascularization in patients with markedly impaired left ventricular function aims at improving overall left ventricular performance, the question arises to what extent is remote and apparently normal myocardium actually normal. Characteristically, such normal myocardium is identified on the blood flow images as myocardium with the highest blood flows. However, especially in markedly dilated left ventricles with diffusely reduced wall motion, such myocardium may indeed be remodeled and not necessarily able to improve contractile function. Tissue histology of such myocardium has revealed increased connective tissue often with diffuse fibrosis.[47] Furthermore, a recent study published in only preliminary form noted attenuated responses of blood flow and glucose utilization to low dose dobutamine stimulation in such myocardium.[48] Thus, identification of remodeled remote myocardium becomes diagnostically challenging. If excess scar formation represents a key feature of such myocardium, then the degree of fibrosis may be measured with the perfusable tissue index.[49,50] This index is derived by determining the extravascular "myocardial mass" from PET transmission and C-11 or O-15 carbon monoxide-labeled red cell blood pool emission images while the myocardial mass capable of rapidly exchanging water can be determined from O-15-labeled water PET emission images. The concept underlying the water perfusable tissue index is that only living myocytes, but not scar or fibrous tissue, are capable of rapidly exchanging water. If there is little if any excessive fibrosis, then the water perfusable myocardial mass equals the total myocardial mass; hence, the water perfusable tissue index will approach unity. If, however, excessive scar tissue formation exists, then the ratio of water perfusable to total myocardial mass declines as a function of the fraction of diffusely distributed scar tissue. While still unexplored, this approach may prove useful for distinguishing between normal and remodeled remote left ventricular myocardium.

Clinical Implications of Blood Flow Metabolism Imaging

Clinically more important than postrevascularization outcomes of segmental function is the effect of therapeutic revascularization by either bypass grafting or coronary angioplasty on (1) global left ventricular function; (2) congestive heart failure related symptoms; and (3) survival. This is because the assessment of myocardial viability is most critical in patients with poor left ventricular function and a high perioperative mortality and morbidity. At the same time, it is those patients who, if surgical revascularization is successful, are likely to benefit most. If blood flow metabolism imaging with PET can answer these clinical questions, it is likely to decisively alter the operative risk-benefit ratio.

Global Left Ventricular Function

The surgical gain in global left ventricular function in the presence of viable myocardium has been pointed out first by Tillisch and colleagues.[20] Patients with at least two myocardial segments (out of a total of 7, or 30%) revealed postsurgical improvement in left ventricular

TABLE 4

Effect of Revascularization and Left Ventricular Ejection Fraction

Author	Pts	n	Extensive mismatch region Pre-LVEF	Post-LVEF	P	n	Small or no mismatch region Pre-LVEF	Post-LVEF	P
Tillisch et al, 1986	17	11	30 ± 11	45 ± 14	<0.05	6	30 ± 11	31 ± 12	NS
Marwick et al, 1982	24	9	37 ± 11	40 ± 9	NS	15	38 ± 13	38 ± 13	NS
Carrel et al, 1992	21	21	34 ± 14	52 ± 11	<0.01	—	—	—	—
Lucignani et al, 1992	14	13	38 ± 5	48 ± 4	<.001	—	—	—	—
Depré et al, 1995	23	*	43 ± 18	52 ± 15	<.001	*	35 ± 9	23 ± 8	NS

* Values not given; n indicates number of patients with and without mismatches.

ejection fraction. Conversely, there was no such improvement in patients without or with only small amounts of mismatch. Thus, the postrevascularization gain in left ventricular function appears to depend on the amount of myocardium that is still viable. As summarized in Table IV, other investigators confirmed these initial findings.[24,25,36,51] If sufficient amounts of viable myocardium were present, then the left ventricular ejection fraction improved; conversely, no improvement occurred when only a small amount of viable myocardium or only a match was observed. The rate of the postrevascularization improvement in global left ventricular function may greatly vary between patients. In one case for example, a patient with severe depression of left ventricular function prior to surgery, demonstrated over a 1-year follow-up period progressive left ventricular ejection fraction from 16% to 40%.[52] The variable rate of functional recovery may be attributable to the morphological alterations in the reversibly dysfunctional myocardium, if observations on regional function can be extrapolated to global left ventricular function. In one study, the rate of functional recovery was found to be correlated inversely with the tissue fraction of "de-differentiated" cells.[53]

Relief from or Improvement of Congestive Heart Failure Symptoms

Di Carli et al[54] reported in a retrospective study that congestive heart failure symptoms markedly improved or even resolved in about

80% of patients with large blood flow metabolism mismatches after they had undergone surgical revascularization. The percentage of patients with such symptomatic improvement markedly exceeded that in patients with mismatches but not submitted to revascularization as well as to that in patient without mismatches, independent of pharmacological or revascularization treatment. Recently, this particular issue has been explored.[55] The prerevascularization blood flow-metabolism mismatch was compared with the long-term improvement in physical activity. It applied a specific scale that expressed physical activity in metabolic units.[56] Patients were submitted to a structured interview prior to and at an average of 25 ± 14 months after coronary artery bypass grafting. As depicted in Figure 6 there was a direct and statistically significant correlation between the extent of the blood flow metabolism mismatch and the postrevascularization change in physical activity. This improvement in the specific activity was most prominent in patients with a blood flow metabolism mismatch that affected at least 20% or more of the left ventricular myocardium.

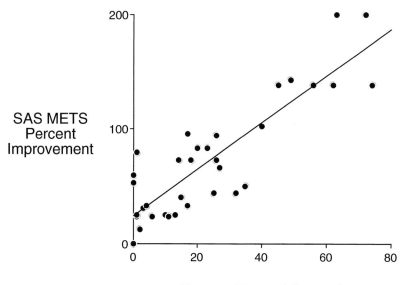

FIGURE 6. Correlation between the improvement in physical activity after revascularization and the extent of a blood flow metabolism mismatch. The physical activity was expressed in metabolic units (METS) as determined by the specific activity scale (SAS). Note the significant correlation between the extent of the blood flow metabolism mismatch and the improvement in physical activity. (Reproduced with permission from Reference 55.)

Blood Flow-Metabolism Mismatches and Future Mortality and Morbidity

Several studies have demonstrated the association between blood flow-metabolism mismatch and increased cardiac morbidity and mortality.[54,57,58] The cardiac event rate, including myocardial infarction and cardiac death, was consistently highest in patient groups with blood flow-metabolism mismatches treated conservatively. Whereas one study found mismatches as an independent predictor of a nonfatal cardiac event and the left ventricular ejection fraction as an independent predictor of death[59] two other studies noted the blood flow metabolism mismatch as an independent predictor of cardiac deaths.[54,58] Different patient populations most likely accounted for these differences. The first study included patients with a wide range of left ventricular functional depression, and the other two studies included only patients with severely depressed left ventricular ejection fractions. For example, in one of the two studies, the left ventricular ejection fraction averaged 26% in all patient subgroups, that is, patients without mismatches treated surgically or conservatively or with mismatches again treated conservatively or with interventional revascularization. In fact, in this study patients without mismatches revealed an about 85% cumulative

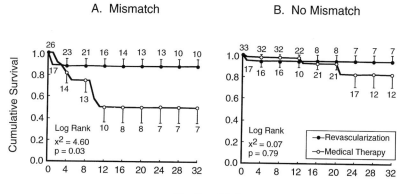

FIGURE 7. Long-term survival in patients with severely reduced left ventricular ejection fraction according to the blood flow metabolism findings on positron emission tomography and treatment. Note the poor cumulative survival of patients with a blood flow metabolism mismatch **(A)** treated conservatively and the significantly better survival in patients with mismatches yet submitted to surgical revascularization. As shown in **B**, also, note the generally better survival of patients without blood flow metabolism mismatches. (Reproduced with permission from Reference 55.)

survival over a 32-month period as compared with only about 50% survival in patients with extensive mismatches (Figure 7).[54] Both patient groups had been treated conservatively. However, the cumulative 32-month survival of patients with mismatches was strikingly improved to about 90% if patients had been submitted to surgical revascularization.

Summary and Conclusions

This chapter suggests that blood flow metabolism mismatches on PET identify patients at high risk for cardiac morbidity and mortality. At the same time, the data indicate that blood flow metabolism patterns identify those patients who are likely to benefit most in terms of left ventricular function, symptomatic relief and survival. This would significantly affect the decision-making process on the most cost-effective and most appropriate therapeutic approach. In support of this notion, preliminary data have demonstrated that PET imaging of blood flow metabolism patterns can in fact identify those patients who will derive significant benefits from surgical revascularization instead of the markedly more complex and costly cardiac transplantation or instead of intensive pharmacologic treatment. In this respect, PET could lead to a reduction in the cost of health care delivery.

Editorial Comment

While the ability of PET to assess perfusion and metabolic function of the myocardium has been well documented, MRI and MRS have the potential to evaluate perfusion-metabolism matches and mismatches. However, MR is in its infancy with such methodology and considerable research is needed to develop and document the utility of MR for this application. In the nearer term, SPECT imaging of F-18 2-fluoro 2-deoxyglucose might be more effectively combined with sestaMIBI or thallium-201 imaging to detect perfusion-metabolic matches or mismatches. SPECT technology has lower resolution than PET, and it could provide another approach to assessment of viability. Again, more development and research are required.

Acknowledgments

The author wishes to thank Eileen Rosenfeld for her skillful assistance in preparing this manuscript and Diane Martin for preparing the illustrations.

References

1. Bergmann SR, Fox KAA, Rand AL, et al. Quantification of regional myocardial blood flow in vivo with $H_2^{15}O$. *Circulation*. 1984;70:724–733.
2. Gould KL, Goldstein RA, Mullani NA, et al. Noninvasive assessment of coronary stenoses by myocardial perfusion imaging during pharmacologic coronary vasodilation. VIII. Clinical feasibility of positron cardiac imaging without a cyclotron using generator-produced rubidium-82. *J Am Coll Cardiol*. 1986;7:775–789.
3. Schelbert HR, Phelps ME, Hoffman EJ, et al. Regional myocardial perfusion assessed with N-13 labeled ammonia and positron emission computerized axial tomography. *Am J Cardiol*. 1979;43:209–218.
4. Bergmann SR, Herrero P, Markham J, et al. Noninvasive quantitation of myocardial blood flow in human subjects with oxygen-15-labeled water and positron emission tomography. *J Am Coll Cardiol*. 1989;14:639–652.
5. Araujo L, Lammertsma A, Rhodes C, et al. Noninvasive quantification of regional myocardial blood flow in coronary artery disease with oxygen-15-labeled carbon dioxide inhalation and positron emission tomography. *Circulation*. 1991;83:875–885.
6. Krivokapich J, Smith GT, Huang SC, et al. N-13 ammonia myocardial imaging at rest and with exercise in normal volunteers: Quantification of absolute myocardial perfusion with dynamic positron emission tomography. *Circulation*. 1989;80:1328–1337.
7. Hutchins G, Schwaiger M, Rosenspire K, et al. Noninvasive quantification of regional blood flow in the human heart using N-13 ammonia and dynamic positron emission tomographic imaging. *J Am Coll Cardiol*. 1990;15:1032–1042.
8. Kuhle W, Porenta G, Huang S-C, et al. Quantification of regional myocardial blood flow using 13N-ammonia and reoriented dynamic positron emission tomographic imaging. *Circulation*. 1992;86:1004–1017.
9. Muzik O, Beanlands RSB, Hutchins GD, et al. Validation of nitrogen-13-ammonia tracer kinetic model for quantification of myocardial blood flow using PET. *J Nucl Med*. 1993;34:83–91.
10. Bol A, Melin JA, Vanoverschelde J-L, et al. Direct comparison of [^{13}N] ammonia and [^{15}O] water estimates of perfusion with quantification of regional myocardial blood flow by microspheres. *Circulation*. 1993;87:512–525.
11. Nitzsche E, Choi Y, Czernin J, et al. Noninvasive quantification of myocardial blood flow in humans: a direct comparison of the N-13 ammonia and the O-15 water technique. *Circulation*. 1996;93:2000–2006.
12. Phelps ME, Schelbert HR, Mazziotta JC. Positron computed tomography for studies of myocardial and cerebral function. *Ann Intern Med*. 1983;98:339–359.
13. Ratib O, Phelps ME, Huang SC, et al. Positron tomography with deoxyglucose for estimating local myocardial glucose metabolism. *J Nucl Med*. 1982;23:577–586.
14. Burt R, Perkins O, Oppenheim B, et al. Direct comparison of fluorine-18-FDG SPECT, fluorine-18-FDG PET and rest thallium-201 SPECT for detection of myocardial viability. *J Nucl Med*. 1995;36:176–179.
15. Gambhir SS, Schwaiger M, Huang SC, et al. Simple noninvasive quantification method for measuring myocardial glucose utilization in humans em-

ploying positron emission tomography and fluorine-18 deoxyglucose. *J Nucl Med.* 1989;30:359–366.

16. Choi Y, Brunken RC, Hawkins RA, et al. Factors affecting myocardial 2-[F-18]fluoro-2-deoxy-D-glucose uptake in positron emission tomography studies of normal humans. *Eur J Nucl Med.* 1993;20:308–318.

17. Schwaiger M, Schelbert HR, Ellison D, et al. Sustained regional abnormalities in cardiac metabolism after transient ischemia in the chronic dog model. *J Am Coll Cardiol.* 1985;6:336–347.

18. Camici P, Araujo LI, Spinks T, et al. Increased uptake of ^{18}F-fluorodeoxyglucose in postischemic myocardium of patients with exercise-induced angina. *Circulation.* 1986;74:81–88.

19. Marshall RC, Tillisch JH, Phelps ME, et al. Identification and differentiation of resting myocardial ischemia and infarction in man with positron computed tomography 18F-labeled fluorodeoxyglucose and N-13 ammonia. *Circulation.* 1983;67:766–778.

20. Tillisch J, Brunken R, Marshall R, et al. Reversibility of cardiac wall motion abnormalities predicted by positron tomography. *N Engl J Med.* 1986;314:884–888.

21. Vanoverschelde J-L, Wijns W, Depre C, et al. Mechanisms of chronic regional postischemic dysfunction in humans: New insights from the study of noninfarcted collateral-dependent myocardium. *Circulation.* 1993;87:1513–1523.

22. Tamaki N, Yonekura Y, Yamashita K, et al. Positron emission tomography using fluorine-18 deoxyglucose in evaluation of coronary artery bypass grafting. *Am J Cardiol.* 1989;64:860–865.

23. Tamaki N, Ohtani H, Yamashita K, et al. Metabolic activity in the areas of new fill-in after thallium-201 reinjection: Comparison with positron emission tomography using fluorine-18-deoxyglucose. *J Nucl Med.* 1991;32:673–678.

24. Carrel T, Jenni R, Haubold-Reuter S, et al. Improvement of severely reduced left ventricular function after surgical revascularization in patients with preoperative myocardial infarction. *Eur J Cardiothorac Surg.* 1992;6:479–484.

25. Lucignani G, Paolini G, Landoni C, et al. Presurgical identification of hibernating myocardium by combined use of technetium-99m hexakis 2-methoxyisobutylisonitrile single photon emission tomography and fluorine-18 fluoro-2-deoxy-D-glucose positron emission tomography in patients with coronary artery disease. *Eur J Nucl Med.* 1992;19:874–881.

26. Marwick T, MacIntyre W, Lafont A, et al. Metabolic responses of hibernating and infarcted myocardium to revascularization: a follow-up study of regional perfusion, function, and metabolism. *Circulation.* 1992;85:1347–1353.

27. Gropler RJ, Geltman EM, Sampathkumaran K, et al. Comparison of carbon-11-acetate with fluorine-18-fluorodeoxyglucose for delineating viable myocardium by positron emission tomography. *J Am Coll Cardiol.* 1993;22:1587–1597.

28. Knuuti M, Saraste M, Nuutila P, et al. Myocardial viability: Fluorine-18-deoxyglucose positron emission tomography in prediction of wall motion recovery after revascularization. *Circulation.* 1994;90:2356–2366.

29. vom Dahl J, Eitzman D, Al-Aouar A, et al. Relation of regional function, perfusion, and metabolism in patients with advanced coronary artery disease undergoing surgical revascularization. *Circulation.* 1994;90:2356–2366.

30. Marzullo P, Parodi O, Sambuceti G, et al. Residual coronary reserve identi-

fies segmental viability in patients with wall motion abnormalities. *J Am Coll Cardiol.* 1995;26:342–350.

31. Czernin J, Porenta G, Müller P, et al. Perfusion defect extent determines LV function in patients with PET ischemia. *Circulation.* 1991;84:II-474.
32. Sun K, Czernin J, Krivokapich J, et al. Effects of dobutamine stimulation on myocardial blood flow, glucose metabolism and wall motion in PET mismatch regions. *J Am Coll Cardiol.* 1994;25:117A.
33. Gewirtz H, Fischman A, Abraham S, et al. Positron emission tomographic measurements of absolute regional myocardial blood flow permits identification of nonviable myocardium in patients with chronic myocardial infarction. *J Am Coll Cardiol.* 1994;23:851–859.
34. Tamaki N, Kawamoto M, Tadamura E, et al. Prediction of reversible ischemia after revascularization: Perfusion and metabolic studies using positron emission tomography. *Circulation.* 1995;91:1697–1705.
35. Maes A, Flameng W, Nuyts J, et al. Histological alterations in chronically hypoperfused myocardium: Correlation with PET findings. *Circulation.* 1994;90:735–745.
36. Depre C, Vanoverschelde J-L J, Melin J, et al. Structural and metabolic correlates of the reversibility of chronic left ventricular ischemic dysfunction in humans. *Am J Physiol.* 1995;268:H1265–H1275.
37. Schwarz E, Schaper J, vom Dahl J, et al. Myocardial hibernation is not sufficient to prevent morphological disarrangements with ischemic cell alterations and increased fibrosis. *Circulation.* 1994;90:I-378.
38. Sun D, Jguyen N, DeGrado T, et al. Ischemia induces translocation of the insulin-responsive glucose transporter GLUT 4 to the plasma membrane of cardiac myocytes. *Circulation.* 1994;89:793–798.
39. Schwaiger M, Sun D, Deeb G, et al. Expression of myocardial glucose transporter (GLUT) mRNAs in patients with advanced coronary artery disease (CAD). *Circulation.* 1994;90:I-113.
40. Chan A, Czernin J, Brunken R, et al. Effects of dietary state on the incidence of myocardial blood flow-metabolism mismatches in patients with chronic coronary artery disease. *J Am Coll Cardiol.* 1993;21:129A.
41. Nienaber C, Brunken R, Sherman C, et al. Metabolic and functional recovery of ischemic human myocardium after coronary angioplasty. *J Am Coll Cardiol.* 1991;18:966–978.
42. Knuuti M, Yki-Järvinen H, Voipio-Pulkki L, et al. Enhancement of myocardial [fluorine-18] fluorodeoxyglucose uptake by a nicotinic acid derivative. *J Nucl Med.* 1994;35:989–998.
43. Hoffman EJ, Huang SC, Phelps ME. Quantitation in positron emission computed tomography. *J Comput Assist Tomogr.* 1979;3:299–308.
44. Parodi P, Schelbert HR, Schwaiger M, Hansen H, Selin C, Hoffman EJ. Cardiac emission computed tomography: Underestimation of regional tracer concentrations due to wall motion abnormalities. *J Comput Assist Tomogr.* 1984;8:1083–1092.
45. Perrone-Filardi P, Bacharach SL, Dilsizian V, et al. Regional left ventricular wall thickening. *Circulation.* 1992;86:1125–1137.
46. Baer F, Voth E, Schneider C, et al. Comparison of low-dose dobutamine-gradient-echo magnetic resonance imaging and positron emission tomography with [18F] fluorodeoxyglucose in patients with chronic coronary artery disease. A functional and morphological approach to the detection of residual myocardial viability. *Circulation.* 1995;91:1006–1015.
47. Schaper J, Froedi R, Hein S, et al. Impairment of the myocardial ultrastruc-

ture and changes of the cytoskeleton in dilated cardiomyopathy. *Circulation.* 1991;83:504–514.

48. Sun K, Czernin J, Krivokapich J, et al. Effects of dobutamine stimulation on myocardial blood flow, glucose metabolism and wall motion in PET mismatch regions. *J Am Coll Cardiol.* 1994;SE:127A.

49. Iida H, Rhodes C, de Silva R, et al. Myocardial tissue fraction—Correction for Partial Volume Effects and Measure of Tissue Viability. *J Nucl Med.* 1991;32:2169–2175.

50. Yamamoto K, Iwase S, Mano T. Responses of muscle sympathetic nerve activity and cardiac output to the cold pressor test. *Jpn J Physiol.* 1992;42: 239–252.

51. Besozzi MC, Brown MD, Hubner KF, et al. Retrospective post therapy evaluation of cardiac function in 208 coronary artery disease patients evaluated by positron emission tomography. *J Nucl Med.* 1992;33:885.

52. Luu M, Stevenson L, Brunken R, et al. Delayed recovery of revascularized myocardium after referral for cardiac transplantation. *Am Heart J.* 1990;119: 668–670.

53. Vanoverschelde J, Melin J, Depre C, et al. Time-course of functional recovery of hibernating myocardium after coronary revascularization. *Circulation.* 1994;90:I-378.

54. Di Carli M, Davidson M, Little R, et al. Value of metabolic imaging with positron emission tomography for evaluating prognosis in patients with coronary artery disease and left ventricular dysfunction. *Am J Cardiol.* 1994; 73:527–533.

55. Di Carli M, Farbod A, Schelbert H, et al. Quantitative relation between myocardial viability and improvement in heart failure symptoms after revascularization in patients with ischemic cardiomyopathy. *Circulation.* 1995;92:3436–3444.

56. Goldman L, Hashimoto B, EF C, Loscalzo A. Comparative reproducibility and validity of systems for assessing cardiovascular functional class: Advantages of a new specific activity scale. *Circulation.* 1981;64:1227–1234.

57. Tamaki N, Kawamoto M, Takahashi N, et al. Prognostic value of an increase in fluorine-18 deoxyglucose uptake in patients with myocardial infarction: Comparison with stress thallium imaging. *J Am Coll Cardiol.* 1993;22: 1621–1627.

58. Eitzman D, Al-Aouar Z, Kanter H, et al. Clinical outcome of patients with advanced coronary artery disease after viability studies with positron emission tomography. *J Am Coll Cardiol.* 1992;20:559–565.

59. Lee K, Marwick T, Cook S, et al. Prognosis of patients with left ventricular dysfunction, with and without viable myocardium after myocardial infarction. *Circulation.* 1994;90:2687–2694.

## Chapter 17

Measurement of Coronary Blood Flow at Rest and During Stress

Hajime Sakuma, MD and
Charles B. Higgins, MD

X-ray angiography has been the traditional method for the evaluation of coronary arterial stenoses. However, assessment of the coronary angiogram as a means of predicting the physiological significance of a coronary arterial stenosis is imperfect[1] because the luminal area of irregular or complicated stenoses cannot be precisely depicted with projectional angiography. Moreover, the diameter of the adjacent arterial segment is frequently abnormal in patients with coronary artery disease, rendering the measurement of the morphological reduction in luminal diameter equivocal.

The functional significance of coronary artery stenosis can be evaluated by measuring coronary flow reserve (CFR), that is, the ratio of maximal hyperemic coronary flow to the baseline coronary flow.[2] Wilson et al[3] reported that CFR measured by the intravascular Doppler ultrasonic catheter was closely related to percent area stenosis and minimal cross-sectional area in the coronary arteries in patients with single discrete coronary stenoses. Joye et al[4] measured CFR with Doppler flow wire and showed that CFR less than 2.0 had high sensitivity (94%) and specificity (95%) in predicting the hemodynamic significance of coronary arterial stenoses in patients with coronary artery disease, using stress thallium-201 SPECT as a standard. Another study using transesophageal Doppler ultrasound demonstrated that CFR greater than 2.1 had a sensitivity of 86% and a specificity of 79% for ruling

From: Higgins CB, Ingwall JS, Pohost GM, (eds). *Current and Future Applications of Magnetic Resonance in Cardiovascular Disease.* Armonk, NY: Futura Publishing Company, Inc.; © 1998.

out critical coronary stenoses in the left anterior descending arteries as defined by coronary angiograms.[5]

Magnetic resonance imaging (MRI) can potentially provide a non-invasive method for measuring blood flow and vasodilator flow reserve in the coronary arteries. However, coronary flow measurement with MRI has been very difficult because the coronary artery demonstrates both cardiac and respiratory motion while the luminal diameter of the vessel is less than 3 to 4 mm.

Methods for Quantification of Coronary Blood Flow with Magnetic Resonance Imaging

Both phase contrast and time-of-flight (TOF) methods have been used in the past several years for measurement of coronary blood flow using MRI. Coronary flow measurement with the TOF approach was reported by Poncelet et al.[6] They obtained a series of single-shot echoplanar images (EPI) with a progressive delay time between a 90° radiofrequency (RF) pulse for large slab saturation and another 90° RF pulse for EPI imaging. A TOF model was used to derive coronary flow velocities from wash-in curves. Edelman et al[7] measured coronary blood flow velocity using a phase contrast method. Electrocardiogram (ECG)-gated magnitude and phase images were acquired during diastole, using a fast gradient-echo sequence with velocity-encoding gradients and a segmented k-space data acquisition. Although initial studies[7,8] measured flow velocities in the coronary arteries at a single temporal phase in the cardiac cycle per breath-hold data acquisition, phase contrast cine MRI can provide coronary blood flow measurements at multiple phases in the cardiac cycle during a single breath-hold period.[9–11]

Fast Phase Contrast Cine Magnetic Resonance Imaging

Coronary blood flow was measured in humans using fast phase contrast cine MRI.[10] Velocity measurements in the coronary arteries were performed with a 1.5-T clinical magnetic resonance (MR) imager (Signa Advantage, GE Medical Systems, Milwaukee, WI). Conventional gradient configurations with a maximum gradient strength of 110 mT/m and maximum gradient slew rate of 27 mT/s were used. Scout images on transaxial imaging planes were obtained to demonstrate the left main coronary artery and proximal portion of the left anterior descending (LAD) artery. Breath-hold cine MR images were then acquired on single oblique imaging planes that corresponded to the long-axis view of the left ventricle.

Flow velocity in the coronary artery was measured with a breath-hold phase contrast cine MR sequence (FastCard-PC, GE Medical Systems, Milwaukee, WI).[9] Double-oblique FastCard-PC images in a plane perpendicular to the LAD artery were acquired with a slice thickness of 5 mm, repetition time (TR) of 16 ms and echo time (TE) of 9 ms, phase-encoding steps of 96 field of view (FOV) of 24 × 18 cm, reconstructed image matrix of 256 × 192, receiver bandwidth of 32 kHz. RF excitation pulses were applied uniformly throughout the scan in order to maintain the spins in the steady state and to avoid the increased signal intensity in the first few temporal images due to the longer T1 recovery period—the so-called "lighting flash" artifact. This also eliminated the need for dummy excitations prior to data collection and enables the acquisition of data immediately after the ECG wave trigger.

Velocity-encoding gradients were applied in the slice-selective direction with velocity window (VENC) of ±100 cm/s. For each k-space view, positive and negative velocity-encoding data were acquired as a sequential pair. Four views of k-space data were collected per segment per RR interval. The true temporal resolution, defined as a data acquisition window in which the motion is averaged over time, was 128 ms, which is given by m × n × TR, where m is a number of flow-encoding sequences for each k-space view and n the a number of views collected per segment. View-sharing reconstruction was used to improve the effective temporal resolution. Images at intermediate temporal phases were generated by using the last n/2 views in each segment of one temporal phase, where n is the number of views per segment. The true temporal resolution, the time required to acquire data for all n views within a segment, is unchanged (128 ms). However, the effective temporal resolution, the temporal separation between each image, can be halved (64 ms).

Fast phase contrast cine imaging data were acquired for 24 heartbeats under a suspended shallow inspiration. Magnitude and phase-difference cine images with 7 to 13 temporal phases were reconstructed. After obtaining the baseline measurement, 0.56 mg/kg of dipyridamole was injected into the antecubital vein over 4 minutes. Approximately 3 to 4 minutes after the injection of dipyridamole, flow velocity in the LAD artery was measured again to evaluate the augmentation of coronary blood flow velocity with pharmacological stress. CFR was calculated as the ratio of hyperemic to baseline coronary blood flow velocity in the LAD artery. Coronary flow volume in the coronary arteries was not measured because limited spatial resolution of the images relative to the small size of the coronary artery made the accuracy of flow volume measurement questionable.

Healthy volunteer

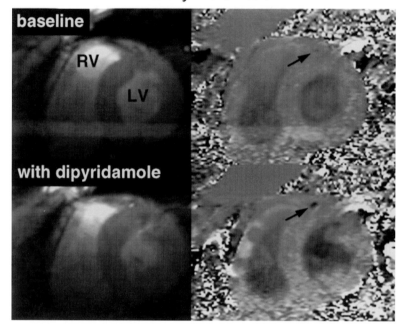

FIGURE 1. Magnitude **(left)** and phase-difference **(right)** images acquired with fast phase contrast cine MR sequence at baseline state and after dipyridamole in a healthy volunteer. Flow in the LAD artery was augmented after dipyridamole injection, which is shown as a darkening of the LAD signal on the phase-difference image (arrows).

Magnetic Resonance Assessments of Coronary Flow Reserve in Healthy Volunteers and Patients with Coronary Artery Disease

Figure 1 shows magnitude and phase-difference images acquired at baseline and after dipyridamole injection in a healthy volunteer. Blood flow in the LAD was shown as a dark signal on the phase-difference images, and increased flow velocity after dipyridamole injection was evident as a substantial darkening of the LAD signal on the phase-difference image. Coronary flow velocity curves in this normal volunteer were plotted at baseline and after dipyridamole injection by measuring relative flow velocity in a region of interest (ROI) placed within the LAD artery compared with the velocity in the surrounding myocardium (Figure 2). For the study depicted in Figure 2, diastolic peak

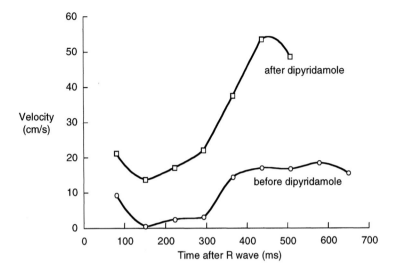

FIGURE 2. Corrected LAD flow velocity curves in a normal volunteer measured in the baseline state and after dipyridamole. The number of the cardiac phases acquired after dipyridamole injection was decreased because of the increased heart rate. Diastolic peak velocity in the LAD artery showed more than threefold increase after administration of dipyridamole.

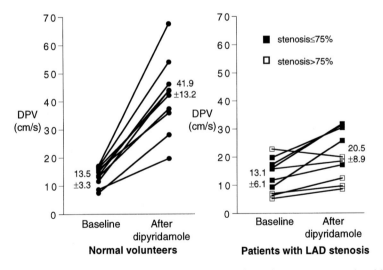

FIGURE 3. Diastolic peak velocity measured by fast phase contrast cine MRI at baseline state and after dipyridamole in normal volunteers **(left)** and in patients with LAD stenosis **(right)**. The diastolic peak velocity (DPV) in the patients' group was significantly lower than that in healthy subjects after dipyridamole administration ($P < .01$).

velocity was 16 cm/s at baseline and increased to 54 cm/s with dipyridamole injection, resulting in a CFR of 3.4.

MR measurements of diastolic peak velocity before and after dipyridamole injection in normal volunteers are summarized in Figure 3.
The average diastolic peak velocity in LAD of a group of normal subjects was 13.5 cm/s ± 13.2 after dipyridamole. The average CFR was
approximately 3.1 in normal volunteers. The normal CFR of 3.1 measured by MRI is consistent with the normal CFR ratios reported by
using other modalities. In the studies using intravenous dipyridamole
or adenosine as a vasodilator, normal CFR was 3.1 to 4.8 by intracoronary Doppler,[12–14] 3.2 by transesophageal Doppler ultrasound,[15,16] and
3.0 by positron emission tomography.[17]

Fast phase contrast cine MR images at baseline state and after dipyridamole injection acquired in a patient with significant LAD stenosis
are shown in Figure 4. Flow velocity in the LAD was slightly increased
after dipyridamole injection, which was recognized as darkening of the
LAD signal on the phase-difference images. The LAD flow velocity
curves before and after dipyridamole injection in this patient are dem-

Patient with LAD stenosis

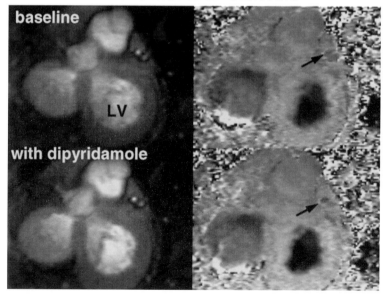

FIGURE 4. Magnitude **(left)** and phase-difference **(right)** images acquired with
fast phase contrast cine MR sequence at baseline state and after dipyridamole
in a patient with a 75% stenosis of the LAD. Flow in the LAD slightly increased
after the injection of dipyridamole (arrows).

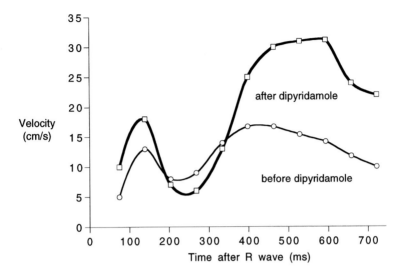

FIGURE 5. Corrected LAD flow velocity curves in the patient shown in Figure 4 measured at baseline state and after dipyridamole. Diastolic peak velocity in the LAD showed less than twofold increase after the administration of dipyridamole.

onstrated in Figure 5. The diastolic peak velocity was 17 cm/s at baseline, and increased to 32 cm/s after dipyridamole injection, resulting in a CFR of 1.8, which is lower than the normal CFR in healthy subjects.

The diastolic peak velocity in the LAD of patients with significant LAD stenosis was compared with those in healthy volunteers (Figure 3). At baseline state, the average diastolic peak velocity was 13.5 cm/s $\pm$ 3.3 in healthy volunteers, and 13.1 cm/s $\pm$ 6.1 in patients with LAD stenosis. There was no statistical significance between the average velocities in the normal group and the patient group before dipyridamole injection. After the administration of dipyridamole, the diastolic peak velocity in the patients increased to 20.5 cm/s $\pm$ 8.9, which was significantly lower than that (41.9 cm/s $\pm$ 13.2) in healthy volunteers (P <.01).

In order to validate MR assessments of CFR in patients with coronary arterial stenosis, the CFR in 14 patients with varying degrees of stenosis in the LAD arteries were measured by intracoronary Doppler flow wire before and after pharmacological stress, and the CFR with Doppler flow wire were compared with those obtained with MRI. Pharmacological stress was induced by intravenous injection of dipyridamole for both MR and Doppler measurements. Figure 6 shows the correlation between the CFR measured by fast phase contrast cine MRI and Doppler flow wire in 14 patients. This initial study demonstrated

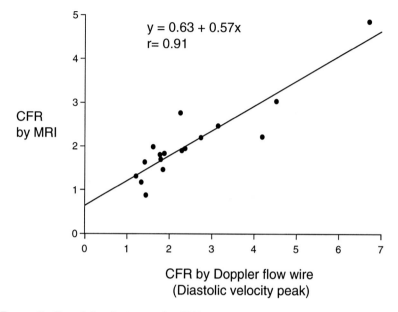

FIGURE 6. Correlation between the CFR measured by fast phase contrast cine MRI and the CFR measured by Doppler low wire during angiography.

that there is good correlation between MR and Doppler measurements of the CFR, with a correlation coefficient of 0.91.

Magnetic Resonance Quantification of Volume Flow in Coronary Arteries

As mentioned in the previous section, the CFR ratio in healthy volunteers and patients with coronary artery disease was calculated as the ratio of hyperemic to baseline coronary flow velocity when the standard gradient system was used. The CFR ratios measured by Doppler flow-wire and transesophageal Doppler ultrasound are based on flow velocity measurements, and have been proven to be effective in clinical assessment of functional significance of the coronary artery stenosis. Therefore, MR assessment of the CFR ratio calculated from flow velocities can be useful as well for the evaluation of functional significance of the coronary artery stenosis in patients. However, MR also has the potential for providing direct measurements of flow volume in the coronary arteries by integrating mean velocity and area of the vessel over the cardiac cycle.

Before attempting to measure absolute blood flow volume in the coronary artery, potential sources of errors in flow volume measurement with MRI have to be considered. Intravoxel averaging of flowing blood signal and static tissue signal at vessel edge is a major source of error. Flowing spins demonstrate greater signal than static spins due to the TOF effect. Therefore, flow volume may be significantly overestimated if the voxel size is not small enough compared with the vessel diameter. Limited temporal resolution in the cardiac cycle is another significant source of error. If temporal resolution in the cardiac cycle is not sufficient, blurring of the vessel may result in an inaccurate flow volume assessment.

Recently, nonresonant high-speed gradients have been used; these gradients can provide better temporal and spatial resolutions in fast phase contrast cine MRI compared with those acquired with the standard gradients. With an increased maximal gradient amplitude and a faster rise time, a smaller field of view (16 cm vs. 24 cm), shorter TE (4.5 ms vs. 9 ms), shorter TR (13 ms vs. 16 ms), and better temporal resolution (104 ms vs. 128 ms) can be achieved by using high-speed gradients, which can improve the accuracy of MR flow volume measurement in the coronary arteries.

In order to evaluate the accuracy of measurements of absolute flow volume in the coronary arteries with fast phase contrast cine MRI, coronary flow volume was evaluated in open-chest dogs using flow meter measurements for comparison. Seven beagle dogs were mechanically ventilated in the magnet. A perivascular transit-time ultrasound flow probe was placed around the proximal LAD artery. Fast velocity-encoded cine MR images were acquired with a Signa Horizon high-speed prototype system (GE Medical Systems, Milwaukee, WI). A velocity-encoding gradient was applied in slice-selective direction with maximal velocity of ±1 m/s. Two lines of k-space were collected per trigger segment, and 9 to 15 cine cardiac phases were reconstructed with the data acquired within 25 seconds. MR flow measurements were repeated every 2 minutes. Flow meter measurements were obtained between MR scans. After acquiring several baseline data, dipyridamole was administered.

Figure 7A shows magnitude and phase-difference images of the LAD artery in the diastolic phase in the baseline state, and Figure 7B shows images at maximal hyperemic state after dipyridamole injection. Flow in the LAD was indicated as a dark signal on the phase difference image, which was substantially increased after dipyridamole injection. For quantification of flow volume ROIs were defined that encompassed the arterial lumen of the LAD and another ROI in the adjacent myocardium for each cardiac phase. Corrected LAD velocity was obtained as a relative velocity compared with adjacent myocardium. MR flow volume was calculated by integrating LAD flow velocity and area of

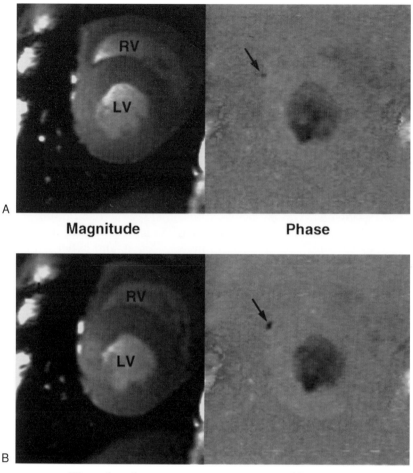

FIGURE 7. Magnitude **(left)** and phase-difference **(right)** image of the LAD in diastole at baseline state **(A)** and at maximal hyperemic state after dipyridamole injection **(B)** in an open chest dog.

the vessel for each of the images corresponded to multiple phases of the cardiac cycle.

Serial measurements of LAD flow volume by MRI and ultrasonic flow meter are presented in Figure 8. The LAD flow volume was rapidly increased with dipyridamole injection and then gradually decreased over time. The flow volume measured with MRI was very close to the value obtained with flow meter. Figure 9 shows the correlation between flow volumes measured by MRI and flow meter. Correlation coefficient

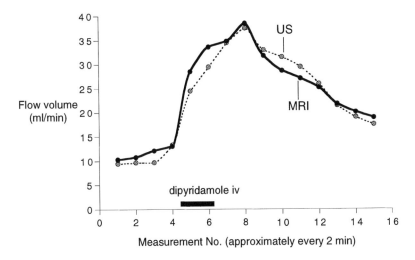

FIGURE 8. Serial measurements of coronary flow volume by MR and ultrasonic flowmeter after dipyridamole injection. MR flow volume at each point was calculated by integrating corrected LAD flow velocity and area of the vessel.

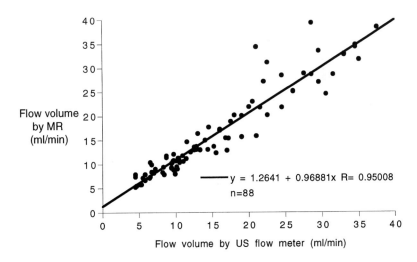

FIGURE 9. Correlation between MR and ultrasound flowmeter measurements of coronary flow volume in seven dogs. Correlation coefficient was 0.95 for the 88 data points.

between MR and ultrasound flow meter measurements was 0.95 and slope of the linear regression line was 0.97 for 88 data points acquired in 7 dogs.

Conclusions

Fast phase contrast cine MRI is a noninvasive technique that can provide assessment of coronary flow velocity and CFR in humans. The CFR measured by MRI in patients with coronary artery disease were significantly lower than the CFR in normal volunteers, and correlated well with the CFR measured by Doppler flow wire. With the use of high-speed gradients, coronary flow volume measurements by MRI correlated closely with ultrasound flow meter measurements in open-chest dogs. With further refinement of MR technology and more wide-spread clinical experience, MRI may eventually be recognized as a comprehensive technique for the evaluation of the presence and physiological significance of coronary arterial stenoses.

References

1. White CW, Wright CB, Doty DB, et al. Does visual interpretation of the coronary angiogram predict the physiological importance of a coronary stenosis? *N Engl J Med.* 1984;310:819–825.
2. Gould KL, Lipscomb K, Hamilton GW. Physiologic basis for assessing critical coronary stenosis: instantaneous flow response and regional distribution during coronary hyperemia as measures of coronary flow reserve. *Am J Cardiol.* 1974;33:87–94.
3. Wilson RF, Marcus ML, White CW. Prediction of the physiologic significance of coronary arterial lesions by quantitative lesion geometry in patients with limited coronary artery disease. *Circulation.* 1987;75:723–732.
4. Joye JD, Schulman DS, Lasorda D, et al. Intracoronary Doppler guide wire versus stress single-photon emission computed tomographic thallium-201 imaging in assessment of intermediate coronary stenoses. *J Am Coll Cardiol.* 1994;24:940–947.
5. Redberg RF, Sobol Y, Chou TM, et al. Adenosine induced coronary vasodilation during transesophageal Doppler echocardiography. Rapid and safe measurement of coronary flow reserve ratio can predict significant left anterior descending coronary stenosis. *Circulation.* 1995;92:199–196.
6. Poncelet BP, Weisskoff RM, Wedeen WJ, et al. Time of flight quantification of coronary flow with echo-planar MRI. *Magn Reson Med.* 1993;30:447–457.
7. Edelman RR, Manning WJ, Gervino E, Li W. Flow velocity quantification in human coronary arteries with fast breath-hold MR angiography. *J Magn Reson Imaging.* 1993;3:699–703.
8. Keegan J, Firmin D, Gatehouse P, Longmore D. The application of breath-hold phase velocity mapping techniques to the measurement of coronary artery blood flow velocity Phantom data and initial in vivo results. *Magn Reson Med.* 1994;31:526–536.

9. Foo TKF, Bernstein MA, Aisen AM, et al. Improved ejection fraction and flow velocity estimates using view sharing and uniform TR excitation with fast cardiac techniques. *Radiology*. 1995;195:471–478.
10. Sakuma H, Blake LM, Amidon TM, et al. Coronary flow reserve: Noninvasive measurements in humans with breath-hold velocity-encoded cine MR imaging. *Radiology*. 1996;198:745–750.
11. Clarke GD, Eckels R, Chaney C, et al. Measurement of absolute epicardial coronary artery flow and flow reserve with breath-hold cine phase-contrast magnetic resonance imaging. *Circulation*. 1995;91:2627–2634.
12. Wilson RF, White CW. Intracoronary papaverine: An ideal coronary vasodilator for studies of the coronary circulation in conscious humans. *Circulation*. 1986;73:444–451.
13. Wilson RF, Wyche K, Christensen BV, et al. Effects of adenosine on human coronary arterial circulation. *Circulation*. 1990;82:1595–1606.
14. Rossen JD, Quillen JE, Lopez AG, et al. Comparison of coronary vasodilation with intravenous dipyridamole and adenosine. *J Am Coll Cardiol*. 1991; 18:485–491.
15. Iliceto S, Marangelli V, Memmola C, Rizzon P. Transesophageal Doppler echocardiography evaluation of coronary blood flow velocity in baseline condition and during dipyridamole-induced coronary vasodilation. *Circulation*. 1991;83:61–69.
16. Redberg RF, Sobol Y, Chou TM, et al. Adenosine induced coronary vasodilation during transesophageal Doppler echocardiography: Rapid and safe measurement of coronary flow reserve ratio can predict significant left anterior descending coronary stenosis. *Circulation*. 1995;92:190–196.
17. Czemin J, Muller P, Chan S, et al. Influence of age and hemodynamics on myocardial blood flow and flow reserve. *Circulation*. 1993;88:62–69.

Chapter 18

Physiological and Biochemical Information from Water in Cardiac Magnetic Resonance Imaging

Robert S. Balaban, PhD

Proton magnetic resonance imaging (MRI) provides outstanding views of cardiac anatomy *in vivo*. However, the information content of MRI goes well beyond the anatomy shown in the high-resolution image of the canine heart in Figure 1. The contrast and signal intensity of this gradient-recalled echo image of the heart also reflects information on perfusion, water molecular dynamics and diffusion, chemical exchange, tissue oxygenation, macromolecular dynamics and surface chemistry, as well as paramagnetic content.

The magnetic resonance (MR) image is mostly composed of signal originating from water protons. This approximately 100 M water proton signal is the major constituent of tissues resulting in the ability of insensitive nuclear magnetic resonance (NMR) methods to create high-resolution (<1 mm in-plane) images of the heart. The one exception to this rule is adipose tissue. Adipose tissue is composed mostly of fat, with little water. Thus, the proton MR signal from adipose originates mostly from fat protons. Water is the solvent of the heart cell. As the solvent, water contributes to the structure of most of the proteins and macromolecules, provides the media for the cystosolic distribution of metabolites and ions, and participates in numerous biochemical reactions. Each of these processes influence the nature of the water proton MR signal from the heart. The water proton MR signal can be sensitized during the image acquisition phase to isolate many of these physiologic

From: Higgins CB, Ingwall JS, Pohost GM, (eds). *Current and Future Applications of Magnetic Resonance in Cardiovascular Disease.* Armonk, NY: Futura Publishing Company, Inc.; © 1998.

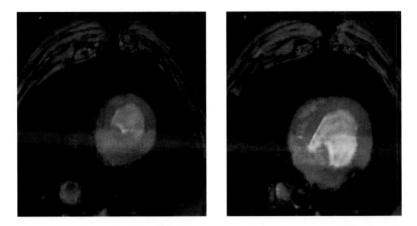

FIGURE 1. High-resolution proton MRI of canine heart at 4 T. Gradient-recalled echo sequence. TE 14 ms. TR 400 ms. Resolution 0.4 × 0.4 × 3mm. (Data from Reference 11.)

interactions. These basic interactions of water in the cytosol and vascular system result in the tissue contrast observed in MRI that significantly adds to the diagnostic value of MRI.

Figure 2 is a diagram of the different types of physiologic information available from water proton MRI of the heart. These parameters include blood oxygenation, tissue perfusion, water hydrodynamics, water self-diffusion rates and direction, macromolecular surface interactions that include surface chemistry and mobility, metabolite chemical exchange, and tissue paramagnetic content. Blood vessel velocity measures[1,2] and myocardial motion or strain measures[3-5] have not been included in this discussion because these topics have been extensively discussed in the literature.

Vascular Oxygenation

Starting in the vasculature that supports cardiac function, how can water MR be sensitized to vascular blood oxygenation? Hemoglobin in its oxygenated state (oxyhemoglobin) is slightly diamagnetic, very similar to normal tissue, and thus it does not significantly modify the MR signal from the heart. However, deoxygenated hemoglobin (deoxyhemoglobin) is strongly paramagnetic and causes a local magnetic field around the red blood cell and surrounding tissue.[6] This magnetic field disrupts the MR signal from water by effectively shifting the resonance frequency of water as it experiences different magnetic field strengths around a deoxygenated red cell. These frequency shifts causes the water

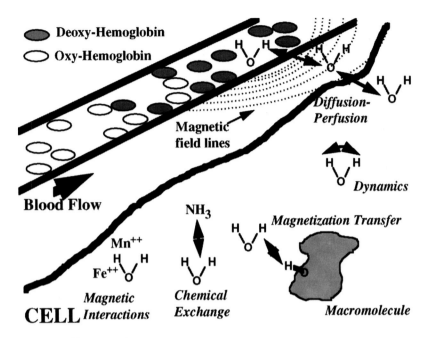

FIGURE 2. Interactions of water detected in proton MRI.

protons signals to be out of phase (i.e., dephasing) in some imaging experiments. This dephasing results in a reduction in the MR signal from these water molecules. Naturally, this effect is more intense in the vascular space and tissue in its immediate vicinity because the magnetic field gradients drop off quickly. The field lines are presented in Figure 2 around the deoxyhemoglobin containing red cells. The deoxyhemoglobin effect is detected in MRI by weighting the image to this dephasing of the water spins caused by the deoxymyoglobin magnetic fields. The dephasing of a spin by bulk or microscopic magnetic field gradients in a sample is often referred to as T2* and is generally associated with a decrease in signal intensity in an acquisition scheme that is sensitive to T2* effects. The most popular approach in detecting deoxyhemoglobin is the use of gradient-recalled echo techniques that emphasize the T2* effects; however, spin-echo sequences can also reveal this information when associated with diffusional motion of water. Because the red cell is moving through the vasculature, and water is rapidly diffusing in and around the vasculature, a large amount of water can be affected, or dephased, by relatively few deoxyhemoglobin molecules. Using this approach, numerous investigators have demonstrated that hypoxic or ischemic regions in the brain can be visualized[7,8] as well as activated regions of the brain.[9,10] In the brain, the effect of local activation of the motor cortex, for example, is associated with a net increase in oxygen tension most likely due to a disproportionally large vascular response to changes in cerebral metabolic activity.

Using a similar approach, it was demonstrated that ischemic or hyperemic regions of the heart can be imaged *in vivo* using gradient-recalled echo MRI.[11] In general, regions that were underperfused had a greater T2* effect from deoxymyoglobin, which decreased the signal intensity in a gradient-recalled echo images. Whereas hyperemia associated with a local infusion of adenosine resulted in an increase in signal intensity due to the decrease in deoxyhemoglobin content. Figure 3 shows an example from this study where the region of the heart that was hyperperfused due to a left anterior descending artery infusion of adenosine was characterized by an increase in signal intensity (>30%) from the decrease in deoxyhemoglobin content. The large effect of hyperemia is partially due to the near complete extraction of oxygen from the blood by the heart under normal conditions, leaving a high concentration of deoxyhemoglobin in the venous vasculature that compromises most of the vascular volume. Thus, deoxyhemoglobin is significantly contributing to the T2* of the heart under control conditions. With a local adenosine infusion, the venous hemoglobin saturation approached 80% resulting in a large decrease in deoxyhemoglobin concentration and corresponding increase in MRI signal intensity. This concept was supported by the observation that ischemia only decreased the signal intensity by approximately 10% despite the complete conversion of all of the hemoglobin to the deoxygenated form.[11] This lack of a large T2* effect with ischemia may also be influenced by the squeezing of blood from the pressurized myocardium during this low-flow condition. This reduction in tissue blood volume will also reduce the concentration of deoxyhemoglobin as would an increase in oxygen tension. Overall, similar results were obtained by Wendland et al[12] who studied the effects of apnea in the heart with gradient-recalled echo EPI imaging. This approach has also been successful in the perfused heart[13] as well as in recent studies on human subjects.[14,15]

In order to obtain quantitative information from T2* data in terms of absolute oxygen tension numerous obstacles must be overcome. Other magnetic susceptibilities in the chest can result in magnetic field gradients that contribute to T2* independent of deoxyhemoglobin. Specifically, the air-water interfaces in the chest are particularly problematic. It is difficult to isolate the sources of different T2* effects without numerous measurements. The total blood volume is critical because the T2* effect is related to the tissue content of deoxyhemoglobin, not oxygen tension directly. That is, deoxymyoglobin content, or T2* can change with blood volume, or capillary hematocrit, without a change

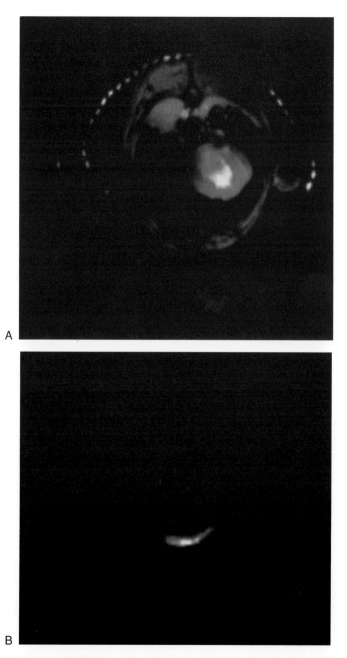

A

B

FIGURE 3. Effect of adenosine-induced increases in coronary flow on MRI signal intensity. **A:** GRE image of an *in vivo* dog heart. **B:** Difference image after the local infusion of adenosine into the left anterior descending artery (LAD) (Data adapted from Reference 11.)

in tissue P_{O_2} or hemoglobin oxygen saturation. It is also important to note that up to 20% of the signal from a voxel within the heart may actually be originating from blood during vasodilatation due to the large volume fraction of blood vessels in heart tissue. The blood volume could also change through the contraction cycle as the wall pressure varies and venous blood is redistributed across the myocardium. The contribution of vascular water with different relaxation rates than tissue can significantly contribute to the signal amplitude changes observed in numerous conditions. These combined effects makes absolute measures of blood volume in the heart critical for the determination of vascular P_{O_2} using T2* measures. In addition, the changes in perfusion or flow rate can also change the apparent spin lattice relaxation rate, as will be discussed, which can also influence these results[11] but can be minimized by the image acquisition parameters. All of these potential vascular effects have major implications in these T2* studies as well as many of the other properties to be discussed. Many of the limitations in quantitating the T2* effects have been presented in the literature as they relate to studies in the myocardium.[11] However, in the major vessels or chambers of the heart where alterations in blood volume, hematocrit, and bulk susceptibility effects are minimal, good estimates of oxygen tensions have been made.[16]

It is important to note that oxygen itself can, directly contribute to the relaxation properties of water, which could be used in a MRI experiment; whether this will prove useful in the heart is still being evaluated. In addition, the concentration of an oxygen isotope,[17] O, can be directly assessed using its specific relaxation effects on water[17,18] providing another potential method of monitoring oxygen tension via water MRI.

Perfusion

Perfusion is another important physiologic parameter that is intimately related to water. Perfusion can be defined as the amount of water moving through a given volume of tissue per unit time. This parameter is critical in determining oxygen and nutrient delivery to the heart muscle. Perfusion can be estimated in MRI studies, without exogenous contrast agents, by taking advantage of the partial saturation of water spins occurring in most imaging studies. This approach is illustrated in Figure 4. The imaging plane in the heart is partially saturated in an imaging experiment because the repetition of the excitation pulses far exceeds the spin lattice relaxation rate (T1) of the tissue water protons. This results in a net decrease in water proton signal intensity from the slice. With perfusion, however, "fresh" in-flowing

Imaging slice is partially saturated by excitation

In-flowing spins replace saturated spins resulting in more net signal

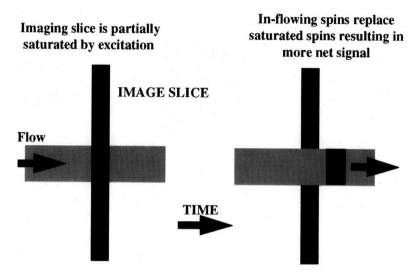

FIGURE 4. Effects of perfusion on water proton MRI signal.

spins will not have experienced the previous excitation pulses and a larger signal will be observed from these in-flowing spins. This perfusion effect is observed as an apparent decrease in the T1 relaxation time because perfusion is recovering the magnetization, rather than nuclear relaxation. Several investigators have shown that this change in apparent T1 with flow can be used to monitor cardiac perfusion *in vitro*.[19,20] Flow related T1 effects have also been observed *in vivo* in the dog with adenosine-induced hyperemia.[11] There are difficulties using this approach. A complete T1 measurement in the presence and absence of in-flow effects is required to quantitate flow and the in-flow effect on T1 is quite small in muscle tissues in comparison to brain or kidney. This latter effect is due to the relatively efficient spin lattice relaxation rate in muscle at low magnetic fields.

Another approach to measuring perfusion is to selectively saturate the in-flowing blood by irradiating the incoming arteries and observing the decrease in signal in the tissue as these saturated spins move into the tissue.[19] This approach can be generalized into a class of procedures called saturation transfer that are used extensively to provide specific information from water. Saturation transfer is a method in which a specific pool of spins is selectively saturated with radiofrequency energy and then transferred via flow, chemical exchange, or dipolar interactions to another pool for detection. In general, this approach is used to transfer information from a small pool to bulk water to take advantage of its large pool size for detection and imaging. For example, in

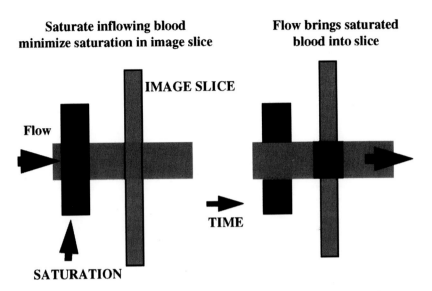

FIGURE 5. Using saturation transfer of in-flowing spins to detect perfusion.

a blood flow measure, the small pool of in-flowing spins is continuously irradiated and these saturated or labeled spins move into the heart tissue via blood flow and diffusion. The saturation label remains in the tissue with a exponential decay equal to the apparent T1 relaxation rate in the tissue. An example of this approach for chemical exchange or dipolar coupling to macromolecules will be described. This method for detecting flow is outlined in Figure 5. In this approach the in-flowing spins are saturated with selective irradiation near the base of the heart, and blood flow delivers these saturated spins to the tissue. With higher flow, a larger portion of saturated spins moves into the myocardium resulting in proportional decrease in signal intensity. With proper corrections and adequate signal-to-noise, this type of approach can provide a quantitative measure of tissue perfusion in the human brain.[21] Whether this will be an effective quantitative tool in the *in vivo* heart has yet to be determined, especially with the complex or collateral flow patterns found in the diseased heart.

Water Diffusion

Regarding the properties of water within the heart cell, water self-diffusion rates and direction can be determined using MRI. This technique relies on basically placing a magnetic field gradient pulse across the heart and then later applying another pulse of opposite direction

Diffusion

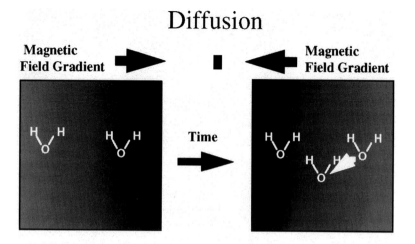

For motionless water molecules, the two opposing gradients cancel. For moving or diffusing water molecules, the gradients do not cancel and MR signal attenuation occurs.

FIGURE 6. Detection of water diffusion or motion using MRI.

but equal amplitude. As seen in Figure 6, water that has moved in the direction of the gradients between the application of the opposing gradients will have a decreased signal intensity because the gradient effects will not cancel. As a function of gradient timing and strength, the actual diffusion coefficient for water can be determined. In the brain, a decrease in this diffusion coefficient has been observed as one of the earliest signals of metabolic compromise[22,23] with ischemia; however, the actual physical mechanism for this effect is unknown. In the heart, this property has mostly been used to determine the fiber orientation in the myocardium because the water diffusion rate would be predictably higher along the muscle fiber orientation.[24,25] No data are currently available on using water diffusion measures in cardiac ischemia, myopathies, remodeling or tissue rejection studies. One of the major challenges in this approach is the large background motion of the myocardium that also results in an apparent diffusion by bulk motion of the water spins. However, several approaches have been developed to overcome this background signal.[25,26]

Finally, diffusion measures are also useful in determining tissue temperatures because the rate of diffusion is temperature sensitive. Using this property, diffusion measures have been suggested as a method of monitoring tissue temperatures during invasive thermal ablation techniques in the vasculature.[27] The chemical shift of water is also temperature sensitive, providing another measure of tissue temperature,[28] although this approach is sensitive to local magnetic field gradients.

Water-Macromolecule Interactions

As water moves within the cystosol it interacts with the macromolecular structure of the tissue. This interaction results in a motion restriction of the water molecule, resulting in shortening of both its nuclear spin-spin (T2) and spin-lattice relaxation times (T1). These are the actual nuclear relaxation rates not influenced by the macroscopic physiologic parameters discussed. Using these basic properties, early investigators were able to demonstrate changes in these relaxation properties in ischemic or remodeled myocardium.[29,30] In general, these effects where in the direction of increasing relaxation times as the ratio of water to macromolecules increased with edema or remodeling of the tissue. The specific mechanisms involved in these gross relaxation effects are still unclear and under investigation.

A specific dipole-dipole interaction of water with macromolecules in the heart results in a decrease in the T1 relaxation rate. This occurs because protons from water are oriented on macromolecules long enough that direct dipole-dipole interactions occur between the macromolecule and water protons. This is analogous to bringing two magnets sufficiently close to each other that they can directly interact through space. This interaction results in a magnetization transfer between the bulk water and the macromolecules. The interaction site on the macromolecules is most likely a chemical exchange site with subsurface hydroxyl groups being the most effective.[31] This specific relaxation pathway can be evaluated directly in MRI using saturation transfer techniques (Figure 7).[31,32] The relatively rigid macromolecules have a rapid spin-spin relaxation rate that results in a broad NMR resonance that is several thousand hertz wide, whereas bulk water is highly mobile resulting in a relatively narrow resonance (20 to 30 Hz). By irradiating several thousand hertz off the bulk water resonance, the macromolecule can be selectively saturated. By the process of saturation transfer, as discussed for perfusion measures, the saturation of the macromolecules now moved into the bulk water protons via the magnetization transfer process at the macromolecule surface. Saturation transfer occurs over many cycles of an exchange process and the label picked up in the exchange persists in the water molecule for seconds due to its rather long T1 relaxation time. Thus, only a few interaction sites (<0.1% of the water protons) can effect the bulk water pool. Whereever an effective coupling between water protons and the macromolecules ex-

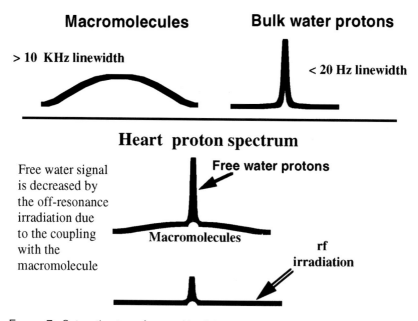

FIGURE 7. Saturation transfer used to detect water-macromolecule interactions in the intact heart.

ists, a large decrease in MR signal will be observed as the saturated macromolecule signal is transferred to the bulk water. In addition, because a major relaxation pathway is eliminated by this process,[31] a significant decrease in T1 relaxation rate occurs with off-resonance irradiation in tissues with significant macromolecule water magnetization transfer. This effect has been shown to be dependent on the surface chemistry and mobility of the macromolecule interaction site.[31]

In the heart, the high concentration of myofilaments and structural elements results in one of the largest magnetization transfer (MT) effects observed.[33] In Figure 8, an example from the human heart is shown where the irradiation of the macromolecules resulted in an approximate 50% decrease in the myocardial signal distinguishing heart wall from fat and blood.[33] Figure 8 shows a control gradient-recalled echo image with little or no T1 weighting. The second image is with an off-resonance irradiation on the macromolecules of the heart. This results in a large decrease in the signal intensity of the myocardium with little or no effect in the vascular space or surrounding fat. The final picture is a negative image highlighting the regions in the chest where a tight coupling between the macromolecules and water is observed. Subsequent animal studies have revealed that the MT effects are related to water content of the myocardium[34] as the relative ratio

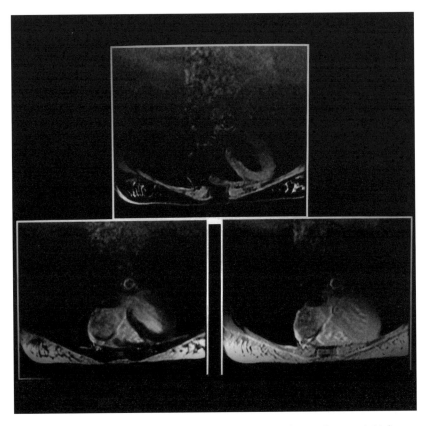

FIGURE 8. Magnetization transfer (MT) in the human heart. Lower right figure is a standard gradient-recalled echo (GRE) image. Lower left image is with irradiation of the macromolecules as discussed in Reference 33. Top image is a negative image of the MT effect highlighting the transfer in the heart and skeletal muscle.

of water to the macromolecular surfaces is critical in determining the rate of magnetization transfer. In addition, this approach can be used to detect the progression of ischemic events under conditions suitable for rapid cardiac MRI.[35] In these later studies, decreases in the MT rate were observed that were independent of water content suggesting a basic change in the surface interaction with the macromolecules with chronic ischemia. Using the action spectrum of the off-resonance irradiation, where the frequency dependency of the off-resonance irradiation on water is determined, the actual spectral characteristics of the macromolecule can be determined[31] revealing some of its motional characteristics. Using this information, it was concluded that the changes in macromolecule/water MT in chronic ischemia were not due to alterations in the overall dynamics of the myocardial macromolecules, but must be due to changes in the local interaction site dynamics and/or surface chemistry.[35] The actual molecular mechanisms involved in MT within heart tissue has not been well established in comparison to lipid and other simple model systems,[3] thus the precise contribution of different macromolecules to the overall effect is still under investigation. However, based on its specificity to macromolecular structure and dynamics, it may prove to be a valuable probe in the investigation of myocardial remodeling.

Due to the influence of water-macromolecule MT on T1, this approach has also been used to magnify blood inflow effects on the apparent T1 of the heart[20] as discussed.

Water and Metabolites

Water is also in chemical exchange with other metabolites in the cell. Any metabolite with an exchangeable proton will exchange magnetization with water, although hydroxyl, carbonyl, or amine groups could in principle be monitored using saturation transfer techniques. The only window of opportunity is that the exchange rate must be fast enough so that the saturation transfer can result in a significant transfer to the bulk water and not too fast so that the MR can not detect the two molecules as separate species.[36] By specifically irradiating the chemical shift position of a low-concentration metabolite to saturate its spin, the associated saturation transfer, via chemical exchange, can result in a large specific decrease in the water resonance. Due to the continual nature of the saturation transfer process, this can result in a several 1000-fold enhancement of a metabolites signal by observing through its exchange with water. Using this approach specific images of ammonia and urea have been created *in vivo*[37] as well as *in vivo* in the kidney.[38] Target metabolites for this type of approach in the heart may include creatine, which is an important molecule in the myocardial energetics or ammonia, which is one of the final products of adenosine breakdown. However, no studies on this approach have yet been presented in the literature on the heart.

Water and Intrinsic Metals

Water magnetization is also sensitive to the concentration of paramagnetic or ferromagnetic molecules in the heart. This sensitivity is the basis of most exogenous contrast agents in use today to study numerous aspects of vascular and myocardial function, However, the intrinsic source of iron from degradation of myoglobin in the severely damaged myocardium may be detectable or the deposition of iron in hemochromotosis.[39] More importantly, the conversion of hemoglobin from oxyhemoglobin to the strongly paramagnetic form of methemoglobin[40] in arteries, heart ventricles, or valves may serve as a measure of the stage or age of blood clots. This approach may prove useful in characterizing clots with regard to clinical risks.

Summary

Extensive physiologic and biochemical information on the heart is available from water proton MRI. By being aware of the potential artifacts and complications, the versatile MRI data acquisition schemes can be tailored to reflect specific information from each of these physiologic processes providing the investigator or clinician with unique and valuable information. It is also important to note that the exploitation of these properties is still under development and many improvements in the quantitative nature of these data as well as the discovery of new approaches to extract physiologic information from the water MR signal is forthcoming.

References

1. de Roos A, Doornbos J, van der Wall EE, van Voorthuisen AE. Magnetic resonance of the heart and great vessels. *Nat Med.* 1995;1:711–713.
2. Pelc NJ, Sommer FG, Li KC, et al. Quantitative magnetic resonance flow imaging. *Magn Reson Q.* 1994;10:125–147.
3. Zerhouni EA. Myocardial tagging by magnetic resonance imaging. *Coron Artery Dis.* 1993;4:334–339.
4. O'Dell WG, Moore CC, Hunter WC, et al. Three-dimensional myocardial deformations: calculation with displacement field fitting to tagged MR images. *Radiology.* 1995;195:829–835.
5. Pelc NJ, Drangova M, Pelc LR, et al. Tracking of cyclic motion with phase-contrast cine MR velocity data. *J Magn Reson Imaging.* 1995;5:339–345.
6. Thulborn KR, Waterton JC, Matthews PM, Radda GK. Oxygenation dependence of the transverse relaxation time of water protons in whole blood at high field. *Biochim Biophys Acta.* 1982;714:265–270.
7. Ogawa S, Lee TM, Nayak AS, Glynn P. Oxygenation-sensitive contrast in magnetic resonance image of rodent brain at high magnetic fields. *Magn Reson Med.* 1990;14:68–78.
8. Turner R, Jezzard P, Wen H, et al. Functional mapping of the human visual cortex at 4 and 1.5 tesla using deoxygenation contrast EPI. *Magn Reson Med.* 1993;29:277–279.
9. Kwong KK, Belliveau JW, Chesler DA, et al. Dynamic magnetic resonance

imaging of human brain activity during primary sensory stimulation. *Proc Natl Acad Sci USA.* 1992;89:5675–5679.

10. Ogawa S, Tank DW, Menon R, et al. Intrinsic signal changes accompanying sensory stimulation: functional brain mapping with magnetic resonance imaging. *Proc Natl Acad Sci USA.* 1992;89:5951–5955.

11. Balaban RS, Taylor JF, Turner R. Effect of cardiac flow on gradient recalled echo images of the canine heart. *NMR Biomed.* 1994;7:89–95.

12. Wendland MF, Saeed M, Masui T, et al. First pass of an MR susceptibility contrast agent through normal and ischemic heart: gradient-recalled echo-planar imaging. *J Magn Reson Imaging.* 1993;3:755–760.

13. Atalay MK, Reeder SB, Zerhouni EA, Forder JR. Blood oxygenation dependence of T1 and T2 in the isolated, perfused rabbit heart at 4.7T. *Magn Reson Med.* 1995;34:623–627.

14. Li D, Dhawale P, Rubin PJ, et al. Myocardial signal response to dipyridamole and dobutamine: Demonstration of the BOLD effect using a double echo gradient-echo sequence. *Magn Reson Med.* 1996;36:16–20.

15. Neimi P, Poncelet BP, Kwong KK, et al. Myocardial intensity changes associated with flow stimulation in blood oxygenation sensitive magnetic resonance imaging. *Magn Reson Med.* 1996;78–82.

16. Li KC, Wright GA, Pelc LR, et al. Oxygen saturation of blood in the superior mesenteric vein: in vivo verification of MR imaging measurements in a canine model. Work in progress. *Radiology.* 1995;194:321–325.

17. Meiboom S. Nuclear magnetic resonance study of the proton transfer in water. *J Chem Phys.* 1961;34:375–382.

18. Ronen I, Navon G. A new method for proton detection of H2(17)O with potential applications for functional MRI. *Magn Reson Med.* 1994;32:789–793.

19. Williams DS, Grandis DJ, Zhang W, Koretsky AP. Magnetic resonance imaging of perfusion in the isolated rat heart using spin inversion of arterial water. *Magn Reson Med.* 1993;30:361–365.

20. Prasad PV, Burstein D, Edelman RR. MRI evaluation of myocardial perfusion without a contrast agent using magnetization transfer. *Magn Reson Med.* 1993;30:267–270.

21. Pekar J, Sinnwell T, Ligeti L, et al. Simultaneous measurement of cerebral oxygen consumption and blood flow using 17O and 19F magnetic resonance imaging. *J Cereb Blood Flow Metab.* 1995;15:312–320.

22. Rother J, de Crespigny AJ, D'Arceuil H, et al. Recovery of apparent diffusion coefficient after ischemia-induced spreading depression relates to cerebral perfusion gradient. *Stroke.* 1996;27:980–986; discussion 986–987.

23. Marks MP, de Crespigny A, Lentz D, et al. Acute and chronic stroke: navigated spin-echo diffusion-weighted MR imaging. *Radiology.* 1996;199:403–408.

24. Garrido L, Wedeen VJ, Kwong KK, Kantor HL. Anisotropy of water diffusion in the myocardium of the rat. *Circ Res.* 1994;74:789–793.

25. Reese TG, Weisskoff RM, Smith RN, et al. Imaging myocardial fiber architecture in vivo with magnetic resonance. *Magn Reson Med.* 1995;34:786–791.

26. Edelman RR, Gaa J, Wedeen VJ, et al. In vivo measurement of water diffusion in the human heart. *Magn Reson Med.* 1994;32:423–428.

27. Cline HE, Schenck JF, Watkins RD, et al. Magnetic resonance-guided thermal surgery. *Magn Reson Med.* 1993;30:98–106.

28. Young IR, Hand JW, Oatridge A, Prior MV. Modeling and observation of temperature changes in vivo using MRI. *Magn Reson Med.* 1994;32:358–369.

29. McNamara MT, Higgins CB: Magnetic resonance imaging of chronic myocardial infarcts in man. *AJR.* 1986;146:315–320.
30. Scholz TD, Martins JB, Skorton DJ. NMR relaxation times in acute myocardial infarction: Relative influence of changes in tissue water and fat content. *Magn Res Med.* 1992;25:1120–1124.
31. Balaban RS, Ceckler TL. Magnetization transfer contrast in magnetic resonance imaging. *Magn Reson Q.* 1992;8:116–137.
32. Wolff SD, Balaban RS. Magnetization transfer imaging: practical aspects and clinical applications. *Radiology.* 1994;192:593–599.
33. Balaban RS, Chesnick S, Hedges K, et al. Magnetization transfer contrast in MR imaging of the heart. *Radiology.* 1991;180:671–675.
34. Scholz TD, Ceckler TL, Balaban RS. Magnetization transfer characterization of hypertensive cardiomyopathy: significance of tissue water content. *Magn Reson Med.* 1993;29:352–357.
35. Scholz TD, Hoyt RF, DeLeonardis JR, Ceckler TL, Balaban RS: Water-macromolecular proton magnetization transfer in infarcted myocardium: A method to enhance magnetic resonance image contrast. *Magn Reson Med.* 1995;33:178–184.
36. Alger JR, Shulman RG. NMR Studies of enzymatic rates in vitro and in vivo by magnetization transfer. *Q Rev Biophys.* 1984;17:83–124.
37. Wolff SD, Balaban RS. NMR imaging of labile proton exchange. *J Magn Reson.* 1989;85:164–169.
38. Scharen-Guival VLM, Sinnwell TM, Balaban RS, Wolff SD. Imaging of proton-water chemical exchange in the kidney using saturation transfer. *Proc Int Soc Magn Res Med.* 1996;1:470. Abstract.
39. Blankenberg F, Eisenberg S, Scheinman MN, Higgins CB. Use of cine gradient echo (GRE) MR in the imaging of cardiac hemochromatosis. *J Comput Assist Tomogr.* 1994;18:136–138.
40. Duewell S, Kasserra CE, Jezzard P, Balaban RS. Evaluation of methemoglobin as an autologous intravascular contrast agent. *Magn Reson Med.* 1996; 35:787–789.

## Part 4

Magnetic Resonance Angiography

Chapter 19

Magnetic Resonance Angiography of the Aortic Arch and Carotid Arteries

Charles M. Anderson, MD, PhD

Magnetic Resonance Angiography of the Aortic Arch and Carotid Arteries

Magnetic resonance angiography (MRA) is particularly well suited to the study of the carotid arteries.[1,2] This aptitude results from the relatively fast flow of blood in the carotid and cerebral arteries, the availability of high sensitivity head and neck imaging coils, and the fact that the head may be held motionless for many minutes. The principal advantage of carotid MRA with respect to conventional x-ray angiography (XRA) is that it is noninvasive. Catheter angiography of the carotid arteries carries a 1% to 4% incidence of stroke, and a nonnegligible incidence of renal failure or contrast reaction.[3,4] Complications in MRA are exceptionally rare. In addition, the cost of MRA is a fraction of that of catheter angiography. As a result of these advantages, the use of conventional angiography has declined significantly wherever MRA is available.

The Extracranial Carotid Arteries

Magnetic Resonance Angiography Protocols for the Carotid Artery

The most widely used method for MRA of the carotid arteries is the time-of-flight (TOF) or flow-related enhancement method. This can

From: Higgins CB, Ingwall JS, Pohost GM, (eds). *Current and Future Applications of Magnetic Resonance in Cardiovascular Disease.* Armonk, NY: Futura Publishing Company, Inc.; © 1998.

be performed either by sequential thin two-dimensional slices[5] or by a three-dimensional slab[6] acquired in the transverse plane. Based on the experience of several investigators, one may make several recommendations about the parameters to be used with these methods.

Sequential Two-Dimensional Time-of-Flight

When acquiring two-dimensional time-of-flight carotid angiograms, slices should have velocity compensation in both the slice selection and frequency-encoding directions. The thickness of the slices should be less than 3 mm so as to reduce the stair-step appearance of sagittal reconstruction from thick axial slices. A further reduction in this artifact can be achieved by overlapping the slices slightly. For example, acquiring 2-mm thick slices every $1\frac{1}{2}$ mm will give an apparent resolution of $1\frac{1}{2}$ mm while enjoying the greater signal-to-noise ratio of a thicker slice. The pixel size can be reduced in-plane by using a small field of view.

The echo time should be minimized to reduce intravoxel phase dispersion from turbulence. Echo times of 8 ms are available on several brands of machine.

The flip angle in the acquired slice should be adjusted so as to minimize pulsatility artifact while achieving the greatest background suppression possible. Usually this is at about $35°$ to $60°$. However, it will vary from instrument to instrument. The repetition time should be at least 30 ms and could be as high as 45 ms in slow flow situations.

Jugular venous signal is suppressed by a so-called traveling or "walking" presaturation band placed above each slice; the position of the saturation band is incremented with the position of the acquired slice. This saturation band will remove signal from arteries when the direction of flow is reversed, so one might repeat the acquisition without a superior saturation band if, for example, subclavian steal phenomenon is suspected.

The set of slices should ideally extend as far cranially as the base of skull. This permits certain identification of antegrade flow in the intrapetrous portion of the internal carotid artery (ICA). If slices are not obtained as high as this, a branch of the external carotid artery (ECA), such as the ascending pharyngeal artery, might be mistaken for a patent ICA when in fact the ICA is occluded.

Three-Dimensional Time-of-Flight

When acquiring a three-dimensional TOF data set, many of the same recommendations for parameters are relevant. One should select a relatively small field of view and a very thin slice in order to reduce loss of signal from intravoxel phase dispersion.[7] A pixel that is 0.8 × 0.8 × 0.8 mm provides very good results. Increasing the matrix size to 256 × 512 improves conspicuity of small vessels by decreasing partial volume averaging. Rectangular field of view, in which both the field of view and matrix size are decreased in the phase-encoding direction, is well suited to MRA in that fewer phase-encoding steps speed the acquisition without significantly sacrificing resolution.

The echo time should be minimized[8] but should be selected so that fat and water are out of phase. This is so that the signal from fat is minimized. For example, it may be possible to achieve a 5-ms echo time on a 1.5-T instrument using asymmetric echoes.[9] However, at this echo time, fat and water are in phase and the fat signal is appreciable. This may overwhelm the signal from the vessel and the maximum intensity projection. For a 1.5-T machine, 7 ms will be out of phase. At 1 T, about 11 me would be a good choice for an echo time that is out of phase.

Flip angle might vary from 20° to 30°. Since small flip angles are used, ghosting is never a problem. The flip angle may be increased with position across a three-dimensional TOF slab so that the influence of blood saturation on vessel contrast is reduced.[10]

The choice of orientation of the three-dimensional slab has important implications for blood saturation. A transverse slab has the advantage that blood need only flow across the slab and, therefore, is unlikely to become saturated. In coronal and sagittal acquisitions, the vessel passes for a long distance in the excited volume and distal saturation is always present to some degree. For this reason, acquisition in transverse orientation may be performed with a short repetition time (TR) (25 to 35 ms), and acquisition in sagittal or coronal orientation requires a relatively long TR; for example, 70 ms.

A recent trend is to acquire a series of thin overlapping transverse three-dimensional slabs—a technique called multiple overlapping thin slab acquisition (MOTSA).[11] Here, a series of three-dimensional TOF volumes are acquired, each one consisting of only 10 to 20 slices, and overlapping the previous set. As a result of the narrow width of the volumes, blood saturation is reduced.

Comparison of Two-Dimensional and Three-Dimensional Time-of-Flight Techniques

There has been considerable controversy regarding the relative advantages of two-dimensional and three-dimensional TOF carotid angiography. It is not possible to state that one is clearly better than the other. Instead, each has its own advantages. For example, the two-dimensional TOF method can visualize vessels that are flowing more slowly. This is important when differentiating between a very high-grade stenosis and complete occlusion of the vessel. This differentiation has important clinical ramifications. A vessel that is completely oc-cluded is not amenable to any surgical correction. However, even a small stream of blood beyond a critical stenosis will permit repair of the affected vessel with an endarterectomy and graft.

A great advantage of three-dimensional TOF is that it is sensitive to blood flow in any direction. For this reason, tortuous vessels are better visualized using the three-dimensional method than the two-dimensional method. In addition, if the ICA leaves the bifurcation at a 90° angle to the common carotid artery, the blood may become partially saturated by two-dimensional acquisition but will be well-visualized by three-dimensional acquisition. A second advantage of the three-dimensional TOF method is that it has inherently greater resolution. The detection of fine detail, such as the presence of an ulcer or a small

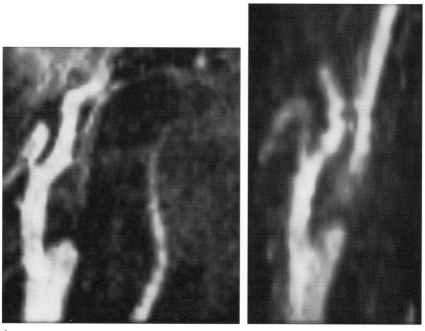

A   B

FIGURE 1. MRA by two-dimensional TOF and three-dimensional TOF of a nearly occluded proximal ICA. **A:** By three-dimensional TOF the ECA is seen with good resolution, but the ICA is barely visible. **B:** By two-dimensional TOF, the ICA is clearly seen beyond a tight stenosis, despite slow flow velocity.

aneurysm, is expected to be better on three-dimensional than on two-dimensional acquisition.

Three-dimensional acquisition is less susceptible to turbulent dephasing artifacts than is two-dimensional. Therefore, the residual lumen in the vicinity of a tight stenosis might be better estimated by three-dimensional rather than two-dimensional TOF.

A complete protocol should include both two-dimensional and three-dimensional TOF acquisitions. The two-dimensional series is used to locate the bifurcation and to differentiate a patent vessel from one that is nearly occluded (Figure 1). The 3D series is acquired to grade the percent diameter stenosis and visualize plaque.

Phase-Contrast Angiography

A projected view of the entire carotid artery and much of the intracranial vasculature may be quickly acquired by placing a 2 to 4 cm thick sagittal two-dimensional phase contrast[12] slab over each carotid vessel in turn. Phase contrast is excellent at visualizing slowly flowing vessels without suffering from saturation. Distal intracranial branches or aneurysms of the carotid artery may be better visualized than with three-dimensional TOF. The disadvantage of the phase-contrast method for carotid bifurcation assessment is that there is often considerable artifactual signal loss within the bulb that may simulate a plaque. Some practitioners use two-dimensional phase contrast in addition to TOF to provide a large field-of-view survey of the carotid artery.

Interpretation

Several points should be observed when interpreting magnetic resonance angiograms. First, it is mandatory to examine the individual slices in addition to the maximum intensity projection (MIP) calculated images.[13,14] These slices have greater contrast than the MIP and will more closely depict the vessel wall contour. If sagittal slices or sagittal reformations are available, they may be inspected to find plaque, which will be seen as a dark or intermediate signal intensity within the dark line of the muscular wall. Individual slices will disclose the presence of metal clip artifacts. Most importantly, the tendency to overestimate the severity of turbulent lesions is greatly reduced on source images.

Flow separation artifact may be encountered in patients with capacious bulbs. In this phenomena, the laminar flow of blood leaves the wall, resulting in strong inflow of relaxed blood in the laminar part, but stagnant saturated blood in the separated part. As a result, the bulb may appear narrowed. Flow separation may also be seen when blood is deflected from the wall by a plaque, resulting in apparent lengthening of the stenosis.

Saturation of slowly flowing blood will effect vessel contrast. The vessel will appear narrowed distally as it traverses the slab. Saturation is worse with three-dimensional than with two-dimensional acquisition. When differentiating a critical stenosis and complete occlusion, it is important to acquire two-dimensional transverse images.

The Significance of Carotid Bifurcation Stenosis

Recent multicenter trials, notably the North American Symptomatic Carotid Endarterectomy Trial (NASCET),[15] the European Carotid Surgery Trial (ECST),[16] and the Asymptomatic Carotid Atherosclerosis Study (ACAS),[17] have concluded that the risk of stroke is correlated with the degree of arterial stenosis of the proximal internal carotid artery (ICA) as measured from conventional contrast angiograms.[18] These trials did not assess the ability of noninvasive imaging to predict those at risk for stroke MRA and computed tomographic angiography (CTA) were not included in the study designs. Doppler ultrasound study (DUS) was obtained for many patients in the NASCET study, but there was little standardization in the protocol for those measurements.[19] Standardized DUS was included in the ACAS trial, but these results have yet to be announced. Therefore, the predictive value of noninvasive testing is assumed, but not proven by an outcome trial.

The lack of good outcome data can be addressed in two ways. First, new multicenter studies could be undertaken in order to determine whether the parameters measured by noninvasive testing might be as predictive or more predictive of stroke as is XRA. These parameters might include the cross-sectional lumen area at the lesion, elevation of blood velocity as a result of the lesion, presence of turbulent flow, or the size of the plaque. A more specific test for stroke risk would be desirable because many patients with narrow x-ray derived diameters will not subsequently incur a stroke. For example, in the ACAS study, only 10% of patients with stenoses exceeding 60% went on to have a stroke. Clearly factors other than vessel diameter alone are contributing to the probability of stroke. Unfortunately, no large-scale outcome studies of MRA are under way.

A second way to address the lack of outcome data is to prove that MRA is highly correlated with measurements of XRA. If XRA is predictive of stroke, then so is MRA. In fact, numerous such comparisons have been made.[20–36] These experiments are difficult to summarize, because each had its own experimental design.[37] The studies evaluated a variety of imaging techniques, especially two-dimensional and three-dimensional TOF. They used different cutoff values to define severe stenoses. Some studies categorized the severity of stenosis by "eyeball" estimation, others by objective measurement of diameters from the film.[38] In each of these studies all discrepancies were arbitrarily attributed to an error in MRA.

One consistent finding was that MRA was exceptionally sensitive for the detection of stenotic disease. The chief difficulty encountered by these investigators was that the degree of stenosis often appeared exaggerated. This resulted from disorderly blood flow within and beyond a stenosis.[39] Of those publications within the last year that sought to identify a 70% to 99% stenosis, Turnipseed[40] found a 100% sensitivity and 88% specificity; Siker[30] a 73% sensitivity and 86% specificity; Laster[33] a 93% sensitivity and 97% specificity; Mittl[35] a 92% sensitivity and 76% specificity (worst error was a 64% stenosis thought to be >70%); and Anderson[36] a 92% sensitivity and 95% specificity. The tendency to overestimate disease was especially problematic when signal in the vicinity of a stenosis disappeared altogether so that the vessel appeared interrupted, a phenomenon often called a "flow gap." Flow gaps were assigned to the >70% stenotic surgical category, yet some lesions less than 70% stenotic could result in flow gap.[23,29,35] This finding has led some authors to advocate the use of MRA as a screening procedure for the presence of stenosis, but not as a definitive replacement for XRA.[1,41]

The tendency to overestimate stenosis has been addressed by three recent publications that measured the degree of stenosis from individual slices rather than from rendered angiographic projections. These slices were either the original transverse sections, or they were reformatted sections longitudinal to the vessel. On individual slices, the plaque could often be visualized directly (Figure 2). Anderson[36] found that three patients with flow gaps on projection were incorrectly placed in the surgical category, but none were incorrectly categorized when read from source images. Huston[29] discovered that specificity for a 50% stenosis improved from 67% to 86% when read from source images. DeMarco[34] found that interpretation from source images eliminated the overall tendency to overestimate stenosis. A *t*-test between projected MRA and XRA showed significant differences, but no significant difference between source image MRA and XRA.

When compared with DUS, MRA has demonstrated similar accuracy in identifying surgical candidates by the NASCET recommendation, some studies found MRA slightly better[26,27,29] others found DUS to have a small advantage.[24,28,30] These differences are probably not significant, and might be related to details in the experimental protocols. Pan[42] compared DUS, MRA, and XRA with diameters measured

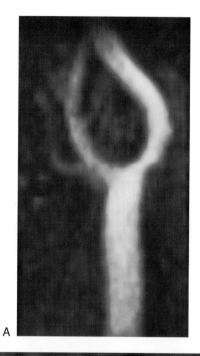

A

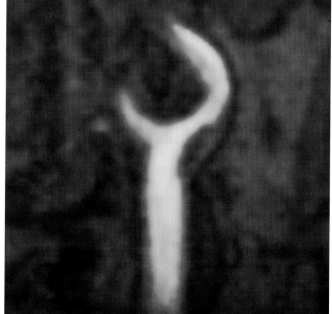

B

from endarterectomy specimens, and discovered that DUS and MRA each correlated better with the endarterectomy specimen than did XRA. This discrepancy was attributed to the fact that the smallest diameter was often missed by XRA when the stenosis was elliptical or complex in shape. An increasing number of investigators are advocating the use of DUS, with MRA confirmation, in lieu of XRA for the selection of endarterectomy candidates.[40,43] If DUS and MRA agree and explain the patient's symptoms, an XRA is not performed. This algorithm has gained greater acceptance with the advent of capitated payment for medical services.

Phase-contrast flow volume rates compare well with Doppler ultrasound derived rates.[44] It is uncertain how this information should be incorporated into the surgical decision.

Internal Carotid Artery Occlusion

The differentiation of near and complete occlusion is important because revascularization procedures of the chronically occluded ICA are ineffective. Recent publications comparing two-dimensional TOF and conventional angiography show complete concordance, however, the total number of patients in these studies was only several hundred.[29,34,36,40] Three-dimensional TOF is not capable of making this distinction. As a result of saturation of blood signal in the distal ICA, blood flow beyond a critical stenosis may not be visible on three-dimensional TOF.

Occluded vessels may rarely appear patent on MRA in two situations. A large, dominant vasovasonum collateral may be mistaken for a patent ICA, a very rare phenomenon. Also, a clot in a recently thrombosed vessel might appear bright (after several weeks it becomes very dark). This appearance has been described in deep venous thrombosis, and could potentially affect carotid studies as well. It may be identified by applying an inferior saturation band and repeating a two-dimensional TOF slice. The vessel should disappear if it is patent.

The best way to detect a patent ICA is by transverse two-dimensional TOF slices at the level of the carotid canal in the base of skull

◄───

FIGURE 2. Residual carotid lumen better seen on reformatted section. **A:** A three-dimensional TOF angiogram displays narrowing of the proximal ICA. **B:** On a sagittal section reformatted from the transverse images, blood in the residual lumen is seen more brightly. Degree of stenosis is less overestimated. In addition, plaque that appears as gray material in bulb, as well as muscular wall (dark line), are visualized.

(Figure 3). At this location, the vessel may be positively identified, and it may be differentiated from, for example, an ascending pharyngeal branch of the external carotid artery. Lack of flow at this level implies an occlusion at the bifurcation because there are no branches of the ICA between these points. Reverse flow of the ICA is very rare. Therefore, absence of the ICA on MRA is almost always the result of occlusion rather than a steal phenomenon. Reverse flow may be discovered by repeating a two-dimensional TOF slice without the superior saturation band. The ability of two-dimensional TOF to determine occlusion and three-dimensional TOF to avoid turbulence artifact have led some to advocate the use of both two-dimensional and three-dimensional TOF in the standard carotid protocol.[1,36,44-46]

Until the advent of color-coded Doppler, sonography was often incapable of detecting a compromised but patent ICA. New studies are warranted to document the improvement in DUS for this indication. A recent study showed MRA was more accurate than DUS.[35] XRA is generally accurate, but may fail if a nonselective arch injection is made, or if an insufficient volume of contrast is used.[47] Whereas none of the modalities is infallible, they are each fairly accurate, and one may assume a correct diagnosis if two of the techniques (MRA, DUS, XRA) agree.

Other Carotid Diseases

Carotid artery dissection is characterized by a hemorrhage in the carotid wall, often with narrowing of the lumen as a result of mass effect or an initial flap. The hemorrhage may involve just the media, or may extend to the adventitia. The site of dissection is often distal to the accessible range of an ultrasound transducer. MRA may be very helpful in locating a dissection, by detecting a focal change in the caliber of the lumen.[48] The absence of stenosis, however, does not rule out this disease. The diagnosis of dissection is more often made by identifying the hemorrhage on transverse spin-echo MRI images. The use of fat-saturation sequences prevents bright hemorrhage from being mistaken for bright fat.

Carotid ulcers have been implicated as a potential nidus for emboli formation. Several studies have sought to correlate the presence of ulcers with the incidence of stroke, with varying success. The identification of ulcers on conventional angiograms is not a simple matter.[49] The space between two adjacent plaques may mimic an ulcer, and vice versa. Furthermore, even if an ulcer is correctly recognized, the status of the endothelial layer is unknown. MRA is no better than XRA, and is often less able to visualize an ulcer if blood flow in the crater is slower

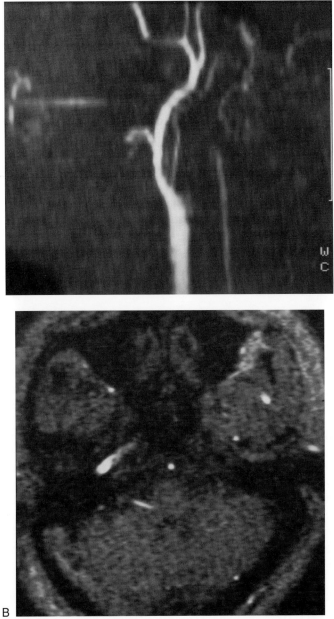

FIGURE 3. ICA occlusion confirmed by two-dimensional TOF section. **A:** The ICA is not seen on two-dimensional TOF maximum intensity projection (MIP) of the left carotid bifurcation, suggesting occlusion. **B:** Occlusion is confirmed by inspecting TOF section at the level of the carotid canal. Inflow signal is present on the right, missing on the left.

than that of the main lumen. For the time being, and until outcome trials have demonstrated a benefit to the identification of ulcers, there is little interest in this entity among MR angiographers.

Plaque characterization and composition has also been proposed as an etiology of stroke. Again, this theory has not been consistently supported by clinical studies. High-resolution MRA of endarterectomy specimens, correlated with histology sections, have shown unique appearances for different constituents of plaque, including calcium, fat, hemorrhage, and fibrosis.[50] Display of this level of anatomic detail is best performed with voxels that are less than 0.3 mm across, a resolution that is not practically attainable *in situ*. Perhaps with a new generation of neck imaging coils one can achieve this type of plaque characterization.

MRA is not the study of choice for fibromuscular hyperplasia, unless the findings are pronounced. The undulations of the carotid wall may be smaller than the slice thickness, or mistaken for slice misregistration, in ED TOF. Three-dimensional TOF provides a more accurate portrayal, but the greater rate of inflow in the center of the vessel in comparison to blood near the wall may cause the undulations to be under appreciated.

The Aortic Arch and Carotid Origins

The most common cause of transient ischemic attacks (TIAs) and stroke in the carotid artery is a stenosis at the bifurcation and bulb, but other carotid sites may be responsible including stenosis or occlusion at the origin of common carotid or vertebral arteries. If significant disease is not found at the bifurcation on an ultrasound examination, but the Doppler waveform appears dampened or flow directions are reversed, an origin or siphon stenosis should be considered. Proximal disease is suggested by a tardus parvus waveform[51] (ie, delayed and dampened peak systolic velocities). In some instances a stenosis at the bifurcation may be missed by Doppler if a proximal carotid stenosis dampens velocities within a significant stenosis of the ICA or bulb. Furthermore, a tandem proximal lesion may lead to compensatory elevated velocities on the contralateral side, simulating a contralateral bifurcation stenosis.

Magnetic Resonance Angiography Protocols for the Aortic Arch

Motsa

The simplest and most consistent approach is a series of overlapping transverse three-dimensional TOF slabs (Figure 4).[52] These slabs

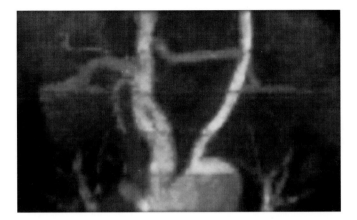

FIGURE 4. Angiogram of the aortic arch vessels obtained by the MOTSA technique. The left subclavian artery is occluded at its origin. A graft extends from the right common carotid artery to the distal left subclavian artery. The downgoing portion of the subclavian artery is not seen because of superior saturation bands.

may be 16 or 32 partitions thick, and should be overlapped by 30% to 50%.

After a set of coronal spin-echo localizers, the lowest TOF slab is prescribed to include the innominate artery origin. One should avoid setting the lowest slab too far inferior because blood in the arch will become saturated before it enters the cephalic vessels. Typical parameters might be TR = 40 ms, flip angle = 20°, FOV = 20 cm, matrix = 192 × 256 (fewer phase-encoding steps may be taken if asymmetric FOV is available), partition thickness = 1 mm. The TE should be selected to place fat and water out-of-phase.

The second slab should be set to overlap the first. For example if 32 partitions are selected, and the partitions are 1-mm thick, the second set could be centered exactly 20 mm higher. This is repeated for 4 to 7 sets, or until the right carotid origin is visualized.

A superior presaturation band is placed above each slab to remove jugular signal. Care must be taken not to miss the diagnosis of subclavian steal of the vertebral arteries. If a vertebral artery is appears missing, several transverse two-dimensional TOF slices should be acquired without a presaturation band, or with an inferior presaturation band, so that patency of the vessel may be established.

Interpretation

A small volume is selected for projection. Otherwise mediastinal and subcutaneous fat may obscure the vascular anatomy. A single refommatted coronal or sagittal slice may be calculated through each origin. In that way angiographic contrast is maximized and mural plaque may be visualized directly. Reformations are also useful for assessing small vessels such as vertebral artery origins. Inspection of the individual slices without projection reveals much greater detail than does the final MIP.

The transverse and downswing of the subclavian artery becomes saturated and is not well visualized. If the goal of the study is to find distal subclavian artery disease, slices or slabs should be oriented sagitally. Flow in grafts may also become saturated, unless care is take to specify an appropriate acquisition origin, and to avoid presaturating the graft by a saturation band. It also helps to set a relatively large Stand-off distance between the acquired slab and the superior saturation band.

A small amount of turbulence at the origin of the left subclavian artery is normal and may be readily differentiated from real stenotic disease by inspecting individual slices. Turbulence is rarely encountered at the origin of the left common caratid artery or innominate artery perhaps because blood has a "straight shot" as it ascends the aorta and enters these proximal vessels. However, it must turn to leave the distal transverse arch and enter the left subclavian artery. This turbulence may predispose to plaque formation, and may explain why disease is most commonly found in the proximal left subclavian artery, where it results in a subclavian steal and possibly posterior circulation symptoms. Disease affecting the innominate or carotid origins are less common, but may result in hypoperfusion or emboli to the anterior circulation.

The Significance of Proximal Carotid Artery Stenosis

While the risk of stroke for patients with severe siphon stenosis is very high,[53] embolization from proximal carotid artery stenosis is thought to be unusual.[54] Nevertheless, these lesions may become flow-limiting or occlude. When they do, they cause changes in the direction of flow in the neck. For example, disease of the subclavian arteries proximal to the vertebral arteries results in a subclavian steal; blood flow reverses in the ipsilateral vertebral artery to provide perfusion to the arm, thereby Stealing blood from the posterior circulation. This may lead to marginal perfusion and loss of consciousness brought on by standing up or turning the head (although not all patients are symptomatic). Similarly, occlusion of the proximal carotid arteries may result in reverse flow of the external carotid to feed the internal carotid artery. Or occlusion of the innominate artery may result in reverse flow of the right ICA to feed the right arm.

Correction of an occlusion or tight stenosis at the arch is often approached extrathoracically by a graft rather than by an endarterectomy (which involves a thoracotomy), unless the stenosis is thought to be a source of emboli. Grafts for proximal occlustion of the left subclavian artery typically extend from a common carotid artery to the distal subclavian artery, or from axillary to axillary artery. The thrombosis rates for these grafts is about 4.5%.[55] Another common procedure that does not involve graft material is a transposition, in which the left subclavian artery is reimplanted on the common carotid artery, or if the proximal left common carotid artery is the site of disease, it is implanted on the left subclavian artery.

Direction of blood flow and patency of most grafts may be assessed by either MRA or Doppler ultrasound.

Arch stenotic lesions are often associated with bifurcation lesions.[56] The precise incidence depends on the definition of severe stenosis used by the x-ray angiographer. In one study, proximal disease was found in 1.8% of patients with bifurcation stenosis, and the incidence of tandem siphon stenosis in patients with bifurcation stenosis was 6%.[57]

Some surgeons maintain that no other imaging beyond Doppler ultrasound is required before surgery.[57] They argue that disease is primarily found at the bifurcation, and that the incidence of tandem lesions is very small.[58] Furthermore, the presence of a tandem lesion may not affect surgical outcome for most patients.[59]

Other surgeons disagree with this conclusion. A flow-limiting origin stenosis ipsilateral to a symptomatic bifurcation stenosis is considered a contraindication to endarterectomy.[55] Surgeons often insist on an x-ray angiogram prior to endarterectomy both to confirm the results of Doppler ultrasound and to find tandem lesions. The use of a confirming modality seems prudent because there are occasionally instances when a Doppler study indicates a significant stenosis and the conventional angiogram reveals little or no disease. Conversely if a proximal lesion is present, the Doppler study might not show elevated velocities at a bifurcation lesion. With the availability of MRA, confirmation may be made noninvasively.

Intracranial Occlusive Disease

The petrous carotid, siphon, circle of Willis, proximal cerebral, as well as the distal vertebral and basilar arteries may be acquired simultaneously by a MOTSA three-dimensional TOF acquisition using the head coil. This study is often requested for symptomatic patients who have normal carotid bifurcations by DUS, or who are thought to have basilar insufficiency or other posterior circulation symptoms. Stenotic and occlusive lesions of the major vessels are visible by this technique. Sites that are commonly affected are the confluence of the vertebral arteries, the midbasilar artery, the siphons, and points of bifurcation of the cerebral arteries.[60–62] Small, terminal arterial branches are below the resolution of the technique, so that occlusions of these vessels are not commonly visible. Likewise vasculitis is not well depicted. A recent study comparing MRA and XRA of 131 patients showed a 85% and 88% sensitivity and a 96% and 97% specificity for detection of stenoses in the intracranial internal carotid and middle cerebral arteries, respectively.[63]

The availability of MRA has dramatically reduced the number of catheter angiograms performed for suspected occlusive disease of the distal vertebral and basilar arteries, for basilar dolocoectasia, and to delineate branches of the basilar artery that may come in contact with the fifth or seventh cranial nerves in patients with hemifacial spasm and trigeminal neuralgia.[64] Use of MRA is desirable because selective studies of vertebral arteries are particularly prone to complications such as dissection or release of emboli. The ascendancy of MRA has been so swift that few studies have been performed to define the concordance of MRA and XRA. Such studies are not forthcoming because XRA is now rarely performed in addition to an MR study.[65] MRA, however, opens up a new and more relevant area of research. Now that posterior circulation screening may be done without the fear of complications, the relation between the myriad symptoms thought to be symptomatic of vertebrobasilar disease may be correlated with anatomic studies, so that the clinical diagnosis made be rendered more specific.

When interpreting vertebral studies, one should keep in mind anatomic variants, such as dominance of one vessel, or the termination of a vessel at the posterior inferior cerebellar artery, with the contralateral vertebral supplying the basilar artery.

A caution is also warranted when studying the carotid siphons. Here, flow changes direction several times in rapid succession, leading to unusual velocity profiles, and to the so-called flow displacement artifact.[66] Different software implementations of TOF suffer from this artifact to varying degree. Before interpreting siphon pathology on a routine basis, the angiographer should test the sequence on normal volunteers.

The circle of Willis provides a ready path for collateral perfusion of the brain in the event of reduced flow in a carotid or vertebral artery. The surgeon may wish to know the direction of flow in the circle in order to learn the hemodynamic significance of a lesion, to judge whether an infarct could have resulted from a lesion in a certain vessel, or to assess what portion of the brain is at risk during a surgical procedure. The direction of flow in, for example, the posterior communicating artery or the A1 segment of the anterior cerebral artery, may be determined by acquiring transverse 2D PC slices with flow encoding in the right-left, then in the anteroposterior, directions.[67] Alternatively, one may place a saturation band over one of the vessels of the neck, while acquiring a three-dimensional TOF angiogram of the circle. Any cerebral vessel that disappears from the image is fed by that saturated vessel.[68]

MRA has greatly aided the diagnosis of pediatric cerebrovascular diseases such as sickle cell, Williams and other vascular syndromes, and stroke. The brisk cerebral flow encountered in children permits excellent MR angiograms, with the result that the prevalence of XRA for infants and young children has been considerably reduced.[69]

Future Trends

The use of noninvasive imaging for the selection of carotid endarterectomy candidates is now well established. Much work remains to be done, however, to better define the relation between the noninvasive techniques. Should DUS or MRA be performed first? Which patients require additional imaging when an abnormality is suspected? Will the new technique of CTA, in which a high-resolution spiral CT of the neck is acquired after peripheral injection of iodinated contrast, be performed instead of MRA? These questions will be answered by outcome studies involving large numbers of patients.

There is room for technical improvement of MRA as well. For example, use of gadolinium contrast has led to exciting advances in aortic and extremity arteriography, which now can be performed in less than 3 minutes. Perhaps a rapid angiogram of the arch, neck, and head vessels could be acquired after injection of gadolinium through a peripheral vein. Early experience with this method has shown that jugular vein enhancement obscures the carotid, but one could remove the vein through postprocessing.

Improvements in lumen depiction are also likely to emerge in the next 2 years. The now widespread availability of high-strength gradients allows better flow compensation and immunity from turbulent signal loss in a tight stenosis. It also permits high-resolution acquisition. This will permit more confidence in measuring stenosis and in identifying ulcers.

Recent studies have used MRA to examine flow patterns of blood in normal and abnormal carotid vessels, and have proposed mechanisms for plaque formation based on these patterns of flow. These studies support the popular hypothesis that plaque develops at areas of low blood velocity at the wall. This information could one day lead to earlier identification of those at risk for development of stenosis, or may lead to surgical procedures that reduce the incidence of restenosis.

Plaque may be imaged at high resolution in resected endarterectomy specimens. These images show plaque contents such as calcium, fat, and fibrous tissue. There is hope that such high-resolution images may be obtained *in situ* as well. Phase-array imaging coils have demonstrated impressive improvements in sensitivity for neck imaging. These studies might be used to monitor regression of plaque with therapy, or could identify those whose plaque is likely to undergo necrosis.

Despite the need for additional data, it is already clear that MRA has a role to play in the assessment of cerebrovascular disease. It has already greatly reduced the number of conventional angiograms performed, and will likely displace even more studies in the future. As physicians learn to interpret these examinations, they should keep foremost in mind the precept that MRA is not XRA. That is to say, MRA is not intended to look precisely like an XRA, but rather displays a wealth of information regarding blood velocities and flow patterns. Someday this information may prove essential for predicting the course of vascular disease.

References

1. Atlas SW. MR angiography in neurologic disease. *Radiology.* 1994;193:1–16.
2. Anderson CM, Edelman RR, Turski PA. *Clinical Magnetic Resonance Angiography.* New York: Raven Press; 1993:181–340.
3. Hankey GJ, Warlow CP, Sellar RJ. Cerebral angiographic risk in mild cerebrovascular disease. *Stroke.* 1990;21:209–222.
4. Grzyska U. Freitag J. Zeumer H. Selective arterial intracerebral DSA: Complication rate and control of risk factors. *Neuroradiology.* 1990;32:296–299.
5. Keller PJ, Drayer BP, Fram EK, et al. MR angiography with two-dimensional acquisition and three-dimensional display. *Radiology.* 1989;173: 527–532.
6. Masaryk TJ, Modic MT, Ruggiere PM, et al. Three-dimensional (volume) gradient echo imaging of the carotid bifurcation: preliminary clinical experience. *Radiology.* 1989;171:801–806.
7. Haacke EM, Wielopolski PA, Masaryk TJ, et al. Optimizing blood vessel contrast in fast three-dimensional magnetic resonance imaging. *Magn Reson Med.* 1990;14:202–221.
8. Schmalbrock P, Yuan C, Chakeres DW. Volume MR angiography: Methods to achieve very short echo times. *Radiology.* 1990;175:861–865.
9. Lin W, Haacke EM, Smith AS. Lumen definition in MR angiography. *J Magn Reson Imaging.* 1990;1:327–337.
10. Purdy DE, Cadena G, Laub G. The design of variable tip angle slab selection (TONE) pulses for improved 3D MR angiography. In: Book of Abstracts: Society of Magnetic Resonance in Medicine 11th Annual Meeting. Berkeley, CA: Society of Magnetic Resonance in Medicine; 1992:882. Abstract.
11. Parker DL, Yuan C, Blatter DD. Mr angiography by multiple thin slab 3D acquisition. *Magn Reson Med.* 1991;17:434–451.

12. Dumoulin CL, Souza SP, Walker MF, Wagle W. Three-dimensional phase contrast angiography. *Magn Reson Med*. 1989;9:139–149.
13. Rossnick S, Laub G, Braeckle R. Three dimensional display of blood vessels in MRI. In: Proceedings of the IEEE Computers in Cardiology. New York: Institute of Electrical and Electronic Engineers; 1986:193–195.
14. Anderson CM, Saloner D, Tsuruda JS, et al. Artifacts in maximum intensity projection display for MR angiograms. *AJR*. 1990;154:623–629.
15. Barnett HJM. North American symptomatic carotid trial collaborators. Beneficial effect of carotid endarterectomy in symptomatic patients with high-grade carotid stenosis. *N Engl J Med*. 1991;325:445–453.
16. European Carotid Surgery Trialist's Collaborative Group. MRC European carotid surgery trial: Interim results for symptomatic patients with severe (70–99%) or with mild (0–29%) carotid stenosis. *Lancet*. 1991;337:1235–1243.
17. Executive Committee for ACAS. Endarterectomy for asymptomatic carotid artery stenosis. *JAMA*. 1994;273:1459–1461.
18. Barnett HJM, Warlow CP. Carotid endarterectomy and the measurement of stenosis. *Stroke* 1993;24:1281–1284. Editorial.
19. Hobson RW, Strandness DE. Carotid artery stenosis: what's in the measurement? *J Vasc Surg*. 1993;18:1069–1070. Editorial.
20. Litt AW, Eidelman EM, Pinto RS, et al. Diagnosis of carotid artery stenosis: Comparison of 2DFT time-of-flight MR angiography with contrast angiography in 50 patients. *AJR*. 1991;156:611–616.
21. Masaryk AM, Ross JS, DiCello MC, et al. 3DFT MR angiography of the carotid bifurcation: potential and limitations as a screening examination. *Radiology*. 1991;179:797–804.
22. Wilkerson DK, Keller I, Mezrich R, et al. The comparative evaluation of three-dimensional magnetic resonance for carotid artery disease. *J Vasc Surg*. 1991;14:803–811.
23. Heiserman J, Drayer B, Fram E, et al. Carotid artery stenosis: Clinical efficacy of two-dimensional time-of-flight angiography. *Radiology*. 1992;182:761–768.
24. Polak JF, Bajakian RL, Oleary DH, et al. Detection of internal carotid artery stenosis—Comparison of MR angiography, color Doppler sonography, and arteriography. *Radiology*. 1992;182:35–40.
25. Kido DK, Panzer RJ, Szumowski J, et al. Clinical evaluation of stenosis of the carotid bifurcation with magnetic resonance angiographic techniques. *Arch Neurol*. 1991;48(5):484–489.
26. Anderson C, Saloner D, Lee R, et al. Assessment of carotid artery stenosis by MR angiography: comparison with x-ray angiography and color-coded Doppler ultrasound. *AJNR*. 1992;13:989–1003.
27. Mattle HP, Kent KC, Edelman RR, et al. Evaluation of the extracranial carotid arteries- correlation of magnetic resonance angiography, duplex ultrasonography, and conventional angiography. *J Vasc Surg*. 1991;3:838–845.
28. Riles T, Eidelman E, Litt A, et al. Comparison of magnetic resonance angiography, conventional angiography and duplex scanning. *Stroke*. 1992;23:341–346.
29. Huston J, Lewis B, Wiebers D, et al. Carotid artery: Prospective blinded comparison of two-dimensional time-of-flight MR angiography with conventional angiography and duplex US. *Radiology*. 1993;186:339–344.
30. Siker M, Furst G, Fischer H, et al. Between-method correlation in quantifying internal carotid stenosis. *Stroke*. 1993;24:1513–1518.

31. Buijs PK, Klop RB, Eikelboom BC, et al. Carotid bifurcation imaging: Magnetic resonance angiography compared to conventional angiography and Doppler ultrasound. *Eur J Vasc Surg* 1993;7:245–251.
32. Blatter DD, Bahr AL, Parker DL, et al. Cervical carotid MR angiography with multiple overlapping thin slab acquisition: comparison with conventional angiography. *AJR.* 1993;161:1269–1277.
33. Laster RE, Ackem JD, Halford HH, et al. Assessment of MR angiography verus arteriography for evaluation of cervical carotid bifurcation disease *AJNR.* 1993;14:681–688.
34. DeMarco JK, Nesbit GM, Wesbey GE, et al. Prospective evaluation of extracranial carotid stenosis: MR angiography with maximum intensity projections and multiplanar reformation compared with conventional angiography. *AJR.* 1994;163:1205–1212.
35. Mittl RL, Broderick M, Carpenter JP, et al. Blinded reader comparison of magnetic resonance angiography and duplex ultrasonography for carotid artery bifurcation stenosis. *Stroke.* 1994;25:4–10.
36. Anderson CM, Lee RL, Levin DL, et al. Measurement of internal carotid artery stenosis from source MR angiograms. *Radiology.* 1994;193:219–226.
37. Bowen BC, Quencer RM, Margosian P, et al. MR angiography of occlusive disease of the arteries in the head and neck: Current concepts. *AJR.* 1994; 162:9–18.
38. Fox J. How to measure carotid stenosis. *Radiology.* 1993;186:316–318.
39. Urchuk S, Plewes D. Mechanism of flow induced signal loss in MR angiography. *J Magn Reson Imaging.* 1992;2:453–462.
40. Tumipseed WD, Kennell TW, Turski PA, et al. Magnetic resonance angiography and duplex imaging: Noninvasive tests for selecting symptomatic carotid endarterectomy candidates. *Surgery.* 1993;114:634–638.
41. Masaryk T, Obuchowski N. Noninvasive carotid imaging: Caveat emptor. *Radiology.* 1993;186:325–331.
42. Pan XM, Saloner D, Reilly LM, et al. Assessment of carotid artery stenosis by ultrasonography, conventional angiography, and magnetic resonance angiography: Correlation with ex vivo measurement of plaque stenosis. *J Vasc Surg.* 1995;21:82–88.
43. Polak J, Kalina P, Donaldson M, et al. Carotid endarterectomy: Preoperative evaluation of candidates with combined Doppler sonography and MR angiography. *Radiology.* 1993;186:333–338.
44. Levine RL, Turski PA, Holmes KA, et al. Comparison of magnetic resonance volume flow rates, angiography, and carotid Dopplers. *Stroke.* 1994;25: 413–417.
45. Pan XM, Anderson CM, Reilly LM, et al. Magnetic resonance angiography of the carotid artery combining two- and three-dimensional acquisitions. *J Vasc Surg.* 1992;16:609–618.
46. Goldberg HI, Atlas SW, Mishkin MM, et al. Comparison of high resolution 3D and 2D time-of-flight MR angiography of carotid artery bifurcation stenosis. *Radiology.* 1993;189:242. Abstract.
47. Batt M, Avril G, Bozzetto C, et al. Atheromatous pseudo-occlusive stenosis of the internal carotid. *J Mal Vasc (France).* 1993;18:233–237.
48. Levy C, Laissy JP, Raveau V, et al. Carotid and vertebral artery dissections: Three-dimensional time-of-flight MR angiography and MR imaging versus conventional angiography. *Radiology.* 1994;190:97–103.
49. Eikelboom BC, Riles TR, Mintzer R, et al. Inaccuracy of angiography in the diagnosis of carotid ulceration. *Stroke.* 1983;14:882–885.

50. Yuan C, Tsuruda JS, Beach KN, et al. Techniques for high-resolution MR imaging of atherosclerotic plaque. *J Magn Reson Imaging.* 1994;4:43–49.
51. Kotval PS. Doppler waveform parvus and tardus: A sign of proximal flow obstruction. *J Ultrasound Med.* 1988;8:435–440.
52. Lewin JS, Laub G, Hausman R. Three-dimensional time-of-flight MR angiography: Applications in the abdomen and thorax. *Radiology.* 1991;179: 261–264.
53. Marzewski DJ, Furlan AJ, St. Louis P, et al. Intracranial internal carotid artery stenosis: long-term prognosis. *Stroke.* 1981;3:821–824.
54. Provan JL. Arteriosclerotic occlusive arterial disease of brachiocephalic and arch vessels. In: Rutherford RB, ed: *Vascular Surgery.* Philadelphia: WB Saunders: 1989:822.
55. Criado FJ. Extrathoracic management of aortic arch syndrome. *Br J Surg.* 1982;69:S45.
56. Blaisdell WF, Clauss RH, Galbraith JG, et al. Joint study of extracranial arterial occlusion IV. A review of surgical considerations. *JAMA.* 1969;209: 1889.
57. Akers DL, Markowitz I, Kerstein M, et al. The evaluation of aortic arch study in the evaluation of cerebrovascular insufficiency. *Am J Surg.* 1987; 154:230.
58. Ranaboldo C, Davies J, Chant A. Duplex scanning alone before carotid endarterectomy: A 5-year experience. *Eur J Vasc Surg.* 1991;5:415–419.
59. Merritt CR, Carroll BA, Mittelstaedt CA, Nyberg DA. *Yearbook of Ultrasound.* St Louis: Mosby; 1992:218.
60. Fujita N, Hirabuki N, Fujii K, et al. MR imaging of middle cerebral artery stenosis and occlusion: Value of MR angiography. *AJNR.* 1994;15:335–341.
61. Warach S, Li W, Ronthal M, et al. Acute cerebral ischemia: Evaluation with dynamic contrast-enhanced MR imaging and MR angiography. *Radiology.* 1992;182:41–47.
62. Wiznitzer M, Ruggiere PM, Masaryk TJ, et al. Diagnosis of cerebrovascular disease in sickle cell anemia by magnetic resonance angiography. *J Pediatr.* 1990;117:551–555.
63. Korogi Y, Takahashi M, Mabuchi N, et al. Intracranial vascular stenosis and occlusion: Diagnostic accuracy of three-imensional, Fourier transform, time-of-flight MR angiography. *Radiology.* 1994;193:187–193.
64. Tien RD, Wilkins RH. MRA delineation of the vertebro-basilar system in patients with hemifacial spasm and trigeminal neuralgia. *AJNR.* 1993;14: 34–36.
65. Wenk KU, Rother J, Schwartz A, et al. Intracranial vertebrobasilar system: MR angiography. *Radiology.* 1994;190:105–110.
66. van Tyen R, Saloner D, Jou LD, Berger S. MR imaging of flow through tortuous vessels: A numerical simulation. *Magn Reson Med.* 1994;31: 184–195.
67. Davis WL, Turski PA, Gorbatenko KG, et al. Correlation of cine MR velocity measurements in the internal carotid artery with collateral flow in the circle of Willis: Preliminary study. *Radiology.* 1993;3:603–609.
68. Edelman RR, Heinrich PM, O'Reilly GV, et al. Magnetic resonance imaging of flow dynamics in the circle of Willis. *Stroke.* 1990;21:56–65.
69. Vogl TJ, Balzer JP, Stemmler J, et al. MR angiography in children with cerebral neurovascular diseases. *AJR.* 1992;159:817–823.

## Chapter 20

Magnetic Resonance Angiography of the Aorta and Peripheral Arteries

E. Kent Yucel, MD

In recent years, the role of magnetic resonance angiography (MRA) in imaging of the aorta and peripheral arteries has been increasingly acknowledged. Recent developments that have improved the clinical applicability of MRA for these applications include cardiac gating, k-space segmentation, and dynamic imaging with enhancement using gadolinium-chelated contrast materials.

Magnetic Resonance Angiography Techniques

MRA of the thoracic aorta can be performed using two-dimensional time-of-flight (TOF) MRA.[1,2] In nongated TOF MRA, ghosting artifacts from the aorta degrade image quality. An earlier approach to dealing with the problem of pulsatility was to perform a cine acquisition with one phase-encoding step during each cardiac cycle. This provided high temporal resolution. However, a single acquisition, encompassing only 1 to 3 slices, requires up to 128 heartbeats using this technique. Therefore, this approach is impractical for imaging the entire aorta. In cardiac-gated MRA, the phase-encoding steps are centered during the period of systolic flow, about 100–400 ms after the QRS complex.[2–6] The acquisition of 12–16 phase encoding steps per heartbeat minimizes ghosting artifacts and allows the scan to be completed in a reasonable time frame (5–10 seconds). Additionally, an inversion

Research support from Philips Medical Systems, North America, is acknowledged.

From: Higgins CB, Ingwall JS, Pohost GM, (eds). *Current and Future Applications of Magnetic Resonance in Cardiovascular Disease.* Armonk, NY: Futura Publishing Company, Inc.; © 1998.

preparation pulse can be added to further suppress background signal.[7,8]

Using newer fast-gradient systems, gated two-dimensional TOF MRA can be implemented with breath-holding. In order to minimize the number of breath-holds required, this method is limited to relatively thick slices acquired in the aortic long-axis plane. Another approach is to acquire approximately 100, 4 to 5-mm thick axial slices during quiet breathing. The thoracic aorta moves very little during breathing, and the lungs themselves produce very little signal. This technique allows more flexibility in postprocessing as the numerous, thin slices permit reformatting using the standard maximum intensity pixel (MIP) projection method into anteroposterior (AP), lateral, or oblique views.

A different approach is the dynamic gadolinium-enhanced (DGE) MRA technique,[9] which involves the infusion of 0.2 to 0.3 mmol/kg dose of a gadolinium-chelated contrast agent during the 1 to 4 minute acquisition period of the three-dimensional gradient-echo scan. For the thoracic aorta, it is generally optimal to use a sagittal oblique acquisition along the aortic long axis (Figure 1). Jugular and brachiocephalic vein enhancement can be quite prominent, but overlapping veins can generally be eliminated by subvolume MIP projections and multiplanar reformations (MPR).

Another method that has been used primarily for the arch and great vessel origins is multislab three-dimensional MRA.[10] This technique uses overlapping thin three-dimensional TOF slabs. The three-dimensional multislab technique allows quite thin slices, and saturation bands can be used to eliminate venous signal. However, the technique suffers from low signal-to-noise and contrast-to-noise, and the overlap between slabs produces a substantial time penalty.

The issues in imaging the abdominal aorta are similar. Cardiac-gated sequences produce a dramatic reduction in the ghosting artifacts. Similarly, DGE MRA produces high-resolution, high-contrast images of the abdominal aorta. With the gated two-dimensional TOF sequence, acquisition in the axial plane is preferred, as in the thoracic aorta. With the DGE MRA acquisition in the coronal plane maximizes coverage of the abdominal aorta.

Experience with MRA of the peripheral vessels has been almost entirely limited to the lower extremity, due to the much higher incidence of clinically significant disease here than in the upper extremity. Imaging of the vasculature of the lower extremity requires coverage of a large anatomic area, more than for any other clinical application of MRA: it must extend from the aortic bifurcation to the feet. For all practical purposes, this has compelled the use of two-dimensional TOF for MRA to the peripheral vessels. Body coil imaging is adequate for the

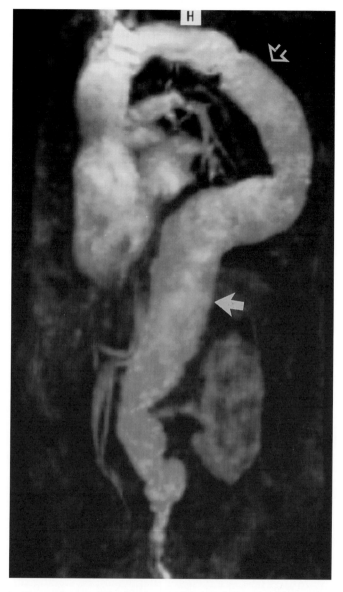

FIGURE 1. Dynamic gadolinium-enhanced three-dimensional MRA of a thoraco-abdominal aneurysm (closed arrow) situated distal to a proximal aortic tube graft (open arrow).

iliac, femoral, and popliteal arteries.[11] Gated sequences reduce ghosting artifacts from normal, pulsatile peripheral arteries. A typical approach would use three acquisitions of 100 to 120 3 to 4-mm axial slices at the pelvis, thigh, and knee. This provides MIP projectional images comparable to the stations of a conventional x-ray arteriographic study of the peripheral circulation. Body coil imaging of the infrapopliteal vessels provides a low-resolution screening image. However, for preoperative imaging the extremity or head coil must be used with slice thickness of 1.5 to 2.5 mm to adequately evaluate the tibial and pedal arteries.

Clinical Applications

Aortic Dissection

In the aorta, MRA can be used for the diagnosis and staging of aortic dissection and evaluation of aortic aneurysms. In aortic dissection, conventional cardiac-gated spin-echo magnetic resonance imaging (MRI) is highly accurate at diagnosing dissection and staging it in terms of the Stanford (A, B) or DeBakey (I, II, III) classifications.[12] MRA has two contributions to make in the evaluation of aortic dissection: identification of slow flow in the false lumen and determination of involvement of branch vessels.

Both the gated two-dimensional TOF techniques and the DGE MRA have provided good results for the evaluation of dissection. DGE MRA has the advantage in detecting extremely slow blood flow. Both methods are able to accurately detect involvement of the arch vessels, mesenteric, renal, and iliac arteries by the dissection. The near-isotropic resolution of three-dimensional imaging used for DGE MRA allows the use of MPR to visualize branch vessels in relation to the intimal flap.

The clinical status of the patient may limit the ability to use MRA in the evaluation of aortic dissection. The environment of the MRI scanner is suboptimal for very sick patients. Access to the patient and hemodynamic monitoring are difficult, and metallic pumps and other life-support devices may not be compatible with the MRI environment. Therefore, MRI is best reserved for diagnosing or staging disease in relatively stable patients, or for follow-up studies to assess aortic diameter, graft integrity, and continued patency of the false lumen.

Penetrating Aortic Ulcer

A disease that can mimic aortic dissection in its clinical presentation is penetrating aortic ulcer.[13] Patients with this condition are usually older than those with typical dissection and have more extensive atherosclerotic plaque in the aorta. In this condition, a focal rupture in mural plaque, usually in the mid-descending thoracic aorta, results in either a focal ulceration communicating with the aortic lumen or an intramural hematoma. Persistent symptoms or enlargement of the ulcer require surgery to prevent progression to aortic rupture. Spin-echo MRI identifies the intramural hematoma; MRA allows ready identification of mural ulceration. DGE MRA is less susceptible to signal loss in areas of stagnant slow, and therefore more accurately delineates luminal contours.

Aortic Aneurysm

Aneurysmal disease can affect any portion of the aorta, although abdominal aortic aneurysms are the most common. In the ascending aorta, the most common cause of aneurysmal disease is cystic medial necrosis, sometimes also associated with Marfan syndrome. In the descending thoracic and abdominal aorta, the most common cause of aneurysmal disease is atherosclerosis. Less common causes include aortitis and mycotic aneurysms.

Imaging of aortic aneurysms is required to determine the extent of the aneurysm and the presence of occlusive disease in major branch vessels. In abdominal aortic aneurysms (AAA), the specific issues that must be addressed are suprarenal extension, accessory renal arteries, patency of the mesenteric and renal arteries, and involvement of the iliac arteries. Spin-echo MRI can accurately measure the size of AAA. However, for determining the relation of the aneurysm to branch vessels and to identify associated occlusive disease, MRA sequences must also be performed.

Both two-dimensional TOF and DGE MRA techniques have been used for the evaluation of AAA.[14–19] DGE MRA has several advantages in AAA evaluation: greater accuracy for detecting accessory renal arteries, lack of saturation effects in the aneurysm itself as well as in the iliac arteries, and faster scan time. DGE MRA for AAA evaluation is best performed in the coronal plan. Sixty-four 1.5 to 2.0-mm slices acquired with a 300 to 400 mm field of view are generally used. A matrix size of 160 or 192 × 256 is adequate to visualize most accessory renal arteries. Careful localization is necessary to ensure coverage of the iliac and common femoral arteries. Image analysis requires the production of MIP projection angiograms from various-viewing angles and review of the source coronal images and MPR.

MRA has been shown to be competitive with conventional angiography for staging the superior and inferior extent of AAA. In some cases, MRA may even be superior to conventional angiography for determining the extent of the aneurysm by virtue of its ability to detect intraluminal thrombus, best seen on the source coronal images. In addition, MRA can determine patency of the celiac, superior mesenteric, renal, and iliac arteries with a high degree of accuracy. Accessory renal arteries can usually be identified. Definitive assessment of inferior mesenteric artery patency may not be possible in large aneurysms due to its small size and extremely anterior location.[15,19] Clinically significant renal artery occlusive disease requires endarterectomy or bypass at the time of aortic surgery, and therefore, its preoperative detection is important. Aneurysmal or occlusive disease of the iliac arteries will lead most surgeons to use an aortobifemoral rather than a tube graft.

Congenital Aortic Abnormalities

Another important area of aortic imaging where MRA can be useful is congenital abnormalities.[6] Many such anomalies can be identified on spin-echo imaging as well, but MRA, either gated two-dimensional TOF or DGE, can be helpful. MIP projection images allow a more straightforward and understandable presentation of the abnormalities rather than simple viewing of tomographic images. In coarctation, MRA can display the collateral circulation around the obstruction. The volumetric data acquired with the three-dimensional DGE MRA allows MPR to be performed in any desired plane to elucidate the pathological anatomy.

Occlusive Arterial Disease

Occlusive disease of the aorta can be the result of atherosclerosis, coarctation, aortitis, or neurofibromatosis. Gated two-dimensional TOF or three-dimensional DGE MRA provide adequate imaging of the site and severity of obstruction. For evaluation of mural plaque in cases of peripheral embolization (blue toe) syndrome, the superior accuracy of DGE MRA for luminal borders is preferred to any two-dimensional TOF method.

The primary clinical indication for angiography of the lower extremities is atherosclerotic occlusive disease. Occlusive disease can be classified as primarily inflow (aortoiliac) or outflow (femoropopliteal) disease. In either case, the task of imaging is to determine where the diseased segment begins and ends, as this determines the length and type of bypass graft used. It is also important to distinguish between focal and diffuse disease, as the former are amenable to percutaneous angioplasty, whereas the latter require bypass grafting.

Two-dimensional TOF MRA is the mainstay of lower extremity vascular imaging. As described above, ghosting artifacts degrade images of normal inflow vessels. Beyond occlusions or severe stenoses, ghosting artifacts disappear due to the change from a highly pulsatile, triphasic flow waveform to a mono- or biphasic pulse wave with markedly diminished amplitude. Ghosting artifacts from normal vessels can be minimized with cardiac-gated TOF techniques.[20] Use of these techniques increases the scan time because a portion of the cardiac cycle is not used for imaging. In reconstituted vessels, cardiac gating is not necessary.

With TOF imaging, horizontal or tortuous arterial segments may show signal loss from progressive spin saturation, which mimics the appearance of a stenosis.[21,22] Inferior saturation bands tracking 15 to 20 mm behind the slice being imaged are used to eliminate venous flow signal in peripheral MRA. These may cause suppression of signal of retrograde flow that can occur in very tortuous vessels, reconstituted vessel segments, and at the outflow from bypass grafts. Another limitation of two-dimensional TOF MRA is its tendency to overestimate the severity of stenosis. Severe stenoses may even produce a complete signal void, indistinguishable from complete occlusion. Fortunately, in the extremities the distinction between focal stenosis and short occlusion is not of crucial importance as both are amenable to angioplasty.

Initial clinical results with-two-dimensional TOF MRA have shown promising results in the femoral, popliteal, and tibial segments.[11,22-28] MRA has even been shown to reveal patent vessels not seen with conventional angiography, which can prevent the need for amputation (so-called angiographically occult vessels). In the femoral and popliteal arteries, MRA can identify angioplasty candidates (Figure 2), and angiographic approach to a femoral angioplasty is completely different than that for a routine diagnostic study. The performance of surgical revascularization using MRA as the only preoperative diagnostic study has been reported.[29,30]

Patients with orthopedic prostheses or surgical clips in proximity to the vessels of interest are not suitable candidates for MRA as these metallic foreign bodies produce artifacts that can obscure nearby vessels.[22] The major problem area with clinical use of two-dimensional TOF for peripheral MRA has been in the iliac arteries, especially when these arteries are ectatic or tortuous.[11,21] DGE MRA has been extremely promising for improved visualization of the iliac arteries, especially when two-dimensional TOF techniques are suboptimal.[31,32] Development of phased-array coils encompassing the entire leg will dramatically improve the efficiency of peripheral MRA.[33,34] Currently, the requirement for multiple repositioning of the coil makes the study time excessive (1.5 to 2.0 hours). Other promising indications for peripheral

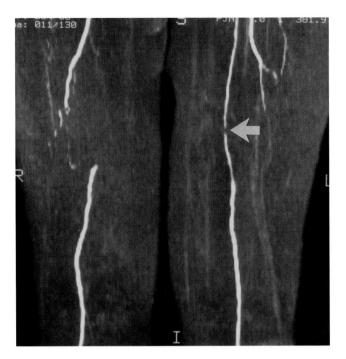

FIGURE 2. Two-dimensional time-of-flight MRA of a patient with atherosclerotic disease. There is occlusion of the right superficial femoral artery (SFA) with reconstitution of the popliteal artery above the knee. There is a focal stenosis of the left SFA suitable for angioplasty (arrow). (Reprinted with permission from Yucel EK. Magnetic resonance angiography. In: Strandness DE, van Breda A, eds: *Vascular Diseases: Surgical and Interventional Therapy*. New York: Churchill Livingstone; 1994.)

MRA include staging of musculoskeletal neoplasms, postoperative evaluation of grafts, and the diagnosis of vascular trauma.[35-40]

References

1. Arlart IP, Guhl L, Edelman RR. Magnetic resonance angiography of the abdominal aorta. *Cadiovasc Intervent Radiol.* 1992;15:43–50.
2. Hartnell GG, Finn JP, Zenni M, et al. MR imaging of the thoracic aorta: Comparison of spin-echo, angiographic, and breath-hold techniques. *Radiology.* 1994;191:697–704.
3. Franck A, Selby K, van Tyen R, et al. Cardiac-gated MR angiography of pulsatile flow: K-space strategies. *J Magn Reson Imaging.* 1995;5:297–307.
4. Selby K, Saloner D, Anderson CM, et al. MR angiography with a cardiac-phase-specific acquisition window. *J Magn Reson Imaging.* 1992;2:637–643.
5. De Graaf RG, Groen JP. MR angiography with pulsatile flow. *Magn Reson Imaging.* 1992;10:25–34.

6. Seelos KC, von Smekal A, Steinborn M, et al. MR angiography of congenital heart disease: Value of segmented two-dimensional inflow technique and maximum-intensity-projection display. *J Magn Reson Imaging.* 1994;4:29–36.
7. Richardson DB, Bampton AEH, Riederer SJ, MacFall JR. Magnetization-prepared MR angiography with fat suppression and venous saturation. *J Magn Reson Imaging.* 1992;2:653–664.
8. Edelman RR, Chien D, Atkinson DJ, Sandstrom J. Fast time-of-flight MR angiography with improved background suppression. *Radiology.* 1991;179: 867–870.
9. Prince MR, Yucel EK, Kaufman JA, et al. Dynamic gadolinium-enhanced three-dimensional abdominal MR arteriography. *J Magn Reson Imaging.* 1993;3:877–881.
10. Parker DL, Yuan C, Blatter DD. MR angiography by multiple thin slab three-dimensional acquisition. *Magn Reson Med.* 1991;17:434–451.
11. Yucel EK, Kaufman JA, Geller SC, Waltman AC. Prospective evaluation of two-dimensional time-of-flight MR angiography in lower extremity athero-sclerotic occlusive disease. *Radiology.* 1993;187:637–641.
12. Nienaber CA, von Kodolitsch Y, Nicolas V, et al. The diagnosis of thoracic aortic dissection by noninvasive imaging procedures. *N Engl J Med.* 1993; 328:1–9.
13. Yucel EK, Steinberg FL, Egglin TK, et al. Penetrating aortic ulcers: Diagnosis by MRI. *Radiology.* 1990;177:779–781.
14. Yucel EK. MR angiography for evaluation of abdominal aortic aneurysm: Has the time come? *Radiology.* 1994;192:321–323.
15. Kaufman JA, Geller SC, Petersen MJ, et al. MR imaging (including MR angiography) of abdominal aortic aneurysms: Comparison with conventional angiography. *AJR.* 1994;163:203–210.
16. Kaufman JA, Yucel EK, Waltman AC, et al. MR angiography in the preoperative evaluation of abdominal aortic aneurysms: A preliminary study. *J Vasc Interv Radiol.* 1994;5:489–496.
17. Durham JR, Hackworth CA, Tober JC, et al. Magnetic resonance angiography in the preoperative evaluation of abdominal aortic aneurysms. *Am J Surg.* 1993;166:173–177.
18. Sallevelt PEJM, Barentsz JO, Ruijs SJHJ, et al. Role of MR imaging in the preoperative evaluation of atherosclerotic abdominal aortic aneurysms. *Radiographics.* 1994;14:87–98.
19. Prince MR, Narasimham DL, Stanley JC, et al. Gadolinium-enhanced magnetic resonance angiography of abdominal aortic aneurysms. *J Vasc Surg.* 1995;21:656–669.
20. Yucel EK, Silver MS, Carter AP. MR angiography of normal pelvic arteries: Comparison of signal intensity and contrast-to-noise ratio for three different inflow techniques. *AJR.* 1994;163:167–201.
21. Snidow JJ, Harris VJ, Trerotola SO, et al. Interpretations and treatment decisions based on MR angiography versus conventional arteriography in symptomatic lower extremity ischemia. *J Vasc Interv Radiol.* 1995;6:595–603.
22. Quinn SF, Demlow TA, Hallin RW, et al. Femoral MR angiography versus conventional angiography: preliminary results. *Radiology.* 1993;189: 181–184.
23. Unger EC, Schilling JD, Awad AN, et al. MR angiography of the foot and ankle. *J Magn Reson Imaging.* 1995;5:1–5.
24. Owen RS, Baum RA, Carpenter JP, et al. Symptomatic peripheral vascular disease: Selection of imaging parameters and clinical evaluation with MR angiography. *Radiology.* 1993;187:627–635.

25. Yucel EK, Dumoulin CL, Waltman AC. MR angiography of lower-extremity arterial disease: Preliminary experience. *J Magn Reson Imaging*. 1992;2: 303–309.
26. Carpenter JP, Owen RS, Baum RA, et al. Magnetic resonance angiography of peripheral runoff vessels. *J Vasc Surg*. 1992;16:807–815.
27. Owen RS, Carpenter JP, Baum RA, et al. Magnetic resonance imaging of angiographically occult runoff vessels in peripheral arterial occlusive disease. *N Engl J Med*. 1992;326:1577–1581.
28. Baum RA, Rutter CM, Sunshine JH, et al. Multicenter trial to evaluate vascular magnetic resonance angiography of the lower extremity. *JAMA*. 1995;274:875–880.
29. Carpenter JP, Baum RA, Holland GA, Barker CF. Peripheral vascular surgery with magnetic resonance angiography as the sole preoperative imaging modality. *J Vasc Surg*. 1994;20:861–871.
30. Cambria RP, Yucel EK, Brewster DC, et al. The potential for lower extremity revascularization without contrast arteriography: Experience with magnetic resonance angiography. *J Vasc Surg*. 1993;17:1050–1057.
31. Snidow JJ, Aisen AM, Harris VJ, et al. Iliac artery MR angiography: Comparison of three-dimensional gadolinium-enhanced and two-dimensional time-of-flight techniques. *Radiology*. 1995;196:371–378.
32. Adamis MK, Li W, Wielopolski PA, et al. Dynamic contrast-enhanced subtraction MR angiography of the lower extremities: Initial evaluation with a multisection two-dimensional time-of-flight sequence. *Radiology*. 1995; 196:689–695.
33. Alley MT, Grist TM, Swan JS. Development of a phased-array coil for the lower extremities. *Magn Reson Med*. 1995;34:260–267.
34. Kojima KY, Szumowski J, Sheley RC, Quinn SF. Lower extremities: MR angiography with a unilateral telescopic phased-array coil. *Radiology*. 1995; 196:871–875.
35. Swan JS, Grist TM, Sproat IA, et al. Musculoskeletal neoplasms: Preoperative evaluation with MR angiography. *Radiology*. 1995;194:519–524.
36. Lang P, Grampp S, Vahlensieck, et al. Primary bone tumors: Value of MR angiography for preoperative planning and monitoring response to chemotherapy. *AJR*. 1995;165:135–142.
37. Turnipseed WD, Sproat IA. A preliminary experience with use of magnetic resonance angiography in assessment of failing lower extremity bypass grafts. *Surgery*. 1992;112:664–669.
38. Manaster BJ, Coleman DA, Bell DA. Pre- and postoperative imaging of vascularized fibular grafts. *Radiology*. 1990;176:161–166.
39. Fillmore DJ, Yucel EK, Briggs SE, et al. MR angiography of vascular grafts in children. *AJR*. 1991;157:1069–1071.
40. Yaquinto JJ, Harms SE, Siemers PT, et al. Arterial injury from penetrating trauma: Evaluation with single-acquisition fat-suppressed MR imaging. *AJR*. 1992;158:631–633.

## Chapter 21

Techniques for Magnetic Resonance Angiography of Coronary Arteries

Dwight Nishimura, PhD, Bob Hu, MD,
Craig Meyer, PhD, Todd Sachs, PhD,
Jean Brittain, PhD, Samuel Wang, MD, PhD,
Pablo Irarrazaval, PhD, Albert Macovski, PhD

The noninvasive imaging of coronary arteries is one of the most important but challenging goals in medical imaging. Given the invasiveness and cost of existing x-ray methods, a noninvasive procedure that correctly identifies the extent of disease in the proximal coronary arteries would be of enormous benefit. We will discuss the more recent methods being developed for magnetic resonance angiography (MRA) of coronary arteries. The unprecedented flexibility of magnetic resonance (MR) results in a wide range of possible schemes to attack the significant problems involved. Recent progress lends considerable optimism that a reliable imaging protocol will soon emerge.

Problems

A formidable array of problems must be overcome to produce coronary artery images with sufficient spatial resolution and contrast, and with minimal flow artifacts. In addition to the small vessel size (< 5 mm diameter), which places significant demands on the spatial resolution and signal-to-noise ratio (SNR) of the imaging sequence, the following problems must be addressed: (1) cardiac and respiratory

From: Higgins CB, Ingwall JS, Pohost GM, (eds). *Current and Future Applications of Magnetic Resonance in Cardiovascular Disease.* Armonk, NY: Futura Publishing Company, Inc.; © 1998.

motion; (2) interfering signals from surrounding vessels, heart chambers, myocardium, and epicardial fat; and (3) substantial susceptibility variation due to the heart/lung interfaces. Although techniques exist to mitigate each of these problems, the challenge is to integrate these techniques to address the problems simultaneously.

Compared with other vascular regions, vessel motion is probably most severe in the case of coronary arteries. Rough estimates of the vessel displacement over the cardiac cycle range from 5 to 10 mm for the major coronary vessels. Compounding matters is the motion of the coronary vessels with respiration. Studies of vessel motion with respiration have indicated a displacement of 1 to 15 mm.[13] Therefore, the extent of vessel motion over the cardiac and respiratory cycles can be comparable to or greater than the coronary vessel diameter.

The presence of surrounding blood and tissue is another significant problem. The imaging method must isolate or suppress the large blood pools and vessels in neighboring regions as well as suppress the myocardium and epicardial fat. Because the flow pathways are more complicated, presaturation techniques, which have proven effective in other vascular regions, have limited effectiveness. Another significant concern pertains to the potential interference from motion artifacts generated by these flowing and moving structures.

A third problem germane to coronary imaging is the pronounced field inhomogeneity due to susceptibility effects from the surrounding lung. This inhomogeneity accentuates T2* decay and signal phase distortion, thereby limiting the amount of signal readout possible from each excitation.

Methods

Given these problems, conventional time-of-flight (TOF) and phase-contrast MRA methods cannot be easily adapted to this region. However, what has emerged over the past 5 years are MR methods relying on the following features: (1) cardiac gating; (2) respiratory compensation; (3) white-blood imaging; (4) fast gradient-echo acquisitions; (5) three-dimensional data sets for volumetric coverage; (6) fat suppression; and (7) other contrast enhancement methods (eg, magnetization transfer,[4,5] T2-magnetization preparation[6]). Interestingly, these methods rely not on flow for adequate vessel contrast but on fat suppression (and other contrast enhancement) along with three-dimensional imaging.

Arguably, the recent improvements and progress in coronary MRA stem from the use of respiratory motion compensation and fast imaging methods. Given the importance of respiratory motion compensation, we will focus on this issue and organize the discussion according to breath-hold and non-breath-hold methods.

Breath-Hold Methods

Thus far, the most commonly used breath-hold method was developed by Edelman et al[7] who applied a fast segmented two-dimensional Fourier transform (2DFT) sequence with fat presaturation on thin sections (about 4 mm thick) oriented to capture the coronary vessel in-plane (Figure 1). The cluster of excitations per cardiac cycle (typically 8 to 10) is usually timed to diastole to minimize vessel motion. Using this method, they and others have achieved encouraging clinical results of the proximal portions of the major coronary arteries.[8-12] For a scan of 16 heartbeats, the typical spatial resolution is 1.4 to 1.8 mm (phase-encode direction) by 1 mm (readout direction). Although multislice versions of this sequence are possible,[13] most implementations involve sequential single-slice acquisitions, with each slice requiring a breath-hold. For multislice imaging, the number of slices achievable is limited because of the relatively long sequence window per cardiac cycle (about 110 ms to acquire 8 phase encodes).

Alternatively, Meyer et al[14] applied a fast spiral-scan technique to coronary imaging (Figure 2). The spiral k-space trajectory, which begins at the origin and emanates outward as it twists, possesses excellent immunity to flow artifacts,[15] making it well suited for cardiac and flow applications. Instead of a fat presaturation pulse, the sequence uses a

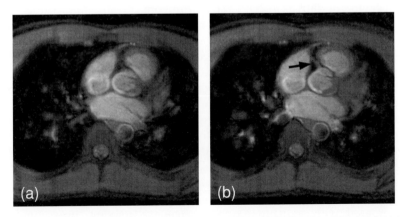

FIGURE 1. Breath-held segmented 2DFT imaging. **(a)** Timing diagram and k-space trajectory. A cluster of excitations is applied each cardiac cycle to acquire a set of phase encodes. **(b)** Left anterior oblique (LAO) section of the right coronary artery (RCA) using a segmented 2DFT sequence.

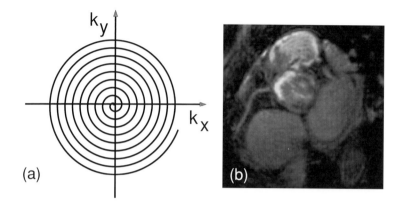

FIGURE 2. Breath-held two-dimensional spiral imaging. **(a)** k-space trajectory for a single spiral interleaf. **(b)** LAO section of the RCA using the spiral sequence.

spectral-spatial readout pulse. Because the spectral-spatial pulse excites only the water component in a thin section, fat is suppressed even in the presence of radiofrequency (RF) nonuniformities. With 20 interleaved spirals on a conventional imager—amounting to a 20 heartbeat scan—breath-hold scans with spatial resolution of about 1.1 to 1.3 mm are achievable (Figure 2b). Because the method offers good temporal resolution (the sequence window is about 35 ms per cardiac cycle), spiral imaging is amenable to a multislice implementation[16] in which 6 to 10 slices can be obtained each breath-hold. One concern with spiral scanning is its off-resonance behavior, which manifests as a blur instead of a geometric shift as in 2DFT. Therefore, some means of off-resonance correction during image reconstruction is desirable to minimize this blur.[17,18]

Another fast-scan method for coronary imaging is echoplanar. Although echoplanar can be used to perform sequential two-dimensional imaging, it is also possible to perform three-dimensional imaging within a single breath-hold by applying a cluster of excitations per cardiac cycle. Such a segmented echoplanar method has been implemented by Wielopolski et al.[19] With 3 breath-holds, this sequence can produce a volumetric data set with 20 partitions. Another approach described by Bornert et al[20] also uses a three-dimensional echoplanar sequence with multiple breath-holds. In this case, the subject initiates the scan when the subject reaches the proper breath-hold position. Compared with sequential two-dimensional imaging, three-dimensional imaging provides better spatial resolution in the slice direction although it is more prone to blood saturation effects.

A different approach to using multiple breath-holds is a method developed by Doyle et al.[21] For each breath-hold, a single phase encode of a multislice acquisition is rapidly acquired. Subsequent breath-holds provide the other phase-encodes for the multislice set. Although substantially more breath-holds are required, the advantage of this method is that the breath-holds are very short (1 second).

Because the above methods require multiple breath-holds for volumetric coverage, the repeatability of the breath-hold positions is important. To address this concern, work by Wang et al[22,23] has focused on combining breath-holding with respiratory monitoring. Respiratory monitoring is typically performed using a so-called navigator echo. Navigator echoes are auxiliary signals acquired along with the regular imaging signals to provide feedback about the presence and extent of motion. In their implementation, a navigator echo monitors the diaphragm position, which correlates well with the largely superior/inferior motion of the heart during respiration.[3] This information about the respiratory position is then fed back to the subject, enabling the subject to hold his or her breath more reproducibly from scan to scan.

Non-Breath-Hold Methods

Although breath-hold methods have generated high-quality coronary images, a single breath-hold places severe limits on the achievable spatial resolution, SNR, and volumetric coverage. Hence a complete examination requires substantial patient cooperation to perform multiple breath-holds in a consistent fashion. As a result, there has been interest in developing methods that allow free breathing during the scan without introducing respiratory artifacts. The extra scan can then be used for better spatial resolution, higher SNR, and/or greater volumetric coverage. Central to this effort has been the use of navigator echoes (or respiratory bellows) to monitor respiratory motion. Although the motion information provided by the navigators can be used for data correction,[24,25] many of the methods use the motion information to assemble the most consistent data set possible.

One use of navigator echoes is respiratory gating.[26,27] During the cardiac-gated acquisition, the navigator echo detects the diaphragm position. If this position is within the specified region, the scanner accepts the raw data; otherwise, the scanner rejects the data and the sequence repeats for the next heartbeat. This approach has been combined with spiral imaging[26] and with segmented 3DFT imaging.[27] Initial studies[27-29] indicate that the respiratory-gated images are comparable to breath-hold images.

Another non-breath-hold approach, investigated by Li et al[30] involves retrospective respiratory gating using navigator echoes. This method does not require real-time decision making by the scanner. After repeating the k-space coverage several times during the scan, a histogram showing the number of phase encodes as a function of diaphragm position is used to determine the effective gating center for image reconstruction. The diaphragm position with the most number of phase encodes in its neighborhood is designated the gating center. Initial results with this method using a segmented 3DFT acquisition have demonstrated excellent vessel visualization and strong immunity to respiratory artifacts.

A third way to use respiratory monitoring for non-breath-hold scanning is a method that involves real-time scan modification.[31] In this method, a complete raw data set is collected as usual during free breathing, with a navigator echo monitoring the diaphragm position of each measurement. Once a full data set is assembled, an image can be reconstructed. A histogram of the respiratory positions is then analyzed in real time to determine the raw data measurement most corrupted by motion (ie, the measurement associated with the respiratory position farthest away from the most common respiratory position in the histogram). As the overscan period begins, the new measurement replaces the most corrupted measurement if the new respiratory position is better than the original. The histogram is then updated in real time to determine the next measurement most corrupted by motion. In this fashion, the histogram of respiratory positions can only narrow with time, leading to a histogram with a diminishing variance. If a real-time image reconstructor is available, then the displayed image will improve continously with a longer overscan period. For a given scan time, the diminishing variance algorithm provides an image with the best consistency in respiratory positions.

Among the applications explored thus far with the diminishing variance algorithm are two-dimensional spiral imaging,[31] three-dimensional spiral imaging,[32] segmented 2DFT,[33] and high-resolution (0.5 mm) two-dimensional spiral imaging.[34] An example of the improved vessel depiction possible with 2D spiral imaging is given in Figure 3. In addition, such non-breath-hold scanning may enhance other methods such as the selective-tagging subtraction method which required a relatively long breath-hold.[35]

In general, the long scan times and patient-friendly nature of non-breath-hold methods are attractive advantages compared with breath-hold methods. However, a concern with non-breath-hold scans is the relative accuracy of the respiratory position estimate and its correlation with coronary vessel position. The achievable spatial resolution may ultimately depend on this factor. Another concern is the longer contiguous scan time that must be tolerated by the subject.

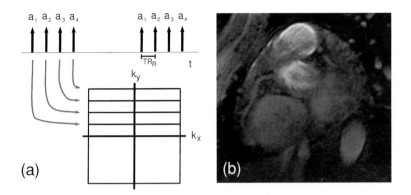

FIGURE 3. Use of navigator echoes to improve coronary vessel depiction. **(a)** two-dimensional interleaved spiral image without respiratory compensation. Average of three complete raw data sets. **(b)** same section with respiratory compensation using the diminishing variance algorithm. Identical scan time as in (a). The RCA (arrow) in (b) is better defined than in (a).

Discussion

Breath-hold imaging stimulated the field of MR coronary angiography. More recent work using respiratory monitoring for non-breath-hold imaging lends considerable optimism that improved imaging protocols will soon emerge.

Critical questions remain, however, with regard to the achievable spatial resolution for adequate stenosis quantification, satisfactory vessel contrast for lesion discrimination, and sufficient volumetric coverage in a reasonable scan time. The logistics of performing the examination can be another important consideration. Protocols for expedient localization and algorithms for rapid image reconstruction and reformatting could play essential roles in promoting the effectiveness of the methods.

Given the rapid progress achieved in MR coronary imaging, it is reasonable to expect continued improvements in image quality. Forthcoming improvements in the gradient subsystem should prove useful in shortening the sequence interval and improving flow compensation. Surface coils appropriately designed for this application will be of significant benefit. Opportunities also exist for improved methods in k-space scanning, respiratory monitoring, contrast enhancement, image reconstruction, and image display. The array of challenges in coronary imaging will likely require the combination of an appropriate set of enhancements.

References

1. Bogren HG, Lantz BMT, Miller RR, Mason DT. Effect of respiration on cardiac motion determined by cineangiography. *Acta Radiologica Diagnosis*. 1977;18:609–620.
2. Cynthia B, Paschal E, Haacke M, Adler LP. The impact of cardiac position inconsistencies due to respiration and beat-to-beat variations. In: *Proceedings of the Tenth SMRM-WIP*. August 1991, p. 1124.
3. Wang Y, Riederer SJ, Ehman RL. Respiratory motion of the heart: kinematics and the implication for the spatial resolution in coronary imaging. In: *Proceedings of the 3rd Society of Magnetic Resonance*. August 1995, p. 1391.
4. Pike GB, Hu BS, Glover GH, Enzmann DR. Magnetization transfer time-of-flight magnetic resonance angiography. *Magn Reson Med*. 1992;25:372–379.
5. Edelman RR, Ahn SS, Chien D, et al. Improved time-of-flight MR angiography of the brain with magnetization transfer contrast. *Radiology*. 1992;184: 395–399.
6. Brittain JH, Hu BS, Wright GA, et al. Coronary angiography with magnetization-prepared T2 contrast. *Magn Reson Med*. 1995;33:689–696.
7. Edelman R, Manning W, Burstein D, Paulin S. Coronary arteries: Breath-hold MR angiography. *Radiology*. 1991;181:641–643.
8. Manning WJ, Li W, Edelman RR. A preliminary report comparing magnetic resonance coronary angiography with conventional angiography. *N Engl J Med*. 1993;328:828–832.
9. Pennell DJ, Keegan J, Firmin DN, et al. Magnetic resonance imaging of coronary arteries: technique and preliminary results. *Br Heart J*. 1993;70: 315–326.
10. Duerinckx AJ, Urman MK. Two-dimensional coronary MR angiography: Analysis of initial clinical results. *Radiology*. 1994;193:731–738.
11. Post JC, van Rossum AC, Hofman MBM, et al. Clinical utility of two-dimensional breath-hold MR angiography in coronary artery disease. In: *Proceedings of the 3rd Society of Magnetic Resonance*. August 1995, p. 1394.
12. Nitatori T, Hachiya J, Korenaga T, et al. Clinical application coronary MR angiography studies of shortening of time for examination. In: *Proceedings of the 3rd Society of Magnetic Resonance*. August 1995, p. 1390.
13. Wielopolski PA, Scharf JG, Edelman RR. Multislice coronary angiography within a single breath hold. In: *Proceedings of the 1st Society of Magnetic Resonance*. April 1994, p. 80.
14. Meyer CH, Hu BS, Nishimura DG, Macovski A. Fast spiral coronary artery imaging. *Magn Reson Med*. 1992;28:202–213.
15. Nishimura DG, Irarrazabal P, Meyer CH. A velocity k-space analysis of flow effects in echo-planar and spiral imaging. *Magn Reson Med*. 1995;33: 549–556.
16. Hu BS, Meyer CH, Macovski A, Nishimura DG. Multislice spiral magnetic resonance coronary angiography. In: *Proceedings of the 2nd Society of Magnetic Resonance*. August 1994, p. 371.
17. Noll DC, Meyer CH, Pauly JM, et al. A homogeneity correction method for MR imaging with time-varying gradients. *IEEE Trans Med Imaging*. 1991; 10:629–637.
18. Irarrazabal P, Meyer CH, Nishimura DG, Macovski A. Inhomogeneity correction using an estimated linear field map. *Magn Reson Med*. 1996;35: 278–282.
19. Wielopolski PA, Manning WJ, Edelman RR. Single breath-hold volumetric

imaging of the heart using magnetization-prepared 3-dimensional segmented echo planar imaging. *J Magn Reson Imaging* 1995;4:403–409.

20. Bornert P, Jensen D. Coronary artery imaging at 0.5 T using segmented 3D echo planar imaging. *Magn Reson Med.* 1995;34:779–485.

21. Doyle M, Scheidegger MB, DeGraaf RG, et al. Coronary artery imaging in multiple 1-sec breath-holds. *Magn Reson Imaging.* 1993;11:3–6.

22. Wang Y, Christy PS, Korosec FR, et al. Coronary MRI with a respiratory feedback monitor: The 2D imaging case. *Magn Reson Med.* 1995;33:116–121.

23. Wang Y, Grimm RC, Rossman PJ, et al. 3d coronary MR angiography in multiple breath-holds using a respiratory feedback monitor. *Magn Reson Med.* 1995;34:11–16.

24. Ehman RL, Felmlee JP. Adaptive technique for high-definition MR imaging of moving structures. *Radiology.* 1989;173:255–263.

25. Brummer ME, Dixon WT, Oshinski JN, Pettigrew RI. Reduction of respiratory motion artifacts in coronary MRA using navigator echoes. In: *Proceedings of the 3rd Society of Magnetic Resonance.* August 1995, p. 748.

26. Sachs TS, Meyer CH, Hu BS, et al. Real-time motion detection in spiral MRI using navigators. *Magn Reson Med.* 1994;32:639–645.

27. Wang Y, Rossman PJ, Grimm RC, et al. Navigator-echo-based real-time respiratory gating and triggering for reduction of respiration effects in three-dimensional coronary MR angiography. *Radiology.* 1996;198:55–60.

28. Hofman MBM, Paschal CB, Li D, et al. MRI of coronary arteries: 2D breath-hold vs 3D respiratory-gated acquisition. *J Comput Assist Tomogr.* 1995;19: 56–62.

29. Oshinski JN, Hofland L, Mukundan S, et al. Respiratory gated coronary magnetic resonance angiography compares favorably with breath-hold imaging. In: *Proceedings of the 3rd Society of Magnetic Resonance.* August 1995, p. 22.

30. Woodard PK, Li D, Dhawake P, et al. Proximal coronary artery stenoses: examination with 3D MR retrospective respiratory gating. In *Proceedings of the AHA Conference on Current and Future Application of Magnetic Resonance in Cardiovascular Disease.* January 1999, p. 80.

31. Sachs TS, Meyer CH, Irarrazabal P, et al. The diminishing variance algorithm for real-time reduction of motion artifacts in MRI. *Magn Reson Med.* 1995;34:412–422.

32. Irarrazabal P, Sachs T, Meyer C, et al. Fast volumetric imaging of the heart. In: *Proceedings of the 3rd Society of Magnetic Resonance.* August 1995, p. 1393.

33. Brittain JH, Sachs TS, Hu BS, Nishimura D. Non-breathheld 2dft-coronary angiography. In: *Proceedings of the 3rd Society of Magnetic Resonance.* August 1995, p. 1395.

34. Meyer CH, Sachs TS, Hu BS, et al. High-resolution spiral coronary angiography. In: *Proceedings of the 3rd Society of Magnetic Resonance.* August 1995, p. 1392.

35. Wang SJ, Nishimura DG, Hu BS, Macovski A. Coronary angiography using fast selective inversion recovery. In: *Proceedings of Ninth Society of Magnetic Resonance Imaging.* 1991;1:166.

## Chapter 22

Magnetic Resonance Angiography of Coronary Arteries
Clinical Results

Warren J. Manning, MD

In the cardiovascular system magnetic resonance (MR) has had its greatest clinical impact in the evaluation of the thoracic aorta for the detection and assessment of aneurysms and dissection.[1] The thoracic aorta, however, is typically 3 to 4 cm in diameter with relatively little bulk motion associated with cardiac and respiratory motion. In contrast, the coronary arteries are only 3 to 4 mm in diameter (or 1/100th the cross-sectional area), more tortuous, and display extensive motion during both the cardiac cycle and with normal respiration. In addition, there is extensive MR signal from surrounding epicardial fat that obscures visualization of the underlying coronary vessels.

Early Attempts at Magnetic Resonance Coronary Angiography of Native Coronary Arteries

Using conventional electrocardiogram (ECG)-gated spin-echo techniques, images of the proximal 1 to 2 cm of the major epicardial coronary arteries (Figure 1) are sometimes seen. Paulin and colleagues[2] used this method in an attempt to identify the coronary ostia in 6 patients who had recently undergone conventional contrast angiography. Despite data acquisition over several minutes and lack of respiratory gating, the presence and origin of both the right and left main coronary

From: Higgins CB, Ingwall JS, Pohost GM, (eds). *Current and Future Applications of Magnetic Resonance in Cardiovascular Disease*. Armonk, NY: Futura Publishing Company, Inc.; © 1998.

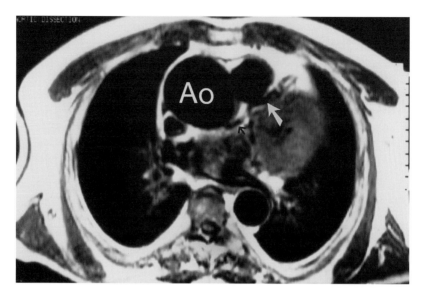

FIGURE 1. Conventional ECG-gated multiphase spin-echo transverse section at the proximal aorta in a patient referred for evaluation of a dilated ascending aorta. Note the left main coronary artery (black arrow) and extension into the left anterior descending (LAD) coronary artery (solid white arrow). (Reprinted with permission from Reference 2.)

artery arteries were identified in 4 of 6 patients. The left, but not the right coronary artery orifice was identified in the remaining 2 patients. Identification of a coronary stenosis, however, was not achieved in any patient.

Current Magnetic Resonance Coronary Angiographic Techniques: Visualization of Normal Anatomy

More recently, visualization of the native coronary arteries has been achieved utilizing MR subtraction methods,[3] three-dimensional techniques,[4] spiral scanning,[5] and segmentation gradient echo sequences.[6,7] A common theme of these MR coronary angiographic methods has included the use of multiple 10 to 20-second breathholds to suppress respiratory motion artifacts.

Currently, the greatest amount of clinical data on MR coronary is available from studies using two-dimensional segmented k-space gradient-echo sequences, first reported in humans by Edelman.[6] With this method, multiple phase-encoding steps are acquired in groups or segments, during a brief period of diastole, in a series of successive

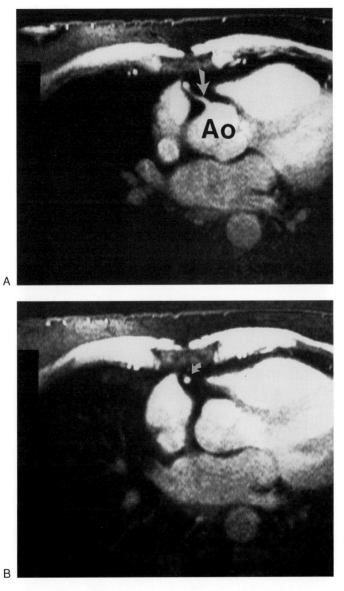

FIGURE 2. Three-mm thick breath-hold transverse MR sections in a healthy volunteer at **(A)** the level of the proximal right coronary artery (RCA; solid white arrow); **(B)** subsequent transverse section of RCA at a more inferior level (white arrow) identifying the vessel in cross section.

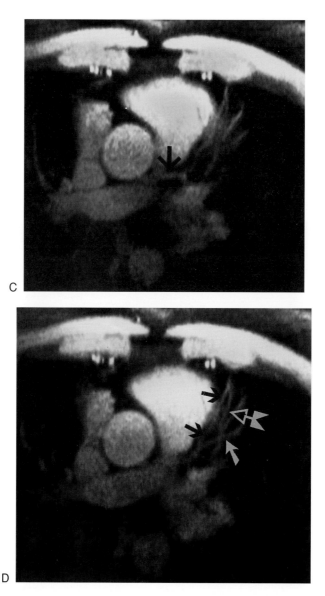

FIGURE 2. *(Continued)* **(C)** Transverse MR section of the left main coronary artery (solid white arrow) continuing on into the d) LAD (black arrows) coronary artery. Note the diagonal branches off the LAD (solid white arrows) and the great cardiac vein (open white arrow); Ao indicates aortic root. (Reprinted with permission from Reference 7.)

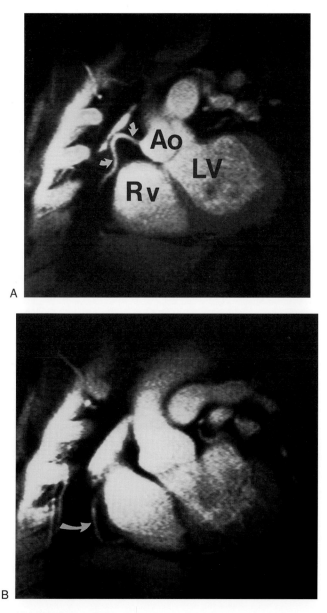

FIGURE 3. **(A–C)** Single oblique magnetic resonance coronary angiography along the long axis of the right coronary artery (curved white arrows) **(D)** single oblique magnetic resonance coronary angiography along the long axis of the left main (solid white arrow) and left anterior descending coronary artery (open white arrow). (Reprinted with permission from Reference 7.)

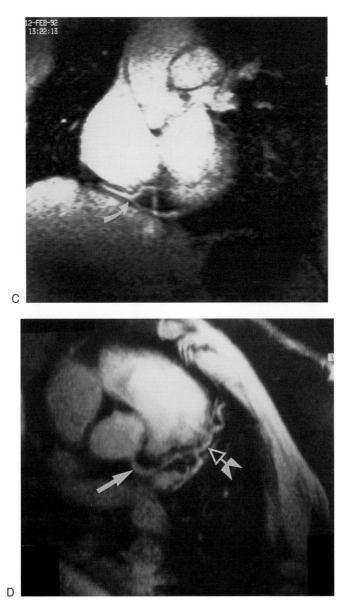

FIGURE 3. *(Continued)*

heartbeats.[6,7] Typically, 128 phase-encoding steps (matrix 128 × 256) are acquired (8 phase-encoding steps per heartbeat for 16 heartbeats) with a field-of-view of 240 mm (in-plane spatial resolution of 1.9 × 0.9 mm) and a 3 to 4 mm slice thickness. Thirty or more breath-hold images are often needed to define the major coronary anatomy.

Typically the coronary ostia are initially identified in the transverse plane (Figure 2) followed by obliquely oriented images acquired along the major or minor axis of the vessels (Figure 3). A cine variation of the sequence with double-oblique imaging planes may allow for visualization of long segments of the left anterior descending and right coronary arteries.[8]

Using this approach, the left main, left anterior descending, and right coronary arteries may be identified in nearly all patients who are able to cooperate with the required breath-hold.[10] The left circumflex coronary artery is more difficult to visualize, and may be identified in 74% to 94% of patients.[10] The lower success rate at visualization of the left circumflex is likely related to the frequent use of an anteriorly placed surface coil as radiofrequency (RF) receiver, and the relatively depressed signal/noise in the area of the posteriorly directed circumflex coronary artery. In addition to these major vessels, diagonal branches of the left anterior descending coronary artery may be identified in up to 80% of subjects and the great cardiac vein in 88% of subjects.[7,9,10]

The entire left main coronary artery is usually seen, while 5 to 8 cm of contiguous segments of the left anterior descending coronary artery and right coronary arteries are seen. Only the proximal 2 to 3 cm of the left circumflex are seen, again likely related to the artery's posterior location and the diminutive size of this vessel as it continues in the atrioventricular groove (Figure 4). Though in plane spatial resolu-

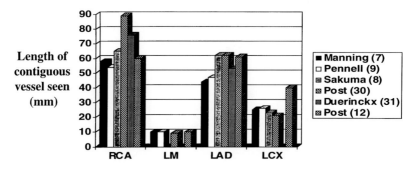

FIGURE 4. Contiguous length of native coronary artery visualized using two-dimensional segmented k-space and three-dimensional MR coronary angiographic techniques. RCA indicates right coronary artery; LM, left main; LAD, left anterior descending; LCX, left circumflex coronary artery.

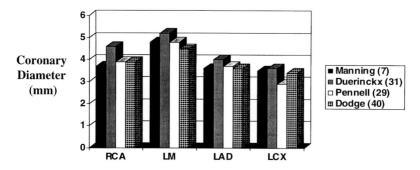

FIGURE 5. MR coronary angiographic determined proximal coronary diameter as compared with angiographic data among normals.[7,29,31,40]

tion is only 1 to 2 mm, proximal coronary artery diameter, as determined by MR, corresponds well to autopsy data. In addition, there has been a good correlation with angiographic data among patients who have had both studies, with a slight overestimation of coronary diameter by MR (Figure 5).[11] This is likely due to partial volume effect and beat-to-beat variability of cardiac motion. Whereas fewer data are available using three-dimensional MR techniques, the extent of coronary vessel visualized appears to be comparable (Figure 4).[4,12,13]

Magnetic Resonance Coronary Angiography for Identification of Anomalous Coronary Arteries

The ability of MR coronary angiography to visualize the proximal/midportions of the native coronary arteries makes it an ideal tool for the identification and delineation of anomalous coronary arteries. Among adults referred for contrast coronary angiography, anomalous origins of the coronary vessels are noted in 0.6% to 1.2% of patients.[14,15] Fortunately, the majority of coronary artery anomalies are not thought to have clinical importance. Origin of a coronary artery from the contralateral side, with subsequent passage between the aorta and pulmonary artery, however, has the potential to impair myocardial perfusion and is associated with sudden death.[16,17] Contrast coronary angiography identifies the presence of an anomalous vessel, but the anatomic course of the aberrant vessel with respect to the aorta and pulmonary artery may sometimes be difficult to discern.

The unique ability of MR to delineate the three-dimensional path of an anomalous coronary artery was recently demonstrated in two blinded studies involving 35 patients with anomalous aortic origins of

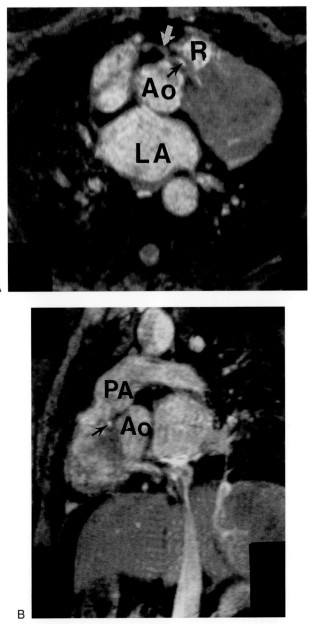

FIGURE 6. Anomalous left main coronary artery from right coronary artery. **(A)** single right-sided coronary artery (white arrow) that gives rise to the left main coronary artery (black arrow) coursing anterior to the aorta (Ao) and posterior to the right ventricular outflow tract (R); **(B)** oblique MR image demonstrating the anomalous vessel in cross section (black arrow).

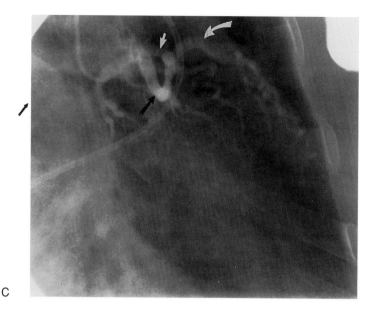

C

FIGURE 6. *(Continued)* **(C)** contrast angiogram showing the left main coronary artery (black arrow) coursing anterior to the aorta and posterior to the pulmonary artery (note the pulmonary artery catheter) before dividing into the left circumflex (straight white arrow) and left anterior descending coronary artery (curved white arrow). PA indicates pulmonary artery. (Reprinted with permission from Reference 19.)

the coronary arteries.[18,19] Overall, MR correctly identified the anomalous coronary vessel in 97% of cases, including all vessels with hemodynamically significant course (Figure 6).

Magnetic Resonance Assessment of Infarct Artery Patency

Among patients with myocardial infarction, restoration of antegrade flow in the infarct artery serves to improve both left ventricular function and survival.[20,21] Whereas contrast coronary angiography is a reliable method for determining infarct artery patency, it is both invasive and costly. Typically, MR coronary angiographic methods are insensitive to the direction of blood flow. Thus, vessels with significant stenoses yet antegrade flow might appear similar to those with occlusions and prominent retrograde blood flow. The combination of MR coronary angiographic methods with a presaturation of the proximal portion of the infarct related offers the opportunity to assess blood flow

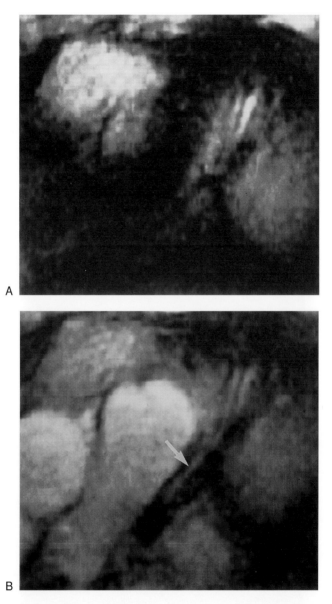

FIGURE 7. Oblique image of the distal left anterior descending (LAD) (white arrow) with **(A)** and without **(B)** presaturation pulses. Loss of signal in the LAD after presaturation **(A)** is consistent with antegrade blood flow in the LAD. In contrast, oblique images of the LAD (white arrow) from another patient with **(C)** and without **(D)** presaturation pulses demonstrates persistence of signal in the distal LAD after presaturation, consistent with retrograde filling of this portion of the vessel. (Reprinted with permission from Reference 22.)

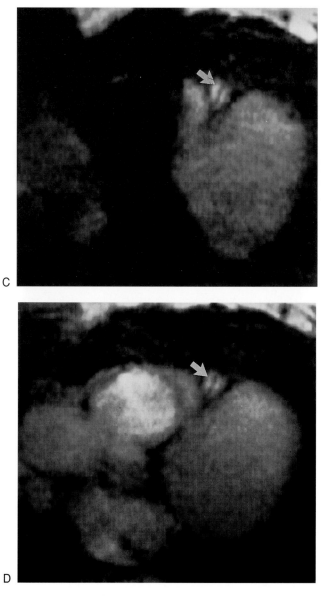

FIGURE 7. *(Continued)*

direction after the infarct related lesion. Such an approach was recently reported by Hundley and colleagues[22] who used a cine gradient echo segmented k-space breath-hold technique to image the infarct artery, and then repeated the sequence with the addition of presaturation pulse proximal to the point of signal dropout so as to saturate signal from blood flowing antegrade through the infarct artery (Figure 7). Thus, if antegrade flow is present, there would be signal loss in the distal vessel, but if there were retrograde blood flow, signal in the distal vessel would remain unchanged. These investigators were successful at characterizing antegrade or retrograde blood flow in all 18 vessels studied.[22] One might expect to obtain similar information by directly measuring blood flow within the coronary vessels using phase velocity methods,[23-25] although this has not been reported.

Identification of Coronary Artery Stenoses by Magnetic Resonance Coronary Angiography

Despite improvements in both prevention and treatment, cardiovascular disease remains the leading cause of death in the United States.[26] In addition, multiple noninvasive tests have been developed to allow for the identification of those with coronary stenoses, but up to 20% of diagnostic coronary angiograms demonstrate no significant stenoses.[27] The ability of MR to noninvasively assess coronary artery integrity would therefore represent an important advance in patient care.

The small caliber of the native coronary arteries (diameter 3 to 4 mm) and relatively limited spatial resolution of current MR coronary angiographic methods (1.5 × 0.9 mm; vs. 0.3 mm for contrast angiography), makes quantitative breath-hold MR coronary angiography improbable using current methods. Despite this limitation, we and others have used the sensitivity of gradient-echo sequences to demonstrate signal voids in areas of turbulence (due to dephasing of protons)/absent flow to identify focal coronary stenoses. A total occlusion or severe stenosis with poor distal blood flow might be expected to appear as an abrupt loss of signal (Figure 8) without visualization of the more distal vessel. In contrast, vessels with severe stenoses but significant antegrade blood flow might be expected to demonstrate a focal loss of signal, followed by bright signal depicting rapid laminar flow in the more distal lumen (Figure 9).

We and others have investigated the ability of MR coronary angiography to identify focal coronary stenoses[28-31] and data for these studies are summarized in Figure 10. Superior results appear to be achieved when the acquisition window is maintained ≤ 100 msec, when imaging is performed in mid-diastole, and when considerable effort is made to

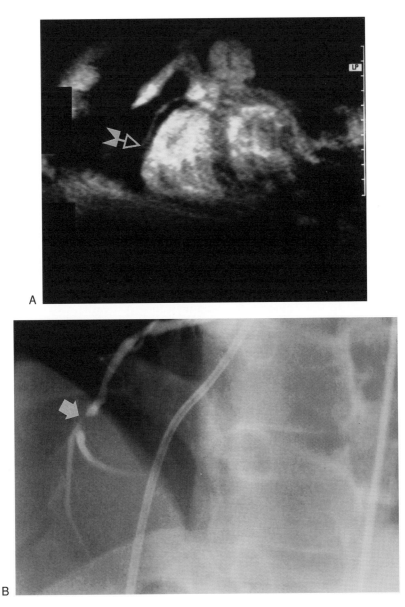

FIGURE 8. **(A)** Oblique sections of the proximal RCA. Note the abrupt loss of signal in the proximal artery (open white arrow). The more distal artery was not visualized in adjacent sections. **(B)** corresponding conventional angiogram demonstrating the subtotal occlusion of the proximal RCA (solid white arrow) with catheter in the right coronary ostium (open white arrow). (Reprinted with permission from Reference 28.)

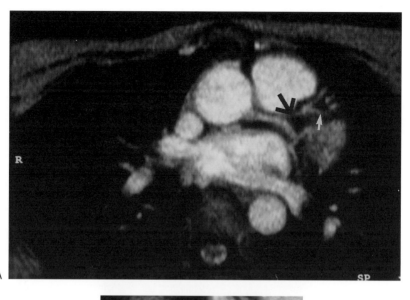

A

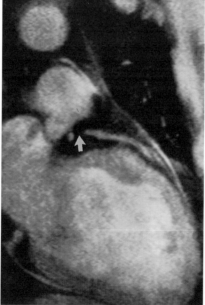

B

FIGURE 9. **(A)** Transverse image demonstrating the left main and left circumflex (LCX) with a signal void (black arrow) in the proximal left anterior descending (LAD). Also note the more distal LAD and diagonal (white arrow) are seen. **(B)** Single oblique magnetic resonance coronary angiography depicting signal void in the proximal LAD (solid white arrow).

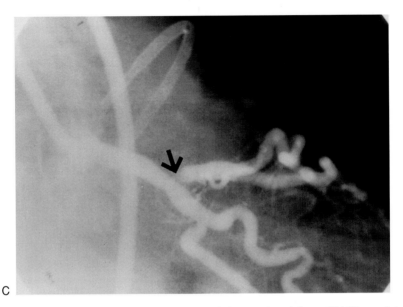

C

FIGURE 9. *(Continued)* **(C)** Corresponding right anterior oblique (RAO) caudal conventional angiogram confirming the tight proximal LAD stenosis (black arrow). (Reprinted with permission from Manning WJ, Edelman RR. MR coronary angiography. *Magn Reson Q.* 1993;9:147.)

teach patients the proper breath-hold technique. In a group of patients with a prevalence of coronary stenoses of 0.74, we found overall sensitivity and specificity of the two-dimensional MR coronary angiographic technique for correctly classifying individual vessels as with (≥ 50% diameter stenosis on conventional contrast angiography) or without disease, was 90% and 92%, respectively. The corresponding positive and negative predictive values were 0.85 and 0.95, respectively.[28] Errors in MR diagnoses are related to multiple causes, including inadequate

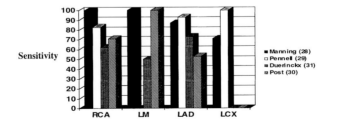

FIGURE 10. Sensitivity data for coronary diameter stenosis from MR coronary angiographic data as compared with angiographic data.[28–31]

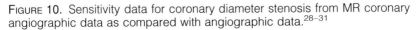

spatial resolution and difficulty with breath-holding leading to image blurring or registration errors. Partial volume averaging may also explain disagreement between methods.

Using a similar approach, Pennell and coworkers[29] graded MR coronary angiographic data as severe (complete signal loss), moderate (partial signal loss) and mild (wall irregularity only) stenoses. They found a significant relation between angiographic diameter stenoses based on these classifications. There was also close agreement on the distance from vessel origin to the site of stenosis between MR and x-ray studies. As expected from similar MR approaches to carotid artery evaluation, the length of stenosis measured by MR exceeded that of conventional contrast angiography.[29] Preliminary data from Rogers and coworkers,[32] however, suggest computer-assisted measurement of coronary flow signal intensity does not correlate with severity of stenoses. A recent study using flow phantoms by Oshinski et al[33] suggests that the magnitude of the turbulent fluctuation velocity, and not merely the presence of turbulence or the Reynolds number was the parameter that determined the extent of signal loss in the area of stenosis.

Future Trends in Magnetic Resonance Coronary Angiography

While the breath-hold magnetic resonance coronary angiography methods appear moderately successful for imaging the coronary arteries and identifying stenoses, such a technique does require patient cooperation. Data suggest that there is significant registration error between breath-holds[34] and a number of novel patient feedback systems have been studied to standardize the breath-hold.[35] Another approach to minimizing respiratory artifacts is the use of navigator echoes to determine the position of the diaphragm in real time, as described by Sachs and coworkers.[36] Frames of data acquired during respiratory motion can be rejected and data required with the next heartbeat. Such a technique is particularly exciting in that it may be combined with three-dimensional approaches, allowing for acquisition of comprehensive cardiac function and coronary data with minimal patient respiratory cooperation. Preliminary data suggest that the use of navigator gating with free-breathing results in image quality similar to that of breath-holding, but with improved patient comfort, superior slice registration, and without sacrifice in time-efficiency.[37] Importantly, the use of navigator gating will permit the development of high-resolution two-dimensional and three-dimensional imaging sequences that were previously impractical using breath-holding. Such an approach should allow for submillimeter spatial resolution and semiquantitative assessment of coronary artery stenoses.

Effect of Intracoronary Stents on Magnetic Resonance Coronary Angiography

The recognition of superior long-term results after percutaneous coronary stent implantation as compared with conventional balloon angioplasty has resulted in the widespread use of intracoronary stents. Typically made from high-grade stainless steel or tantalum, these stents are currently implanted in 10% to 15% of percutaneous revascularization procedures, but their use is expected to more than double before the year 2000. Scott and Pettigrew[38] recently studied intracoronary stents *ex vivo* and found they were not significantly influenced by the magnetic fields currently used for clinical imaging (≤ 1.5 T). Stents are well visualized as a signal void, most directly on MR images without fat saturation.[39] This signal void precludes evaluation of this portion of the vessel for angiographic stenosis.

Conclusion

In conclusion, we are now witnessing the evolution and clinical application of MR coronary angiographic techniques. Currently, such methods may be best applied for the delineation/identification of anomalous coronary arteries and infarct artery patency. It is premature to advocate breathhold MR coronary angiography for the detection of stenoses for clinical use. While breathhold quantitative MR coronary angiography for native coronary stenoses is currently not feasible, the combination of free-breathing with MR navigators may soon allow for enhanced spatial resolution and semiquantitative MR coronary angiography.

References

1. Nienaber CA, von Kodolitsch Y, Nicolas V, et al. The diagnosis of thoracic aortic dissection by noninvasive imaging procedures. *N Engl J Med.* 1993; 328:1–9.
2. Paulin S, von Schulthess GK, Fossel E, Krayenbuehl HP. MR imaging of the aortic root and proximal coronary arteries. *AJR.* 1987;148:665–670.
3. Wang SJ, Hu BS, Macovski A, Nishimura DG. Coronary angiography using fast selective inversion recovery. *Magn Reson Med.* 1991;18:417–423.
4. Li D, Paschal CB, Haacke EM, Adler LP. Coronary arteries: Three-dimen-

sional MR imaging with fat saturation and magnetization transfer contrast. *Radiology.* 1993;187:401–406.

5. Meyer CH, Hu BS, Nishimura DG, Macovski A. Fast spiral coronary artery imaging. *Magn Reson Med.* 1992;28:202–213.

6. Edelman RR, Manning WJ, Burstein D, Paulin S. Coronary arteries: Breath-hold MR angiography. *Radiology.* 1991;181:641–643.

7. Manning WJ, Li W, Boyle NG, Edelman RR. Fat-suppressed breath-hold magnetic resonance coronary angiography. *Circulation.* 1993;87:94–104.

8. Sakuma H, Caputo GR, Steffens JC, et al. Breath-hold MR cine angiography of coronary arteries in healthy volunteers: value of multiangle oblique imaging planes. *AJR.* 1994;163:533–537.

9. Pennell DJ, Keegan J, Firmin DN, et al. Magnetic resonance imaging of coronary arteries; Technique and preliminary results. *Br Heart J.* 1993;70:315–326.

10. Post JC, van Rossum AC, Hofman MBM, et al. Current limitations of two-dimensional breath-hold MR angiography in coronary artery disease. In: Book of Abstracts: Society of Magnetic Resonance 1994. Berkeley, CA: p. 508. Abstract.

11. Scheidegger MB, Vassalli G, Hess OM, Boesiger P. Validation of coronary artery MR angiography: comparison of measured vessel diameters with quantitative contrast angiography. In: Book of Abstracts: Society of Magnetic Resonance 1994. Berkeley, CA: p. 497. Abstract.

12. Post JC, van Rossum AC, Hofman MBM, et al. Respiratory-gated three-dimensional MR angiography of coronary arteries and comparison with x-ray contrast angiography. In: Book of Abstracts: Society of Magnetic Resonance 1994. Berkeley, CA: p. 509. Abstract.

13. Dogherty L, Schnall MD, Holland GA, et al. Fast 3D imaging of coronary arteries using Gd-DTPA enhancement. In: Book of Abstracts: Society of Magnetic Resonance 1995. Berkeley, CA: p. 1397. Abstract.

14. Engel HJ, Torres C, Page HL. Major variations in anatomical origin of the coronary arteries: angiographic observations in 4,250 patients without associated congenital heart disease. *Cathet Cardiovasc Diagn.* 1975;1:157–169.

15. Kimbiris D, Iskandrian AS, Segal BL, Bemis CE. Anomalous aortic origin of coronary arteries. *Circulation.* 1978;58:606–615.

16. Cheitlin MD, De Castro DM, McAllister HA. Sudden death as a complication of anomalous left coronary origin from the anterior sinus of Valsalva. A not-so-minor congenital anomaly. *Circulation.* 1974;50:780–787.

17. Levin DC, Fellows KE, Abrams HL. Hemodynamically significant primary anomalies of the coronary arteries: Angiographic aspects. *Circulation.* 1978;58:25–34.

18. Post JC, van Rossum AC, Bronzaer JGF, et al. Magnetic resonance angiography of anomalous coronary arteries. A new gold standard for delineating the proximal course? *Circulation.* 1995;92:3163–3171.

19. McConnell MV, Ganz P, Selwyn AP, Li W, et al. Identification of anomalous coronary arteries and their anatomic course by magnetic resonance coronary angiography. *Circulation.* 1995;92:3158–3162.

20. The Gusto Angiographic Investigators. The effects of tissue plasminogen activator, streptokinase, or both on coronary-artery patency, ventricular function, and survival after acute myocardial infarction. *N Engl J Med.* 1993;329:1615–1622.

21. ISIS-2 (Second International Study of Infarct Survival) Collaborative Group. Randomized trial of intravenous streptokinase, oral aspirin, both or neither

among 17,187 cases of suspected acute myocardial infarction. *Lancet.* 1988; 2:349–360.

22. Hundley WG, Clarke GD, Landau C, et al. Noninvasive determination of infarct artery patency by cine magnetic resonance angiography. *Circulation.* 1995;91:1347–1353.

23. Edelman RR, Manning WJ, Gervino E, Li W. Flow velocity quantification in human coronary arteries using fast, breath-hold MR angiography. *J Magn Reson Imaging.* 1993;3:699–703.

24. Keegan J, Firmin D, Gatehouse P, Longmore D. The application of breath hold phase velocity mapping techniques to the measurement of coronary artery blood flow velocity: phantom data and initial in vivo results. *Magn Reson Med.* 1994;31:526–536.

25. Poncelet BP, Weisskoff RM, Wedeen VJ, et al. Time of flight quantification of coronary flow with echo-planar MRI. *Magn Reson Med.* 1993;30:447–457.

26. 1993 Heart and Stroke Facts Statistics. American Heart Association: Dallas TX; 1993:3.

27. Johnson LW, Lozner EC, Johnson S, et al. Coronary arteriography 1984–1987: A report of the Registry of the Society of Cardiac Angiography and Interventions: O. Results and complications. *Cathet Cardiovasc Diagn.* 1989;17:5–10.

28. Manning WJ, Li W, Edelman RR. A preliminary report comparing magnetic resonance coronary angiography with conventional angiography. *N Engl J Med.* 1993;328:828–832.

29. Pennell DJ, Bogren HG, Keegan J, et al. Assessment of coronary artery stenosis by magnetic resonance imaging. *Heart.* 1996;75:127–133.

30. Post JC, van Rossum AC, Hofman MBM, et al. Clinical utility of two-dimensional breath-hold MR angiography in coronary artery disease. In: Book of Abstracts: Society of Magnetic Resonance 1995. Berkeley, CA: p. 1394. Abstract.

31. Duerinckx AJ, Urman MK. Two-dimensional coronary MR angiography: analysis of initial clinical results. *Radiology.* 1994;193:731–738.

32. Rogers WJ, Kramer CM, Simonetti OP, Reichek N. Quantification of human coronary stenoses by magnetic resonance angiography. In: Book of Abstracts: Society of Magnetic Resonance 1994. Berkeley, CA: p. 370. Abstract.

33. Oshinski JN, Ku DN, Pettigrew RI. Turbulent fluctuation velocity: The most significant determinant of signal loss in stenotic vessels. *Magn Reson Med.* 1995;33:193–199.

34. Liu YL, Riederer SJ, Rossman PJ, et al. A monitoring, feedback and triggering system for reproducible breath-hold MR imaging. *Magn Reson Med.* 1993;30:507–511.

35. Wang Y, Christy PS, Korosec FR, et al. Coronary MRI with a respiratory feedback monitor: the 2D imaging case. *Magn Reson Imaging.* 1995;33: 116–121.

36. Sachs TS, Meyer CH, Hu BS, et al. Real-time motion detection in spiral MRI using navigators. *Magn Reson Med.* 1994;32:639–645.

37. Khasgiwala VC, McConnell MV, Savord BJ, et al. Comparison of respiratory gating techniques and navigator locations for magnetic resonance coronary angiography. American Heart Association Scientific Conference on Current and Future Application of Magnetic Resonance in Cardiovascular Disease. San Francisco, CA. January 1996.

38. Scott NA, Pettigrew RI. Absence of movement of coronary stents after

placement in a magnetic resonance imaging field. *Am J Cardiol.* 1994;73: 900–901.

39. Duerinckx AJ, Atkinson D, Hurwitz R, et al. Coronary MR angiography after coronary stent placement. *AJR.* 1995;165:662–664.

40. Dodge JT Jr, Brown BG, Bolson EL, Dodge HT. Lumen diameter of normal human coronary arteries: Influence of age, sex, anatomic variation and left ventricular hypertrophy of dilation. *Circulation.* 1992;86:232–246.

## Part 5

Magnetic Resonance Spectroscopy

Quantification of Myocardial Phosphorus Magnetic Resonance Spectroscopy in Humans

Paul A. Bottomley, PhD

The underlying premises of this chapter are that the ratio of the high-energy phosphate metabolites, phosphocreatine (PCr) and adenosine triphosphate (ATP), and their individual concentrations in the myocardium are fundamental properties of the tissue, not the method used to measure them, and that phosphorus (^{31}P) nuclear magnetic resonance spectroscopy (MRS) can measure these quantities. It follows that studies of comparable groups of normal controls from different laboratories should generate comparable numbers. Precautions taken during MRS acquisition along with postacquisition corrections can substantially eliminate interlaboratory differences, resulting in very good and independent agreement on the normal human myocardial metabolite levels.

The ability of ^{31}P MRS to provide noninvasive measurements of regional high-energy phosphate metabolism endows this tool with a unique opportunity to define the levels and ratios of PCr and ATP in the normal human heart, and of probing their alteration in disease states, including ischemia and heart failure. However, full realization of these goals requires a proper accounting of various magnetic resonance (MR) factors on which the body's energy metabolism does not inherently depend. Thus, whereas individual ^{31}P MRS measurements of the PCr/ATP ratio in the normal human heart tend to fall within relatively narrow bounds for a given study, the possible effects of magnetic field

Supported in part by SCOR grant P50HL52315 from the National Institutes of Health.

From: Higgins CB, Ingwall JS, Pohost GM, (eds). *Current and Future Applications of Magnetic Resonance in Cardiovascular Disease.* Armonk, NY: Futura Publishing Company, Inc.; © 1998.

strength, spin-lattice relaxation time (T1), contamination from nonmyo-cardial tissue and other instrumental factors must be excluded before physiologic explanations can be invoked to explain interstudy differences, which can be quite large.[1]

Much of the distortion in the values of myocardial PCr and ATP measured by ^{31}P MR has as its underlying cause compromises made to compensate for the poor sensitivity and low concentrations of the metabolites relative to proton (^{1}H) nuclear magnetic resonance imaging (MRI). Thus, the surface detection coils that are invariably used to maximize the ^{31}P signal-to-noise ratio (SNR) produce highly spatially dependent signal intensity as a result of their nonuniform sensitivity and excitation fields.[1] To maximize SNR, acquisitions are commonly performed under partial saturation conditions with sequence repetition periods, TR ≤ T1 of the metabolite of interest. The effect is not only to attenuate the absolute amount of signal, which is important for absolute quantification, but also to distort the PCr/ATP ratio because the T1s of myocardial PCr and ATP differ significantly.[2] Similarly, to maximize SNR, the size of the selected volume elements (voxels) must be rather large, typically sampling 10 to 30 mL of myocardium,[3] and often poorly defined in one or two dimensions. This raises concerns about contamination from skeletal muscle in the chest, which has a higher PCr content, or liver tissue which has no PCr, and blood in the ventricular chamber, which also has some ATP but no PCr.[1]

We have endeavored to develop robust but practical protocols to deal with these problems and thereby enable measurements of the absolute concentrations and relative ratios of myocardial PCr and ATP in normal subjects and in patients. We summarize progress here.

Spatial Localization

Ensuring that the MRS signals are acquired substantially from the myocardium is a first priority. Two requirements are: (1) an ability to identify the myocardium of interest while the subject is fully engaged in the MRS system and (2) an ability to localize the MRS signals to the identified region of interest. Because most whole-body MRS systems are first and foremost MRI scanners and MRS localization uses MRI gradients anyhow, it has long been a practice to use MRI-guided, MRI-gradient localized MRS in conjunction with surface coil detection.[4] Localization schemes that we have found particularly fruitful are: one-dimensional chemical shift imaging (CSI), which uses nonselective excitation (a hard-pulse) followed by a single pulsed MRI phase-encoding gradient directed perpendicular to the surface coil to spatially encode a series of plane sections parallel to the coil[2,5]; and a three-dimensional

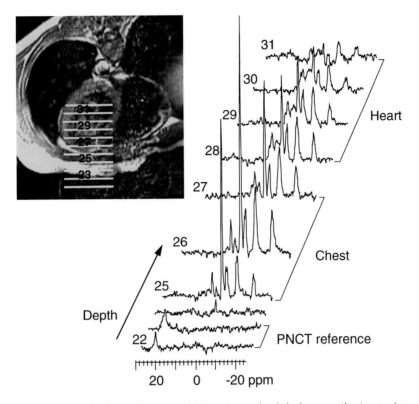

FIGURE 1. A typical cardiac-gated data set acquired during a patient examination for quantifying myocardial metabolite levels. The subject was oriented prone, rotated on the left side. The axial MRI (left) is used to locate the ^{31}P spectra relative to the heart. The ^{31}P spectra (right) were excited by 34.9° BIRP pulses[10] and spatially localized by the one-dimensional CSI method with 1-cm resolution averaging 768 spatially-encoded NMR signals. The acquisition time was 12.4 minutes. Spectra numbered the same derive from the same sections annotated in the image. The PNCT peaks are from phosphonitrilic chloride trimer solution embedded in the coil as a reference. (Adapted with permission from Reference 6.)

CSI method using slice selection, followed by phase-encoding in the other two dimensions.[1,3] A typical one-dimensional CSI data set is illustrated in Figure 1.

The one-dimensional CSI surface coil method affords only the somewhat fuzzy localization affected by the limits of the sensitivity profile of the surface coil in the two nongradient-encoded dimensions. Therefore, it is important to limit the size of the surface coil in order to avoid significant contamination of myocardial MRS metabolites by contributions from neighboring chest muscle and liver: relative to mus-

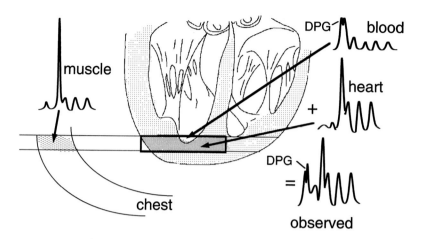

FIGURE 2. The ^{31}P spectrum from a localized voxel (darkest shading) in the anterior wall of the normal heart potentially contains integrated contributions of MRS signals from: ventricular blood with DPG, some ATP but no PCr; myocardium with a PCr/ATP ratio of about 1.8; and, if there are regions of NMR sensitivity that intersect the chest, chest muscle with a PCr/ATP ratio of 5 or so. (Adapted with permission from Reference 1.)

cle, the MRS-detectable PCr and ATP levels in fat and lung are negligible.[4] With 1-cm section resolution and a 6.5-cm diameter receiver coil, the one-dimensional CSI method typically interrogates 10 to 30 mL volumes of myocardium, as estimated by MRI.

The voxel sizes for ^{31}P three-dimensional CSI in the heart are usually set at about 16 to 20 mL (2 cm × 2 cm × 4 cm or 5 cm).[1] MRI-based tissue volumetry suggests that such voxels are typically less than half-filled with myocardium, due to the curvature and complexity of the myocardial anatomy.[3] Often the remainder of the voxel is occupied by pericardial fat, lung, or blood, so the effective resolution for myocardial PCr will typically be around 10 mL.[3] This reduction in effective voxel size and the increased number of phase-encoding steps that must be accommodated, usually necessitates a longer acquisition period for three-dimensional CSI studies compared to the one-dimensional CSI method in order to preserve useful SNR and complete the spatial encoding.

Figure 2 is a sketch of the cardiac voxel showing the main sources of MRS signal contamination.[1] The [PCr] and [ATP] in normoxic skeletal muscle are about 25 and 6 mmol/kg wet weight, respectively,[6] which leads to a PCr/ATP ratio several times higher than the highest ratio of about 2.1 that has been reported for the normal human heart.[1] Canine and human myocardial [ATP] is the same as muscle according to biochemical assay and *in vivo* MRS measurements, respectively.[6] Therefore, any contaminating metabolite signals from chest muscle will increase the [PCr] and PCr/ATP ratio measured by MRS in myocardial voxels. On the other hand, liver contains ATP but no PCr,[4] and its presence will therefore reduce the PCr/ATP ratios. Unfortunately, distortions introduced by skeletal muscle or liver contamination, to which one-dimensional localization methods are most prone, cannot easily be remedied postacquisition, and must be avoided by careful patient positioning, including orientation, and choice of surface coil size. Note that contaminating muscle and liver signals will be attenuated by inhomogeneity in the main magnetic field and phase cancellation the further that they lie from the cylindrical axis of the coil, when separate transmitter and receiver coils are used.[3]

Blood ATP Correction

Blood MRS signals are a common occurrence in voxels that intersect the ventricular chamber. Blood contains no PCr, but can contribute ATP signal, for which a correction can be made. Because the blood [ATP] is much lower than in heart at about 0.46 mmol/kg wet weight (assuming a 40% hematocrit[7]), significant contamination can usually only occur when the myocardium fills but a tiny fraction of the voxel.[6] The presence of blood is indicated by a characteristic doublet in the ^{31}P spectrum at chemical shifts of 5.4 and 6.3 parts per million (ppm) relative to PCr at 0 ppm, due to 2,3-diphosphoglycerate. Because [ATP]/[DPG] = 0.30 ± 0.02, the amount of ATP added by blood can be estimated by quantifying the DPG resonance. The corrected ATP signal is calculated by subtracting the blood ATP from the total observed ATP:

$$\text{(corrected ATP)} = \text{(contaminated ATP)} - 0.15 \times [\text{DPG}],$$

remembering that DPG has two phosphates[1].   [1]

The effect of imposing such a correction on myocardial PCr/ATP ratios is to increase them typically by about 13%.[1] The assumptions underlying the correction is that blood DPG and ATP are MRS-visible to the same extent, and that the ATP/DPG ratio is approximately constant. Even so, provided that while the corrections remain small, large deviations from these assumptions will generally compromise the final PCr and ATP quantification less than neglecting the correction altogether.[1]

Surface Coil Effects

For PCr/ATP ratios, nonuniformity in the surface coil sensitivity across a voxel or between several different voxels is not a problem to

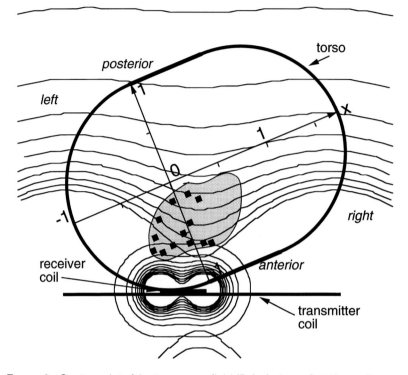

FIGURE 3. Contour plot of the transverse field (B_1) of a large flat 40-cm diameter circular surface transmitter coil and an optimally positioned 6.5-cm diameter detection coil, superimposed on a model of a prone torso of anterior-posterior dimension 0.3 and showing a myocardium (shaded) whose location was determined from MRI measurements averaged from several volunteers. The contours are at 10% intervals relative to the sensitivity at the center of the coils, and were computed from the Biot-Savart Law. The torso is rotated on the left side, as reported previously in patient studies[5]. Axes are marked in units of the radius of curvature of the model, 15 cm. Points in the myocardium circle the left ventricular wall, and the anterior right ventricle. The main magnetic field is directed perpendicular to the page.

the extent that each metabolite in each voxel is affected to the same extent. For measurements of metabolite concentrations in which an external standard is used, any differences in sensitivity at the location of the myocardial voxel and at the location of the standard must be accounted for. This can be done via the use of magnetic field plots of the coil (Figure 3).[3]

Nonuniformity in the excitation field that results in spatially dependent partial saturation due to flip-angle variations is, however, a significant problem because the location of myocardial voxels relative to the surface coil will vary from subject to subject, and because it is often desirable to sample and compare signals from several myocardial voxels in the same subject that would then experience different flip-angles. We have implemented two solutions.

Uniform Excitation Field

The first solution is to use a separate, much larger surface coil for ^{31}P MR excitation such that its excitation field is substantially uniform over the smaller sensitive volume of the receiver coil.[3] Figure 3 is a contour plot of the transverse field (B_1) of a 40-cm diameter circular surface coil computed from the Biot-Savart Law superimposed on a model of a prone torso showing a myocardium whose location was determined from MRI measurements averaged from several volunteers, and depicting the sensitivity profile of a 6.5-cm diameter optimally positioned detection coil. The torso is rotated on the left side, as reported previously in patient studies.[5] The variation in field across the heart is less than ±10% over the anterior myocardium to which the detection coil is sensitive.

Adiabatic Excitation

The second solution is to use adiabatic excitation pulses. Garwood and colleagues[8] describe an adiabatic pulse, BIR-4, capable of producing arbitrary preset flip-angles that are constant over a 10-fold or more variation in B_1-field amplitude. BIR-4 comprises four equally long segments whose frequency is swept tangentially, and whose amplitudes are modulated by a hyperbolic tangent, which results in holes in the pulse between the first and second, and between the third and fourth, segments. The flip-angle, α, is set by introducing phase jumps of $(180° \pm \alpha/2)$ and $-(180° \pm \alpha/2)$ at the two amplitude holes.[8]

Errors in implementing the BIR-4 pulse can arise from system hardware limitations that result in an accumulation of phase error or difficulty in setting the phase when the amplitude is zero. In our experience, errors of up to 10° between the preset and true flip-angle can occur.[9] We have found that this error can be reduced by about an order of magnitude or to within ±1° of the true flip-angle with a two-step cycling of the phase-jump inside the BIR-4 pulse, forming a BIRP (**BIR-4 Phase-cycled**) pulse (Table 1).[9] Because the flip-angle remains constant over a vast range of B_1 values and BIRP pulses are accurately prescribed by the phase jump, the pulses can be used without calibration, simply by ensuring that an adequate amount of transmitter power is available. They can be implemented either by using the same coil

TABLE 1

Difference Between the Nominal and the True Flip-Angles of BIR-4 and BIRP Pulses, for Nominal Flip-Angles from $-90°$ to $+90°$[1]

Pulse duration, amplitude	n	Mean error in flip-angle		Fitted error, δ in flip-angle†	
		BIR-4	BIRP	BIR-4	BIRP
4 ms, 69 μT	14	$-7.4°$	$+1.3°$	$-10.2°$	0.6°
4 ms, 290 μT	10	$-5.5°$	$+0.1°$	$-5.6°$	0.2°
4 ms, 290 μT*	10		0.6°		0.6°
3 ms, 124 μT	17	4.1°	$-0.5°$	5.3°	$-0.5°$
4 ms, 53 μT	38	6.6°	0.2°	7.1°	0.007°
4 ms, 90 μT	20	6.5°	$-0.5°$	6.3°	$-0.3°$
4 ms, 124 μT	18	6.8°	$-0.6°$	6.8°	$-0.97°$
6 ms, 94 μT	20	7.1°	$-1.7°$	9.8°	$-0.9°$
8 ms, 22 μT	21	8.8°	$-0.7°$	11.0°	$-0.1°$

n indicates number of flip-angles measured; * Surface coil excitation and detection. † Signal fitted to $S = S_0 \cdot \sin(\alpha + \delta)$ where $(\alpha + \delta)$ is the true flip-angle, and α is the nominal value.

for excitation and reception, or with a separate larger surface transmitter coil.

The elimination of the need to adjust pulse power during patient studies, and the confidence that the flip-angle is accurately set, are significant advances over earlier methods of setting flip-angles by trial-and-error calibration of a 90° (or other) pulse.

Partial Saturation Effects

Distortion from partial saturation results when TR is short compared to the T1 of myocardial PCr and ATP and the MRS flip-angle is large or is adjusted to maximize SNR.[2] For concentration measurements, corrections that account for the absolute amount of the distortion must be applied. For metabolite ratios, the saturation correction depends on the difference in T1 values of metabolites that comprise the ratio.[2] Thus, measurements of myocardial PCr/ATP would be simplified if T1 (PCr) = T1 (ATP). Unfortunately the evidence is against this.[1,10] The mean values and 95% confidence intervals (bracketed) for the T1 of human myocardial PCr and β-ATP are 4.4 seconds (3.9 seconds, 4.9 seconds), and 2.3 seconds (1.7 seconds, 2.8 seconds), respectively, averaged from data published in six independent studies.[10] The value of the ratio, T1 (PCr)/T1 (β-ATP), is 1.85, with confidence interval (1.6, 2.1). We have implemented two methods for correcting the resultant distortion.

Direct Measurement of Saturation Factors

The first approach is to measure the correction factor, F, directly from the ratio of MRS signals acquired under under fully relaxed conditions, to that acquired under the partially saturated conditions used for the study.[5] This is done for each subject, as part of the MRS protocol. Because T1 is so long, the SNR is inadequate to provide meaningful measurements of F on the fully localized myocardial voxel. A practical solution is to use the unlocalized but uniformly-excited signal detected by the surface coil on the chest.[2] Such a measurement can be done in 5 or 6 minutes and is readily incorporated into patient protocols. Because skeletal muscle in the chest contributes to this measurement, the correction, as applied to the myocardial PCr/ATP ratio, assumes that the T1 ratio, T1 (PCr)/T1(ATP), is essentially the same in skeletal and heart muscle.[2] The average ratio of T1(PCr)/T1(β-ATP) from data published in nine independent studies is 1.80 with 95% confidence interval (1.6, 2.0), not significantly different from the value of 1.85 for the heart T1 ratio listed above.[10] This approach is also validated by localized surface coil measurements of F on 82 subjects gated at the heart rate with the flip-angle adjusted to maximize the PCr signal, which show no significant variation of F with either the amount of muscle contributing to the unlocalized spectrum, or disease state: the mean factor for correcting the PCr/ATP ratio was 1.36 ± 0.03 SE.[2]

Calculation from Known T1s

The second approach is to calculate F, as defined above, from known myocardial T1, TR, and flip-angle (α) values:

$$F = (1 - \cos \alpha.\exp[-TR/T1])/(1 - \exp[-TR/T1]). \qquad [2]$$

For cardiac-gated studies, TR is given by the heart rate and α must be known or measured during the study protocol. The use of preset BIR-4 or BIRP pulses, as described above, avoids having to measure α, and reduces concerns about the effects of B_1 nonuniformity. However, the choice of T1 can be controversial when there are large differences in T1 measurements from different laboratories.[11] This raises three significant problems: (1) if T1 is uncertain, an "Ernst angle," which yields the optimum SNR for a given value of TR cannot be calculated and preset; (2) if T1 is uncertain, what value should be used for calculating the saturation correction; and (3) what error would result in the saturation corrected MRS values due to an inappropriate choice of T1 for a particular strategy of setting α?[10]

We have explored the use of upper (T1u) and lower (T1v) bounds of T1 to deal with its uncertainty.[10] Again, the 95% confidence intervals calculated from a compilation of independent human ^{31}P MRS T1 metabolite values from the literature can be used as these bounds.[10] Two simple strategies for setting α are to use an Ernst angle based on an average T1 or an average Ernst angle:

$$\cos \alpha = \exp - (u + v)/2, \qquad [3]$$

or

$$\alpha = \{\arccos[\exp(-u)] + \arccos[\exp(-v)]\}/2, \qquad [4]$$

where u = TR/T1u and v = TR/T1v. However, over a large confidence interval, these strategies result in greater SNR loss relative to the SNR

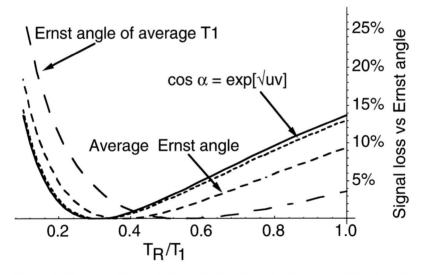

FIGURE 4. The signal loss relative to that achieved with a correct Ernst angle excitation, that results when T1 is uncertain but falls between 0.1 TR and 1.0 TR, for three different strategies for setting the flip-angle: (1) the flip-angle is given by the Ernst angle of the average T1 (equation [3]); (2) the flip-angle is given by the average of the Ernst angles at the two bounds of uncertainty (equation [4]); and (3) the Ernst angle is given by an optimized expression (equation 5). (Adapted with permission from reference 10.)

that would result from use of an Ernst angle if T1 were known, than an optimized angle given by the expression:[10]

$$\cos \alpha_o = \exp(-\sqrt{uv}).$$ [5]

The relative performance of these three strategies is illustrated in Figure 4.[10] With the flip-angle set to α_o, signal loss due to uncertainty in T1 is limited to $\leq 14\%$ for up to a 10-fold uncertainty in T1 with T1 $\leq$ TR, that is, over the entire range $0.1 \leq$ TR/T1 ≤ 1. Moreover, the effect that an uncertainty in T1 of a factor of 2 has on a MRS signal corrected for partial saturation using equation [2] with flip-angle α_o and a value of T1 equal to the mean of the confidence interval, is limited to $\leq 20\%$.[10]

For acquisitions gated at a typical normal heart-rate of TR $= 0.86$ second, the optimum BIRP flip-angle, α_o, for myocardial PCr based on the above confidence intervals is $34.6°$, yielding F(PCr) $= 3.14$. The saturation correction for the PCr/ATP ratio is 1.30,[10] consistent with the empirical measurements of F(PCr/ATP) $= 1.36$ from 82 subjects noted above.[2]

Myocardial PCr/ATP

The measurement of an undistorted or fully corrected PCr/ATP ratio is a significant and useful step along the road to absolute quantification: corrected ^{31}P MR PCr/ATP ratios are reduced in heart failure depending on severity,[12] and during ischemia in patients with coronary

---

TABLE 2

Effect of Saturation and Blood Correction on Some Myocardial PCr/ATP Ratios

Raw ratio	Saturation-corrected	Blood, saturation corrected	Reference
1.3 ± 0.4†			4
	1.6 ± 0.4*		14
1.3	1.7 ± 0.2		3§
	1.7 ± 0.2		5§
1.1	1.6	1.8 ± 0.2	13§
1.2	1.8	1.9 ± 0.2	15§

Raw ratios acquired with NMR pulse flip-angles at or near the Ernst angle for PCr ($=$ arcos[exp{$-$ TR/T1}]) at the heart-rate or with TR $= 1.0$ second†. * Acquired with minimal saturation. § Acquired using CSI MRS localization.

TABLE 3

Published Myocardial PCr/ATP
Ratios Corrected for Saturation
and Blood Contamination

Value	n	Reference
1.80 ± 0.21	12	13
1.93 ± 0.21	17	15
1.8 ± 0.1	6	16
1.95 ± 0.45	19	12
1.65 ± 0.26	9	17
1.85 ± 0.28	11	19
1.80 ± 1.03	11	21
1.80 ± 0.34	8	6
1.23 ± 0.17	6	18

n indicates number of subjects.

artery disease.[5] The effect of applying the blood and saturation corrections on our uniformly excited myocardial PCr/ATP ratio after careful coil positioning is shown in Table 2.[3–5,13–15] The raw PCr/ATP ratios of about 1.3 are increased by 40% to about 1.85.

Considering publications in which both saturation and blood corrections were performed or where blood contamination was negligible,[6,12,13,15–19] there is good agreement on the normal myocardial PCr/ATP value, as summarized in Table 3. The mean value of the (first) eight concordant values is 1.82 ± 0.09 SD, which, given the evidence that tissue ATP and PCr are 100% MR visible,[20] should represent the best current estimate for the true PCr/ATP ratio in the normal human heart.[1]

Metabolite Concentrations

A measurement of the corrected myocardial PCr/ATP ratio can be converted to concentration measurements of PCr and ATP by recording the MRS signal from a concentration standard and accounting for the volume of myocardium contributing to the spectrum.

External Phosphate Reference

The usual approach is to use an external phosphate reference and MRI tissue volumetry with three-dimensional localized MRS.[3,21] The external standard can be placed on the chest during the MRS examination protocol,[3] or MRS measurements can be done on the standard in a separate experiment.[21,22] The concentration estimates must be corrected for any differences in sensitivity of the surface coil in myocardial and reference voxels,[3] and possible differences in coil loading accounted for if separate experiments are done. The concentration of a metabolite, $[p]$ is thus:

$$[p] = \frac{Sp.[r]}{Sr} \cdot \left\{ \frac{Fr.Er}{Fp.Ep} \right\} \cdot \left\{ \frac{V_r \cdot \psi_r \cdot \Phi_r}{V_p \cdot \psi_p \cdot \Phi_p} \right\} \tag{6}$$

where $[r]$ is the concentration of the external reference, S is the integrated MRS signal, V is the volume of sample in the voxel, ψ is the sensitivity, E accounts for signal decay between excitation and detection, F is the saturation factor, and ϕ accounts for signal loss due to the phase shift across voxel for the metabolite voxel (subscripts p) and reference (subscripts r).[3] The absolute fractional error in $[p]$ is the sum of the fractional errors in all of the factors contributing to equation [6].

Water Referencing

Concern about the cumulative error potential in the above approach, and difficulties with MRI-based tissue volumetry due to the large voxels and the complexity of the cardiac anatomy, have led us to an alternative approach that obviates the need for image-based tissue volumetry, and can be incorporated into existing one-dimensional[31]P CSI protocols with only an additional ^{1}H one-dimensional CSI acquisition.[6] If the water resonance in the ^{1}H data set is acquired with the same detection coil (assuming radiofrequency penetration effects are negligible) and if the myocardium is the predominant source of the water signal, the water resonance will have the same spatial resolution characteristics as the ^{31}P data set and moreover its intensity will be proportional to the same volume of myocardium. It can therefore be used as a concentration reference. The metabolite concentration can then be calculated from the ratio of the ^{31}P and water ^{1}H MRS signals from the same voxel:

$$[P] = \frac{Sp.[W].C_{PH}}{S_W} \cdot \left\{ \frac{F_P \cdot E_P}{E_W} \right\} \tag{7}$$

(eq.7)where $[W]$ is the concentration of tissue water protons in the heart (normally, 81 mol/kg), subscripts W refer to the water ^{1}H signal, and C_{PH} is a constant scaling factor accounting for the difference in ^{1}H and ^{31}P NMR sensitivity.[6] C_{PH} is given by the quotient of the ^{1}H signal per proton to the ^{31}P signal per phosphorus nucleus.

   This method depends on S_W being a good estimator of tissue water. For myocardial one-dimensional CSI studies, there are two sources of water signal of nonmyocardial origin that could contribute to the ^1H spectra, and for which corrections can be made. First, pericardial fat is very low in high-energy phosphates but contributes some water. The water signal, S_W, can be corrected for fat by subtracting an amount, $L.S(CH_2)$, where $S(CH_2)$ is the lipid ^1H signal in the spectrum, and L is the water content of fat, which is about 15%.[6] Second, blood could contribute to the water signal without contributing any PCr or much ATP. The ^{31}P DPG signal can be used to correct the water ^1H signal for blood water contributions by inverting equation [7]:

$$S(\text{blood}) = \frac{S(DPG).[W_B].C_{PH}}{2.[DPG]} \cdot \left\{ \frac{F_{DPG} \cdot E_{DPG}}{E_B} \right\}, \qquad [8]$$

where $S(\text{blood})$ and $S(DPG)$ are, respectively, the ^1H water and total ^{31}P DPG signal from blood, and $[W_B] = 89.7$ mol/kg is the water proton concentration of blood, and $[DPG] = 1.64$ mmol/kg.[6,7] The bracketed term in E and F approaches unity for short acquisition delays and when the moving blood has insufficient time to partially saturate. The myocardial ATP signal is again corrected for the small contribution from blood via equation [1]. The fat- and blood-corrected water signal to be substituted in equation [7] is thus:

$$S_W = S(H_2O) - L.S(CH_2) - S(\text{blood}), \qquad [9]$$

where $S(H_2O)$ is the observed water signal.[6] For [PCr] and [ATP] measurements, The combined fat and blood corrections increase one-dimensional CSI estimates of human myocardial [PCr] and [ATP] by

---

TABLE 4

Noninvasive ^{31}P MRS Measurements of Metabolite Concentrations in Normal Human Heart

[PCr]	[ATP]	Reference
11 ± 3	6.9 ± 1.6	3
11.3 ± 3.7	7.4 ± 2.9	22
12.1 ± 4.3	7.7 ± 3.0	21
10.0 ± 2.0	5.8 ± 1.6	6

Concentrations are in mmol/kg wet weight, mean ± SD.

about 17% and 33%, respectively.[6] The method has been validated by blinded phantom studies, and on human muscle.

PCr and ATP concentrations reported to date for the human heart are summarized in Table 4,[3,6,21,22] and are in good agreement.

Conclusions

We have identified some important problems and sources of scatter in human myocardial PCr and ATP measurements by ^{31}P MRS, including those associated with deficiencies in spatial localization and the invariably large voxel sizes, the effects of nonuniformities resulting from the use of surface coils, and partial saturation effects and uncertainty in the myocardial T1 values. We have provided specific practical solutions to overcome or accommodate these problems, including: a method of correcting for blood contamination; the use of large separate transmitter coils or preset adiabatic excitation pulses to provide uniform excitation; methods of correcting for partial saturation via direct measurement of saturation factors, or via computation from known T1 values; and a method of selecting the flip-angle to maximize metabolite SNR and minimize potential error in the saturation-correction when the T1s are uncertain. We have shown that the application of such techniques results in reasonable reproducibility amongst PCr and ATP ratios and concentrations. We look forward to their application to the study of myocardial energy metabolism in normal and patient populations in resting and dynamic protocols.

References

1. Bottomley PA. MR spectroscopy of the human heart: the status and the challenges. *Radiology.* 1994;191:593–612.
2. Bottomley PA, Hardy CJ, Weiss RG. Correcting human heart ^{31}P NMR spectra for partial saturation. Evidence that saturation factors for PCr/ATP are homogeneous in normal and disease states. *J Magn Reson.* 1991;95: 341–355.
3. Bottomley PA, Hardy CJ, Roemer PB. Phosphate metabolite imaging and concentration measurements in human heart by nuclear meagnetic resonance. *Magn Reson Med.* 1990;14:425–434.
4. Bottomley PA. Noninvasive study of high-energy phosphate metabolism in human heart by depth-resolved ^{31}P NMR spectroscopy. *Science.* 1985; 229:769–772.
5. Weiss RG, Bottomley PA, Hardy CJ, Gerstenblith G. Regional myocardial metabolism of high-energy phosphates during isometric exercise in patients with coronary artery disease. *N Engl J Med.* 1990;323:1593–1600.
6. Bottomley PA, Atalar E, Weiss RG. Human cardiac high-energy phosphate metabolite concentrations by 1-D resolved NMR spectroscopy. *Magn Reson Med.* 1996;35:664–670.

7. Minakami S, Suzuki C, Saito T, Yoshikawa H. Studies on erythrocyte glycolysis. I. Determination of the glycolytic intermediates in human erythrocytes. *J Biochem.* 1965;58:543–550.

8. Garwood M, Ke Y. Symmetric pulses to induce arbitrary flip angles with compensation for RF inhomogeneity and resonance offsets. *J Magn Reson.* 1991;94:511–525.

9. Bottomley PA, Ouwerkerk R. BIRP, an improved implementation of low-angle adiabatic (BIR-4) excitation pulses. *J Magn Reson.* 1993;103A:242–244.

10. Bottomley PA, Ouwerkerk R. Optimum flip-angles for exciting NMR with uncertain T_1 values. *Magn Reson Med.* 1994;32:137–141.

11. Bottomley PA. The true values of myocardial high-energy phosphates? Neubauer S, Horn M, Bauer WR, et al. Response. *Magn Reson Med.* 1993; 29:145–147. Letters.

12. Neubauer S, Krahe T, Schindler R, et al. [31]P magnetic resonance spectroscopy in dilated cardiomyopathy and coronary artery disease. *Circulation.* 1992;86:1810–1818.

13. Hardy CJ, Weiss RG, Bottomley PA, Gerstenblith G. Altered myocardial high-energy phosphate metabolites in patients with dilated cardiomyopathy. *Am Heart J.* 1991;122:795–801.

14. Bottomley, PA, Herfkens RJ, Smith LS, Bashore TM. Altered phosphate metabolism in myocardial infarction: P-31 MR spectroscopy. *Radiology.* 1987;165:703–707.

15. Bottomley PA, Weiss RG, Hardy CJ, Baumgartner WA. Myocardial high-energy phosphate metabolism and allograft rejection in patients with heart transplants. *Radiology.* 1991;181:67–75.

16. Menon RS, Hendrich K, Hu X, Ugurbil K. ^{31}P NMR spectroscopy of the human heart at 4T: Detection of substantially uncontaminated cardiac spectra and differentiation of subepicardium and subendocardium. *Magn Reson Med.* 1992;26:368–376.

17. de Roos A, Doornbos J, Luyten PR, et al. Cardiac metabolism in patients with dilated and hypertrophic cardiomyopathy: Assessment with proton-decoupled P-31 MR spectroscopy. *J Magn Reson Imaging.* 1992;2:711–719.

18. van Dobbenburgh JO, Lekkerkerk C, van Echteld CJA, de Beer R. Saturation correction in human cardiac ^{31}P MR spectroscopy at 1.5T. *NMR Biomed.* 1994;7:218–224.

19. Yabe T, Mitsunami K, Okada M, et al. Detection of myocardial ischemia by ^{31}P magnetic resonance spectroscopy during handgrip exercise. *Circulation.* 1994;89:1709–1716.

20. Humphrey SM, Garlick PB. NMR-visible ATP and Pi in normoxic and reperfused rat hearts: a quantitative study. *Am J Physiol.* 1991;260:H6–H12.

21. Yabe T, Mitsunami K, Inubushi T, Kinoshita M. Quantitative measurements of cardiac phosphorus metabolites in coronary artery disease by ^{31}P magnetic resonance spectroscopy. *Circulation.* 1995;92:15–23.

22. Okada M, Mitsunami K, Yabe T, et al. Quantitative measurements of phosphorus metabolites in normal and diseased human hearts by ^{31}P NMR spectroscopy. *Proc SMRM.* 1992;2:2305. Abstract.

## Chapter 24

Phosphorus Magnetic Resonance Studies of Mitochondrial Creatine Kinase
From *In Vitro* to *In Vivo*

F.A. van Dorsten, PhD, T. Reese, PhD,
M. Laudy, MSc, C.J.A. van Echteld, PhD,
M.G.J. Nederhoff, BSc, J. Ton, MSc,
F.D. Laterveer, PhD, F.N. Gellerich, PhD,
and K. Nicolay, PhD

Introduction

Creatine kinase (ATP:creatine phosphotransferase; EC 2.7.3.2) is abundant in tissues that have a high and/or rapidly fluctuating free-energy demand.[1,2] Five different isoenzyme species of creatine kinase (CK) are known, and these are expressed in a tissue-specific manner and subject to subcellular compartmentalization. In heart and especially in skeletal muscle, the most abundant CK species is found in the cytoplasm where it occurs as a dimer. In mature skeletal muscle, the cytoplasmic enzyme is exclusively of the M-type (designated as MM-CK) and in heart, a minor fraction is present as a heterodimer between the M- and B-type species (MB-CK). The B-type isoenzyme dominates in smooth muscle and in brain. In striated muscle, the MM- and MB-

Part of this research was carried out at the Netherlands *in vivo* NMR facility and the Nijmegen SON Research Center which are both supported by the Netherlands Organization for Scientific Research (NWO). F.N. Gellerich gratefully acknowledges a visitors grant from NWO. F.D. Laterveer was supported by the Netherlands Foundation for Chemical Research (SON).

From: Higgins CB, Ingwall JS, Pohost GM, (eds). *Current and Future Applications of Magnetic Resonance in Cardiovascular Disease.* Armonk, NY: Futura Publishing Company, Inc.; © 1998.

dimers partly are freely dispersed in the cytoplasmic phase and partly are found in association with a number of subcellular structures, including the myofibrillar M-band, glycolytic multi-enzyme complexes and the sarcoplasmic reticulum membrane.[1,3] Apart from the MM-, MB- and BB-CK species, there are two different mitochondrial isoforms of CK[2]: (1) the so-called sarcomeric mitochondrial CK (Mi-CK), which is found in muscle and (2) the ubiquitous Mi-CK. Both Mi-CK species are located in the intermembrane space of the mitochondrion and mainly occur as octamers *in vivo*. The octameric enzyme can be readily dissociated into dimers under *in vitro* conditions. It has been suggested that Mi-CK is preferentially located in intermembrane contact sites between inner and outer membrane. Using purified mitochondrial membranes, we have previously shown with the Langmuir-Blodget technique that octameric Mi-CK is capable of forming stable contacts between opposing outer and inner membrane interfaces.[4] Contact formation was shown to be specific for the Mi-CK octamer (ie, dimeric Mi-CK and other abundant intermembrane space proteins appeared ineffective) and to be promoted by the mitochondrion-specific phospholipid cardiolipin.[4,5]

Based on the existence of the different CK isoforms and their subcellular distribution, the following major functions for the CK system have been proposed (for reviews see Refs. 1–3).

The Temporal ATP Buffer Function

At the expense of phosphocreatine (PCr), CK activity keeps adenosine triphosphate (ATP) and adenosine diphosphate (ADP) concentrations and the pH steady under conditions of high cellular activity. This is the textbook example of CK function that has been documented for many tissues.[1,2] The temporal ATP buffering activity could have been supported by a single CK enzyme species, at any location in the cell. The existence of CK isozymes suggests that CK serves more functions.

The Local ATP Buffer Function

It has been suggested that the CK system also functions to maintain the ATP/ADP ratio high at sites of rapid ATP utilization.[1-3] The evidence for this thermodynamic function is based on the finding that CK activity is coupled to that of the myosin adenosine triphosphates (ATPase) and the Ca^{2+}-ATPase of the sarcoplasmic reticulum. Part of the cytosolic CK pool is bound in close proximity to these ATPases.

The Energy Transport Function

The different CK isoenzymes have been suggested to constitute the phosphocreatine shuttle or circuit.[1-3] Phosphocreatine (PCr) is thought to act as a free-energy carrier that connects sites of free-energy delivery with sites of free-energy use through diffusion. The Mi-CK isoform plays a key role in the model[1] in that the coupling of its activity to oxidative phosphorylation yields PCr as an end product of mitochondrial activity. The CK species associated with cytosolic ATPases are at the PCr utilizing/creatine (Cr) producing side of the circuit. The circuit model is partly based on the estimated free-energy transporting capacity of the ATP/ADP couple as compared with that of the PCr/Cr couple. ATP and ADP are expected to diffuse less rapidly through the cytoplasm. More importantly, however, the free concentrations of ADP are several orders of magnitude lower than those of Cr, resulting in a much lower diffusion-dependent transport capacity of ADP relative to Cr. Based on mathematical modelling, Meyer et al[6] suggested that the CK system facilitates the diffusion of free-energy equivalents through the cell and thus may accelerate and smooth transitions between different work states and dampen oscillations in the concentrations of ATP and ADP.[2]

The models of the multifaceted CK function are based on *in vitro* studies on purified enzymes, model membranes, and subcellular organelles and membranes, as well as theoretical considerations. For the *in vivo* case, there is general agreement on the temporal ATP buffering role under energy stress. The other aspects of CK function have so far not been subjected to unambiguous tests in the *in vivo* situation, simply because until recently no appropriate tools to do so were available. As an example, feeding of animals with β-guanidino propionic acid (GPA), a creatine analogue, has been used frequently to assess the importance of the CK system. Chronic PCr and Cr depletion was anticipated to gradually eliminate CK function. Surprisingly, Shoubridge et al[7,8] found that GPA feeding had only moderate effects on heart and skeletal muscle. More recently, Zweier et al[9] reported a significant functional impairment of myocardium from GPA-fed animals at high workloads. In these GPA studies the PCr concentration remained well above the K_m^{PCr} of CK. Furthermore, massive adaptations were seen that greatly detract from the usefulness of creatine analogues in CK function research. Recently, transgenic mouse models of the CK system in striated muscle have been generated by Wieringa and coworkers[10-12] that enable the *in vivo* testing of the various elements of the circuit model in skeletal and heart muscle. A preliminary characterization of such CK mouse mutants yielded the following results. Skeletal muscle from homozygous knock-outs of the cytosolic MM-CK lacks the ability to perform burst exercise. Phosphorus (^{31}P)-nuclear magnetic resonance (NMR) studies showed that PCr hydrolysis on exercise is similar to that in wild-type muscle, implying that Mi-CK is operative in ATP buffering in the mutant.[10] ^{31}P-NMR magnetization transfer showed that CK-mediated flux in the MM-CK knock-out muscle at rest is negligible. Double Mi-CK/MM-CK knock-out mutants exhibit a strong impairment of skeletal muscle performance and gross ultrastructural and biochemical changes.[12]

The present study was aimed at elucidating the kinetic and the functional properties of the mitochondrial isoenzyme of CK under *in vitro* and *in vivo* conditions, using ^{31}P-NMR techniques. *In vitro* studies were done on enzyme purified from an *E. coli* expression system for chicken heart Mi-CK. Both the nonbound and the membrane-bound configuration of Mi-CK were investigated to assess the kinetic consequences of membrane anchoring. *In vivo* studies on Mi-CK were performed in skeletal and heart muscle from transgenic mice that are homozygous for the deletion of MM-CK. This transgenic model not only provides unique tools for specifically assessing Mi-CK function, but also for addressing fundamental bioenergetic issues in the *in vivo* state.

Materials and Methods

Materials

Creatine Kinase Preparations

Chicken heart mitochondrial CK was expressed in *E. coli* and purified as described previously,[13] using procedures developed by Furter et al.[14] The specific activity of the preparations was between 50 and 90 U/mg protein and the purity was >95% as measured by sodium dodecyl sulfate-polyacrylamide gel electrophoresis (SDS-PAGE). Octamer-to-dimer ratio of purified Mi-CK was determined by gel permeation chromatography on a Superose 12 HR10/30 FPLC column (Pharmacia, Sweden).[13] MM-CK from rabbit muscle was obtained from Boehringer (Mannheim, Germany) and used without further purification.

Isolation of Mitochondria

Mitochondria were isolated from rat heart and rat brain essentially as described.[15,16] The respiratory control ratio typically ranged from 6 to 10 for heart mitochondria and from 5 to 7 for brain mitochondria, using 10 mM glutamate/2 mM malate and 10 mM succinate, respectively, as substrates.

Transgenic Mice

Transgenic mice that are homozygous for the deletion of the cytoplasmic, muscle CK isoform were generated as described by Van Deursen et al[10] and were generously provided by Dr. B. Wieringa (Nijmegen University, The Netherlands).

Miscellaneous

Dextran M20 (M_r 15,000–20,000) was purchased from Serva. All other chemicals used were of the highest grade available and were obtained from regular commercial sources.

Methods

Creatine Kinase Activity Assays

The activity of CK was measured by spectrophotometry at 25°C, both in the forward (from PCr to ATP) and reverse direction (from ATP to PCr) as detailed previously.[13] Michaelis-Menten parameters of Mi-CK were determined for PCr, ADP, Cr, and ATP by varying the concentration of one substrate at four different concentrations of the appropriate second substrate.

Mitochondrial Creatine Kinase Binding

Large unilamellar vesicles were made from dioleoylphosphatidylcholine (DOPC), (beef heart) cardiolipin (CL) and a DOPC-CL mixture (4:1 ratio, based on phosphorus) by extrusion of a liposomal suspension through a 0.4 μm filter.[17] Thereafter, the vesicles were diluted to the appropriate concentration in a buffer containing 200 mM mannitol, 25 mM sucrose, 30 mM HEPES, 1 mM EDTA and 0.5 mM β-mercaptoethanol (pH 7.4). Next, in a volume of 100 μL, a fixed amount of Mi-CK (ie, 3–5 μM Mi-CK octamer) was added to a variable concentration of lipid to give a ratio of lipid phosphorus to Mi-CK octamer between 0 and 3000. After 15-minute incubation at 25°C, Mi-CK binding was assessed by ultracentrifugation (30 minutes 436,000 × g) to separate bound from nonbound enzyme. Mi-CK activity was measured in the supernatant and, after resuspension, in the lipid pellet fraction. It was carefully checked that, in the absence of lipid, Mi-CK enzyme did not sediment under the present conditions. Mi-CK binding was determined both in the absence and in the presence of its substrates Cr (10 mM), PCr (10 mM), and ATP (5 mM). In the latter case, $MgCl_2$ was added to a final concentration of 6 mM.

Scattering Assay of Vesicle Aggregation

Mi-CK/membrane interaction was also studied with a light scattering assay that is based on the fact that enzyme-induced aggregation of lipid vesicles causes an increased turbidity. Scattering was measured at 400 nm in the above vesicle binding buffer at 25°C. The lipid concentration was 300 μM while Mi-CK was titrated to different final concentrations.

Respiratory Assay of Mitochondrial Creatine Kinase in Heart Mitochondria

The delivery of adenosine diphosphate (ADP) generated by Mi-CK activity to oxidative phosphorylation was quantified in isolated rat heart mitochondria, essentially as described previously,[18,19] with minor modifications. Briefly, heart mitochondrial suspensions (0.2 mg of protein per milliliter) were incubated at 25°C in a final volume of 1.5 mL of a medium containing 10 mM NaCl, 120 mM MES, 20 mM imidazole, 20 mM taurine, 8 mM $MgCl_2$, 5 mM KH_2PO_4, 0.5 mM dithiothreitol, 30 mM mannitol, 0.5 mM EDTA, 6.8 mM PEP and 25 mM creatine (pH 7.4), supplemented with 10 mM glutamate and 2 mM malate as respiratory substrates and, where indicated, 10% (w/v) dextran M20. Mi-CK stimulated respiration was started by the addition of 4.7 mM ATP. Next, pyruvate kinase was added (final activity 0–340 U/mg mitochondrial protein) to act as an extramitochondrial sink of ADP. Separate incubations were done for each PK activity. Oxygen consumption was measured using an Oroboros oxygraph (Graz, Austria). Respiratory rates were evaluated as the first derivative of the $[O_2]$-time trace. In parallel, samples from identical incubations were quenched in organic solvents for biochemical determinations of ATP, ADP, pyruvate and PCr.[18,19]

In Vitro ^{31}P Nuclear Magnetic Resonance

^{31}P-NMR was done at 121.5 MHz on a Bruker MSL-300 spectrometer, using either a 10-mm broad-band probe (for studies on purified enzymes) or a 20-mm dedicated ^{31}P NMR probe (for studies on mitochondria). Probe temperature was maintained at 25°C. NMR studies on rat brain mitochondrial suspensions (0.8 mg/mL) were performed in a final volume of 8 mL essentially as described,[20] except that the medium additionally contained: NAD$^+$-specific glucose-6-phosphate dehydrogenase (5 U/mL), lactate dehydrogenase (10 U/mL), 1 mM NAD$^+$, 10 mM pyruvate, 1 mM phosphocreatine, 7 mM creatine and, where indicated, 20 mM glucose. Magnetization transfer of purified CK species was done with the steady-state saturation transfer method, as detailed elsewhere,[13] using frequency selective saturation with a low-power (150 μW) continuous wave pulse. Apparent T1 relaxation times of PCr or γ-ATP were measured separately with saturation recovery while continuously saturating γ-ATP or PCr, respectively.

Phosphorus Nuclear Magnetic Resonance of Langendorff-Perfused Mouse Heart

Hearts were excised and perfused according to Langendorff at 100 cm H$_2$O and 37°C. The modified Krebs-Henseleit perfusate contained 5 mM pyruvate and 10 mM glucose as substrates, as well as 20 mM KCl to induce cardiac arrest. ^{31}P-NMR studies were done at 202.4 MHz on a Bruker AM-500 spectrometer. Magnetization transfer through myocardial CK was measured with time-dependent saturation transfer. Saturation times ranged from 0 to 6 seconds and the fixed relaxation delay was 6 seconds. Selective saturation was achieved with a DANTE train of 0.8 μs pulses, separated by a delay of 125 μs. Typically, 64 scans were accumulated.

Phosphorus Nuclear Magnetic Resonance of Mouse Skeletal Muscle In Vivo

Mice were anaesthetized with 1.3% isoflurane in O$_2$/N$_2$O (30:70 (v:v)). Body temperature was maintained by wrapping the animal in a water-heated blanket. The hind leg was positioned in a three-turn solenoidal coil tuned to the ^{31}P frequency of 80.5 MHz. ^{31}P-NMR studies were done on a SIS Co 4.7 T *in vivo* spectrometer. Spectra were acquired at rest with 60 μs radiofrequency pulses using a relaxation delay of 30 seconds and averaging 32 scans. As above, CK mediated-magnetization transfer was measured with the time-dependent saturation transfer method in which variable times of frequency-selective irradiation (range 0.3 to 10 seconds) were used in combination with a fixed relaxation delay (15 seconds).

Nuclear Magnetic Resonance Data Evaluation

The NMR spectra were subjected to time-domain fitting procedures to obtain peak amplitudes. The pseudo-first order, unidirectional rate constants of the CK reaction were determined from the magnetization transfer data essentially as described by Bittl and Ingwall.[21]

Results

Mitochondrial Creatine Kinase *In Vitro*

Muscle-specific cytosolic MM-CK has been studied *in vitro* by a variety of techniques, including ^{31}P-NMR. Recently, we have extended these studies to the purified mitochondrial isoenzyme.[13] As expected, the flux through Mi-CK as measured by ^{32}P-NMR magnetization transfer increased linearly with the added activity (V_{max}) of the enzyme. Interestingly, the ratio of flux-to-$\dot{V}_{max}$ for Mi-CK was twice that of MM-CK under the same conditions (ie, 0.31 and 0.15 for Mi-CK and MM-CK, respectively).[13] This difference is mainly due to the higher apparent affinity of Mi-CK for MgADP (K_m^{ADP} 22 μM) compared to MM-CK (K_m^{ADP} 80 μM). Moreover, the CK fluxes measured by NMR were in quantitative agreement with the fluxes as calculated from the Morrison-Cleland kinetic model,[22] for both isoenzyme species. Our NMR data also suggested that the octameric and dimeric species of Mi-CK give rise to similar steady-state fluxes.

We have recently measured the kinetic consequences of binding of Mi-CK to a membrane interface. These studies were prompted by the notion that most of the Mi-CK is associated with the inner mitochondrial membrane, presumably involving electrostatic interactions between the basic enzyme and the negatively charged phospholipid cardiolipin.[1,4,5] Furthermore, inner membrane association is considered of functional importance for the coupling of Mi-CK activity to oxidative phosphorylation.[2] Mi-CK was incubated in the presence of large unilamellar liposomes, containing cardiolipin. Figure 1 shows the extent of Mi-CK binding as a function of the molar ratio of enzyme octamer to vesicular phospholipid phosphorus. Above a molar ratio of approximately 1000, Mi-CK was completely bound. The cardiolipin content of the vesicles used in this experiment is similar to the cardiolipin content of the inner mitochondrial membrane. Mi-CK appeared to bind with higher affinity to pure cardiolipin vesicles, as expected, and with lower affinity to DOPC membranes. Figure 1 also shows that binding of CK was somewhat less in the presence of a functional substrate mixture.

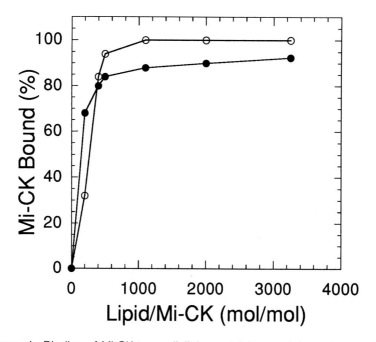

FIGURE 1. Binding of Mi-CK to cardiolipin-containing model membranes. Mi-CK octamer (3 μM) was incubated with varying amounts of DOPC/cardiolipin (4:1 ratio) vesicles. After 15 minutes, samples were centrifuged to separate bound and non-bound Mi-CK, followed by the measurement of enzyme activity in pellet and supernatant. Activity was quantitatively recovered. Open and closed symbols refer to measurements in the absence and presence of CK substrates, respectively. For further details see *Materials and Methods.*

In order to gain further insight into the nature of the membrane interaction of Mi-CK, turbidity measurements were performed. Previously, such light scattering studies have proven useful in assessing the ability of proteins and peptides[23] to induce vesicle aggregation. Figure 2 depicts the effects of Mi-CK addition on the turbidity of suspensions of cardiolipin-containing vesicles and pure DOPC vesicles. Clearly, the enzyme caused a strong vesicle aggregation in the case of the cardiolipin-containing membranes and had no effect for DOPC. Above certain threshold concentrations, the following agents reduced the enzyme-induced increase in scattering: sodium phosphate (pH 7.4) (>25 mM; Figure 2), NaCl (>55 mM) and MgCl$_2$ (>3 mM) (not shown). This effect is probably caused by interference with the electrostatic interaction between enzyme and membrane. In a certain range of intermediate concentrations each of these agents had a cooperative effect on the CK-induced turbidity increase that exceeded the sum of the separate effects of CK or salt addition (see Figure 2 for the case of P$_i$).

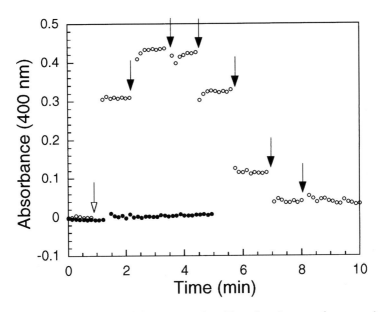

FIGURE 2. CK-induced vesicle aggregation. The absorbance of suspensions of pure DOPC vesicles (closed symbols) and cardiolipin-DOPC (1:4) vesicles (open symbols) was measured at 400 nm. Open arrow: addition of 0.3 μM Mi-CK octamer; closed arrows: successive additions of sodium phosphate (pH 7.4), each equivalent to a final concentration of 10 mM. Further details in *Materials and Methods*.

Under conditions of complete binding and of extensive vesicle aggregation, we have next determined the kinetic properties of membrane-associated Mi-CK, using ^{31}P-NMR and spectrophotometry. Parallel measurements of the T1 of PCr and ATP enabled the quantitation of the flux through CK in the forward and reverse direction. Figure 3 depicts the comparison of the flux for free and bound Mi-CK, as a function of the enzyme activity present. The Michaelis-Menten parameters of Mi-CK, as measured by spectrophotometry, also remained unchanged upon membrane binding, in agreement with the NMR findings.

Mitochondrial Creatine Kinase in Isolated Mitochondria

We have studied the functional properties of Mi-CK extensively in isolated mitochondria from a number of different tissues, including rat heart and brain. One approach consisted of measuring the delivery

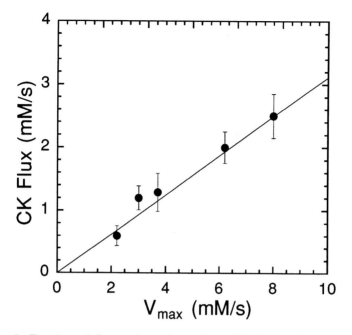

FIGURE 3. Flux through free and membrane-bound Mi-CK. The flux through Mi-CK was measured by ^{31}P saturation transfer as a function of enzyme activity present, as detailed elsewhere.[13] Closed symbols: in the presence of a fixed concentration of Cl-DOPC (1:4) vesicles with the molar ratio of lipid phosphorus to Mi-CK octamer ranging from circa 3000 to 750; solid line: linear regression through data points measured in the absence of vesicles. Further details in *Methods*.

of ADP from Mi-CK to oxidative phosphorylation, using oxygraph techniques. In these experiments, ADP stimulation of mitochondrial respiration is used as an assay of ADP delivery to the mitochondrial matrix. The effect on respiration of the addition of pyruvate kinase (in the presence of phosphoenol pyruvate [PEP] provides information on the fractional ADP delivery to the extramitochondrial compartment. Figure 4 shows the dependence of Mi-CK stimulated respiration of rat heart mitochondria on the activity of pyruvate kinase (PK) in the medium. Interestingly, mitochondrial activity remained well above resting (state 4) rates even when the extramitochondrial ADP scavenging activity was exceedingly high. This suggested that a significant fraction of the ADP generated by Mi-CK in the intermembrane space was delivered to the matrix, as substrate for oxidative ATP synthesis. Similar experiments with exogenous (yeast) hexokinase for extramitochondrial ADP generation (Figure 4) showed that in this case PK was able to suppress respiration to state 4 levels. Biochemical measurements

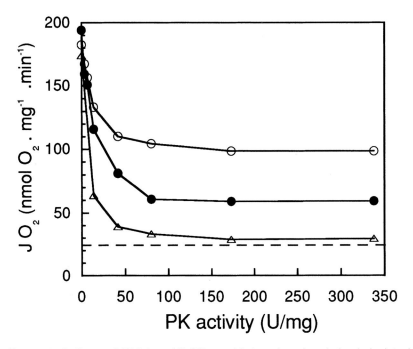

FIGURE 4. Delivery of ADP from Mi-CK to oxidative phosphorylation in isolated rat heart mitochondria. Respiration by rat heart mitochondria was either stimulated through the activity of mitochondrial creatine kinase in the presence of excess creatine (circles) or exogenously-added yeast hexokinase in the presence of glucose (triangles). Pyruvate kinase (in the presence of phosphoenolpyruvate) was added to compete with oxidative phosphorylation for the ADP produced by kinase activity. Mi-CK related respiratory response was measured in the absence (closed circles) and presence of dextran in the medium (open circles). The broken line indicates the rate of state 4 respiration. Other details in *Materials and Methods.*

of steady-state ATP and ADP levels indicated that the extramitochondrial ADP concentration was considerably lower in the case of Mi-CK stimulated respiration as compared to hexokinase stimulated respiration. This experiment was also performed under conditions that mimic the *in vivo* situation in terms of colloid-osmotic pressure. This was achieved by addition of 10% dextran 20. Importantly, in the presence of such macromolecules mitochondrial morphology is similar to that in the intact tissue.[18,19] Figure 4 demonstrates that at physiological oncotic pressures a larger fraction of the ADP produced by Mi-CK escaped phosphorylation by PK and was delivered to oxidative phosphorylation. As expected, ADP routing in the case of extramitochondrial (yeast) hexokinase was insensitive to the presence of dextran (not shown).

Biochemical measurements of ATP and ADP showed that, at a certain rate of respiration, higher extramitochondrial ATP/ADP ratios occur when ADP is regenerated by Mi-CK compared with ADP regeneration by extramitochondrial (yeast) hexokinase. In the presence of dextran, these differences increased. Taken together, these and other data suggest that significant, flux-dependent diffusion gradients of ADP are formed across the outer membrane (see also refs. 15, 18, and 19).

In the above oxygraph experiments on isolated rat heart mitochondria, Mi-CK operated at $\dot{V}_{max}$ by addition of excess Cr and ATP. Using ^{31}P-NMR, we next determined the sensitivity of the (steady-state) mass-action ratio of Mi-CK to changes in the workload exerted on the mitochondria. Figure 5 shows an example of a ^{31}P-NMR experiment in which isolated rat brain mitochondria were used. It should be noted that, through the low mitochondrial density, intramitochondrial phosphates did not significantly contribute to the ^{31}P spectra. Endogenous, outer-membrane bound hexokinase was

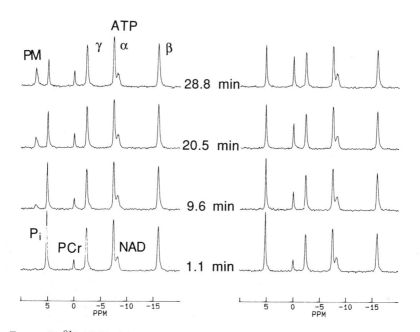

FIGURE 5. ^{31}P-NMR of the mass-action ratio of Mi-CK in isolated rat brain mitochondria. ^{31}P-NMR was used to measure the mass-action ratio of mitochondrial CK in suspensions of rat brain mitochondria (0.8 mg/mL). Measurements were made in the presence (**left**) or absence (**right**) of glucose in the medium. Mitochondria were added at time zero. Assignments: PM, phosphomonoester; P_i, inorganic phosphate; PCr, phosphocreatine. Details in *Materials and Methods*.

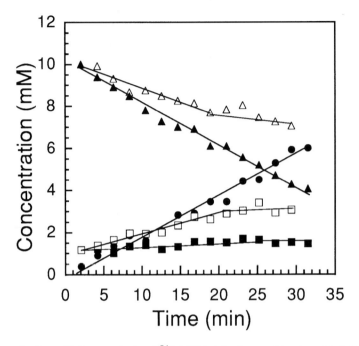

FIGURE 6. Quantitative analysis of ³¹P-NMR data from rat brain mitochondria. Peak intensities in the series of spectra shown partly in Figure 5 were quantitated as detailed elsewhere.[20] Symbols refer to the concentrations of: P_i (triangles), PM (circles), PCr (squares). Open and closed symbols: in the absence and presence of glucose, respectively. See legend to Figure 5 for details.

used as the load enzyme. In the presence of glucose, hexokinase activity led to the formation of a peak in the phosphomonoester region of the ³¹P spectrum. In order to prevent product inhibition of hexokinase by glucose-6-phosphate the medium contained glucose-6-phosphate dehydrogenase and NAD⁺. Therefore, the low-field peak increasing with time in the presence of glucose represents the 6-phosphoglucono-δ-lactone product of the dehydrogenase reaction. The steady-state PCr concentration was considerable higher in the presence of glucose (Figure 6). This implies that the PCr/Cr concentration ratio was lower with the hexokinase load operative and that the enzyme acted as a (local) sensor of the ATP/ADP ratio. These *in vitro* NMR data suggest that Mi-CK in muscle tissue of the MM-CK knock-out mice may be used to report on the effective ADP concentration in the mitochondrial intermembrane space *in vivo*.

Mitochondrial Creatine Kinase in Skeletal Muscle of MM-CK Knock-Out Mice *In Vivo*

In recent years, Wieringa and coworkers[10–12] have developed transgenic mouse models that are homozygous for the deletion of specific members of the CK iso-enzyme family, including the muscle-specific cytosolic MM-CK.[10] Skeletal and cardiac muscle from such MM-CK -/- mice harbour Mi-CK as the only remaining CK species (except

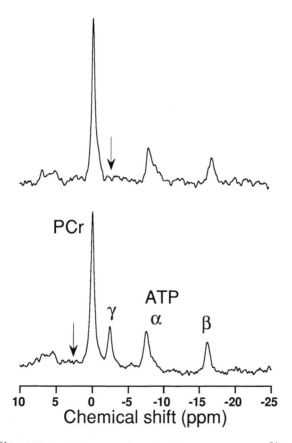

FIGURE 7. ^{31}P-NMR of hind leg muscle in the MM-CK -/- mouse. ^{31}P-NMR spectra were measured from the hind leg muscle of MM-CK -/- mouse during frequency-selective irradiation (arrows) to assess magnetization transfer from PCr-to-ATP mediated by CK. A comparison between the spectrum with control irradiation (**bottom**) and the spectrum with γ-ATP saturated (**top**) demonstrates negligible flux through the CK reaction, as evidenced from the similar intensity of the PCr peaks in the two spectra. Details in *Materials and Methods*.

for a trace of BB-CK in myocardium).[10] CK-mediated flux has been extensively studied by *in vivo* [31]P saturation transfer techniques, both in skeletal and heart muscle. Figure 7 demonstrates that there was no significant flux through Mi-CK in hindleg skeletal muscle from the MM-CK knock-out mouse, in agreement with previous reports.[10] This is probably due to the fact that the activity of Mi-CK was too low to sustain an appreciable flux (see also Figure 3). Electrical stimulation of the MM-CK -/- muscle caused a rapid decrease in the tissue PCr levels, at constant ATP concentration (data not shown; see also ref. 10). This implies, as expected, that the Mi-CK mass-action ratio responded to the reduction in the extramitochondrial phosphate potential, in line with the above studies on isolated mitochondria. At the moderate stimulations and the limited temporal resolution of the NMR data acquisition employed sofar, no remarkable differences if any between wild-type and mutant tissue were observed in terms of rate and extent of PCr hydrolysis during stimulation and recovery during rest. Importantly, however, simultaneous recordings of the twitch force indicated that the mutant tissue had acquired a more aerobic, slow-twitch character, in agreement with previous data.[10] Indications for adaptative changes along these lines were also obtained from the increased specific activities of mitochondrial marker enzymes.[10] Electron microscopy revealed that there was a pronounced proliferation of intermyofibrillar mitochondria. Furthermore, muscle glycogen levels were significantly elevated in the mutant.[10] The adaptive changes, involving increased mitochondrial capacity and glycogen content, are in accordance with the improved endurance relative to wild-type.

Mitochondrial Creatine Kinase in Myocardium from MM-CK Knock-Out Mice

Finally, we have done ^{31}P-NMR studies of isolated hearts from MM-CK -/- mice, perfused according to Langendorff. Both in terms of instrumentation and of NMR signal detection, such experiments are demanding: the wet weight of an adult mouse heart typically is only 125 mg. For sensitivity reasons NMR was done at the highest field available to us for these experiments, ie, 11.8 T. Initial comparative ^{31}P measurements at field strengths of 4.7, 8.4, and 11.8 T demonstrated that the highest signal-to-noise was obtained at the higher field. Broadening effects due to for example chemical shift anisotropy appeared of minimal importance.

As an example, Figure 8 shows ^{31}P spectra of a potassium chloride (KCl)-arrested heart from a MM-CK knock-out mouse. As for the transgenic skeletal muscle, the basal ^{31}P-NMR spectra of wild-type and

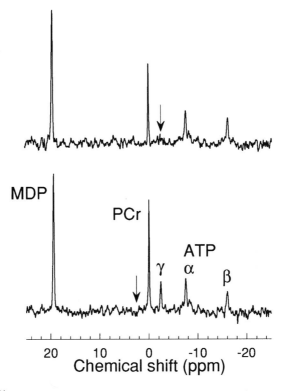

FIGURE 8. ^{31}P NMR of Langendorff-perfused myocardium from the MM-CK -/-mouse. Phosphorus NMR spectra were measured from the KCl-arrested heart of a MM-CK -/- mouse while perfused according to Langendorff. Frequency-selective irradiation (arrows) was used to assess magnetization transfer from PCr-to-ATP mediated by creatine kinase. The PCr peak is considerably lower in the spectrum with γ-ATP saturated (**top**) than in the spectrum with control irradiation (**bottom**), indicative of a significant flux through the CK reaction. MDP: methylene diphosphonate external standard. Details in *Materials and Methods*.

knock-out hearts were essentially indistinguishable. Interestingly, CK-mediated chemical exchange was detectable by saturation transfer, both in normal (not shown) and in transgenic hearts. In the KCl-arrested state, Mi-CK flux in the mutant represented approx. 50% of the flux measured in the wild-type tissue. Biochemical assays indicated that the $\dot{V}_{max}$ of CK in MM-CK -/- heart was approximately 25% of the total CK $\dot{V}_{max}$ in wild-type heart. Recently, Veksler et al[24] have reported that the Mi-CK $\dot{V}_{max}$ in hearts from wild-type and MM-CK -/- mice are essentially identical.

Currently, we are analyzing extensive experiments in which wild-type and transgenic hearts were subjected to different workloads. At each workload, basal spectra and time-dependent saturation transfer data were acquired.

Discussion

We have studied the mitochondrial member of the CK isoenzyme family from striated muscle. A range of *in vitro* and *in vivo* experimental systems and techniques was used to assess the functional properties of Mi-CK. In the presence of cardiolipin-containing membranes, the octameric Mi-CK expressed a strong tendency to simultaneously interact with two opposing membrane interfaces (see model in Figure 9).

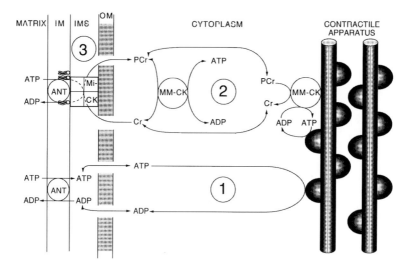

FIGURE 9. Working model of the Mi-CK iso-enzyme. Mi-CK is sandwiched between the inner and outer membrane at intermembrane contact sites. This location allows for functional coupling to the nucleotide carrier and efficient communication with the cytoplasm. Membrane anchoring is partly due to electrostatic interactions between the basic enzyme and the negatively charged phospholipid cardiolipin in the inner membrane. Pathway 1 represents passive diffusion of ATP and ADP, connecting the mitochondrion with a major site of ATP utilization, ie, the contractile apparatus. Pathway 2 depicts the diffusion of PCr and Cr through the cytoplasm to connect sites of PCr delivery/Cr use with sites of PCr use/Cr delivery, exemplified here by M-band localized MM-CK. Pathway 3 represents the activity of Mi-CK which aids in overcoming the ADP diffusion resistance, imposed by the outer membrane, by translating a PCr/Cr signal that is propagated from the cytosol. ANT indicates adenine nucleotide carrier; IM, inner membrane; IMS, intermembrane space; OM, outer membrane.

This corroborates previous findings with other membrane techniques.[1,4,5] This configuration where Mi-CK is sandwiched between two membranes most likely also holds in the enzyme's authentic location in the intermembrane space. Electron microscopy has revealed that Mi-CK occurs in regions where: (1) opposing faces of the outer leaflet of the inner membrane form the cristae membranes; (2) the outer leaflet of the inner membrane and the inner leaflet of the outer membrane come closely together in the (intermembrane) contact sites.[1] It remains to be established whether direct interactions between the Mi-CK enzyme itself and membrane phospholipids are responsible for Mi-CK's localization or that protein-protein interactions between Mi-CK and integral inner and/or outer membrane proteins are involved. Brdiczka and coworkers[25] have recently provided evidence that Mi-CK may form multimolecular complexes with the pore protein (ie, porin) in the outer membrane and the adenine nucleotide carrier in the inner membrane.

We found that the kinetic properties of Mi-CK remained unchanged on binding between two cardiolipin-containing membrane surfaces. This suggests that membrane anchoring *per se* has no direct effect on the functional properties of Mi-CK. For the hexokinase isoenzyme I from brain,[26] we recently reported that binding to the outer surface of the mitochondrial outer membrane does cause a distinct increase in the affinity of the kinase for ATP while not affecting the $\dot{V}_{max}$.[27] The change in K_m^{ATP} is probably due to a conformational change accompanying membrane anchoring. Hexokinase binding to phosphorylating mitochondria led to a further reduction in apparent K_m^{ATP} that was interpreted as an indication for nucleotide channelling (ie, directed metabolite transfer that does not involve complete mixing of ATP and ADP with their bulk extramitochondrial pools) between bound enzyme and the mitochondrial matrix.

Evidence for similar compartmentation phenomena related to Mi-CK is presented in Figure 4, which depicts experiments on isolated heart mitochondria. Part of the ADP resulting from Mi-CK activity was delivered to oxidative phosphorylation and was not phosphorylated by extramitochondrial pyruvate kinase. Interestingly, ADP transport from Mi-CK to the matrix increased further in the presence of 10% dextran, a condition known to induce an *in situ*-like mitochondrial morphology. Similar observations were recently reported for two other mitochondrial kinases, ie, adenylate kinase (like Mi-CK contained in the intermembrane space) and hexokinase isoenzyme I (bound to the external surface of the outer membrane).[19,28] In parallel, we observed that at the same respiratory rate (ie, the same intermembrane space ADP concentration), the extramitochondrial ADP levels were lower in the presence of dextran. From these data, we propose that: (1) the outer membrane represents a diffusion barrier to ADP, restricting its equilibration between the intermembrane space and the extramitochondrial compartment[18,19,28] and (2) ADP diffusion gradients are formed across the outer membrane, in a flux-dependent manner.[18] Among the molecules central to energy metabolism in excitable cells (ATP, ADP, PCr, and Cr), diffusion gradients are only considered relevant for ADP because its steady-state concentration is several orders of magnitude lower than that of the others. Gellerich et al[18] have recently proposed a model in which Mi-CK functions in translating PCr/Cr signals from the cytosol (and thereby indirectly presenting alterations in cytosolic ATP/ADP ratio to the mitochondrial apparatus) and, vice versa, functions in transporting ATP equivalents from the mitochondrion (in the form of PCr). We hypothesize that in particular this function of indirect ADP shuttling into the mitochondrion is one of the major roles of Mi-CK in cellular energy metabolism.[18] The mitochondrial isoenzyme of adenylate kinase may fulfill a similar role,[28] in particular in tissues not harboring the CK system. In the case of adenylate kinase, adenosine monophosphate routing from the cytosol similarly leads to the generation of an ADP signal in the intermembrane space.

The NMR data on isolated mitochondria (Figures 5 and 6) demonstrate that mitochondrial CK indeed acts as a local sensor of the ATP/ADP ratio, which is responsive to altered workload. The measurement of the mass-action ratio enables the estimation of the ADP concentration in the intermembrane space. Evidently, the transgenic mouse homozygous for the deletion of MM-CK offers unique opportunities for assessing the latter parameter in intact cardiac and skeletal muscle.

The MM-CK -/- mice clearly demonstrate that the M-type CK isoenzyme is a nonessential gene product in that the mice are viable and their muscles function. Ultrastructural, biochemical, and functional tests of mutant skeletal muscle have provided evidence for distinct adaptations. In particular, the functional deficit in burst activity implies that MM-CK plays a role in the energy metabolism of fast-twitch muscle. Impaired burst activity may be related to a local accumulation of ADP at the myofibrils, causing product inhibition of the myosin ATPase. In the control tissue this would be prevented by the MM-CK associated with the myofibrillar M-band. The profileration of intermyofibrillar mitochondria may be aimed at shortening the diffusion distances between mitochondrion and myofibril. Ventura-Clappier et al[29] have used skinned fibers from gastrocnemius muscle to assess the potential effects of MM-CK elimination on myofibrillar function. The transgenic material developed similar maximal forces as the wild-type material while also the calcium sensitivity remained unaltered. Because the myosin isoform pattern was also unchanged, these results show that no fundamental remodeling of the myofibrillar system takes place.

Adaptive responses to MM-CK deletion rather occur in the mitochondrial apparatus and the glycolytic complexes.[29]

Veksler et al[24] have recently provided evidence for intriguing adaptive changes in cardiac mitochondria in response to the elimination of MM-CK. Respirometry on skinned ventricular fibers was used to measure the apparent K_m^{ADP} of mitochondrial oxidative phosphorylation in wild-type and mutant material. The K_m^{ADP} was two times lower in the mutant fibers, which suggests that the permeability of the mitochondrial outer membrane to ADP is greatly increased. The structural basis for this remarkable finding remains to be elucidated. Ventura-Clappier et al[29] found a similar upregulation of glycolytic enzymes in ventricular tissue as in fast-twitch tissue. Currently, rigorous functional assessments of intact hearts are not available for MM-CK -/- mice.

Except for the distinct consequences of MM-CK deletion for the NMR-detected flux through skeletal muscle and myocardial CK, the ^{31}P-NMR data available to date have not provided evidence for distinct differences in ADP levels, both at rest and upon stimulation, between wild-type and transgenic striated muscle *in situ*. It is a major challenge to increase the NMR sensitivity to such an extent that the improved time resolution allows measurement of transient responses to more stressful workloads whereby differences in the muscles can be exaggerated.

Koretsky and coworkers (reviewed in ref. 30) have also used transgenic models to assess certain aspects of the functional role of the CK system in cellular energy metabolism. The brain type BB-CK was expressed in liver that was found to be more resistant to hypoxic stress[31] as well as to the adverse effects of fructose load.[32] These findings can be explained from the fact that PCr synthesized through BB-CK activity assured prolonged ATP homeostasis. Perfused BB-CK transfected livers were also used to measure the apparent affinity of mitochondrial oxidative phosphorylation for ADP, using ^{31}P-NMR to estimate cellular ADP levels from the PCr-to-ATP concentration ratio and oxygraph techniques to measure mitochondrial activity.[30] Workloads were varied by varying the fructose content of the perfusate. The cellular ADP concentration increased with increased fructose load and the K_m^{ADP} could be estimated. In contrast, hormonal stimulation of the liver system using phenylephrine that also caused a marked increase in hepatic O_2 use had no significant effect on the ^{31}P-NMR spectra. This demonstrates that the steady-state ADP concentrations remained unchanged in this case.[30] Clearly, mitochondrial activity can be controlled in different ways depending on the physiological condition. These and other studies[30] from Koretsky's group elegantly illustrate the versatility of transgenic mouse models for assessing fundamental bio-energetic questions in the *in vivo* state.

Magnetization transfer studies on striated muscle from MM-CK -/- mice provide the possibility to specifically quantitate the flux mediated by the mitochondrial CK isoenzyme. By comparing our preliminary analysis of the myocardial CK flux data with *in vitro* findings,[13] we tentatively conclude that the flux through Mi-CK in heart corresponds to the flux expected on the basis of Mi-CK activity. In contrast, CK flux in intact skeletal muscle that may be expected to be dominated by MM-CK remained far below expectations (not shown).

Interestingly, using graded MM-CK expression Van Deursen et al[11] were able to show that the flux measured by NMR does not depend on MM-CK enzyme present in a straightforward manner: at expression levels below 50% of wild-type no CK flux was detectable, whereas the flux at 50% expression approached that of wild-type tissue. The basis of the difference in NMR detectability of Mi-CK versus MM-CK flux remains to be elucidated. Van Deursen et al[11] suggested that MM-CK species bound to subcellular structures are silent in NMR flux measurements. Direct evidence to support this proposal is presently not available. Our data on Mi-CK (Figure 3) demonstrate that binding *per se* has no effect on the flux through this CK species.

A working model of Mi-CK functioning in cellular energy metabolism is depicted in Figure 9. We propose that Mi-CK acts as a local sensor of the PCr/Cr ratio and that by responding to changes in this ratio with workload the enzyme indirectly aids in the uptake of ADP across the outer membrane. Its localization at intermembrane contact sites enables Mi-CK to functionally interact with the nucleotide carrier in the inner membrane and positions it in close proximity of the outer membrane porin. The elimination of the cytoplasmic branch of the CK system in MM-CK knock-out mice leads to the proliferation of the mitochondrial compartment, presumably to increase the free-energy delivering capacity of the cell and to compensate for ADP diffusion limitations. Transgenic animal models will continue to serve an important role in the clarification of the functional importance of the members of the CK isoenzyme family, not only in striated muscle but also in other tissues like brain. Current transgenic approaches, although fully specific for the desired gene product, are limited by the fact that the organism is altered early in development. Adaptations may therefore gradually develop and their causal relationship with the genetic defect difficult to define. Novel developments suggest that precise spatial and temporal control of gene expression in the mouse may eventually become possible.[30]

Summary

The functional and kinetic characteristics of the mitochondrial iso-enzyme of Mi-CK were studied with ^{31}P-NMR techniques. Mi-CK was studied in purified form, in isolated mitochondria *in vitro*, in Langendorff-perfused mouse heart and in mouse skeletal muscle *in vivo*. Mi-CK could be specifically investigated in intact muscle through the use of transgenic animals that are homozygous for the deletion of the muscle-specific, cytoplasmic CK isoform. *In vitro* studies showed that the flux through Mi-CK as measured by ^{31}P saturation transfer increases linearly with enzyme activity, can be quantitatively accounted for on the basis of its kinetic parameters and is not affected by membrane binding of the enzyme. Experiments on heart and brain mitochondrial suspensions demonstrated that Mi-CK acts as a local (ie, mitochondrial intermembrane space) sensor of the ATP/ADP concentration ratio and aids in ADP shuttling across the outer membrane. Skeletal and cardiac muscle from transgenic mice that lack the cytoplasmic CK species have ^{31}P-NMR spectra, which are very similar to those from wild-type tissue. CK-related flux is negligible in transgenic skeletal muscle while readily detectable in transgenic myocardium. The NMR data suggest that the ^{31}P-NMR-detected flux through Mi-CK *in vivo* is in accordance with the activity of the enzyme present while the flux mediated by the muscle-specific cytosolic CK species partially escapes detection. Further studies are warranted to assess the functional and physiological consequences of the transgenic transformation of the CK system in intact myocardium.

Acknowledgments

We are indebted to H.-J. Muller and G. van Vliet for their expert technical assistance, to Drs. T. Wallimann and R. Furter for the gift of the E. coli strain expressing Mi-CK, and to Dr. B. Wieringa for making the transgenic mice available.

References

1. Wallimann T, Wyss M, Brdiczka D, et al. Intracellular compartmentation, structure and function of creatine kinase isoenzymes in tissues with high and fluctuating energy demands: the "phosphocreatine circuit" for cellular energy homeostasis. *Biochem J*. 1992;281:21–40.
2. Wyss M, Smeitink J, Wevers R, et al. Mitochondrial creatine kinase: A

key enzyme in aerobic energy metabolism. *Biochim Biophys Acta*. 1992;1102: 119–166.

3. Wallimann T. Dissecting the role of creatine kinase. *Curr Biol*. 1994;1:42–46.

4. Rojo M, Hovius RC, Demel R, et al. Mitochondrial creatine kinase mediates contact formation between mitochondrial membranes. *J Biol Chem*. 1991; 266:20290–20295.

5. Rojo M, Hovius RC, Demel R, et al. Interaction of mitochondrial creatine kinase with model membranes: A monolayer study. *FEBS Lett*. 1991;281: 123–129.

6. Meyer RA, Sweeney HL, Kushmerick MJ. A simple analysis of the phospho-creatine shuttle. *Am J Physiol*. 1984;246:C365–C377.

7. Shoubridge EA, Challiss RAJ, Hates DJ, et al. Biochemical adaptation in skeletal muscle of rats depleted of creatine with the substrate analogue β-guanidino propionic acid. *Biochem J*. 1985;232:125–131.

8. Shoubridge EA, Jeffry FMH, Keogh JM, et al. Creatine kinase kinetics, ATP turnover, and cardiac performance in hearts depleted of creatine with the substrate analogue β-guanidino propionic acid. *Biochim Biophys Acta*. 1985; 847:25–32.

9. Zweier JL, Jacobus WE, Korecky B, Brandesj-Barry Y. Bioenergetic conse-quences of cardiac phosphocreatine depletion induced by creatine analogue feeding. *J Biol Chem*. 1991;266:20296–20304.

10. Van Deursen J, Heerschap A, Oerlemans F, et al. Skeletal muscles of mice deficient in muscle creatine kinase lack burst activity. *Cell*. 1993;74:612–631.

11. Van Deursen J, Ruitenbeek W, Heerschap A, et al. Creatine kinase in skele-tal muscle energy metabolism: a study of mouse mutants with graded reduction in M-CK expression. *Proc Natl Acad Sci USA*. 1994;91:9091–9095.

12. Steeghs KGJ, Benders A, Oerlemans, F, et al. Altered Ca^{2+} responses in muscles with combined mitochondrial and cytosolic creatine kinase defi-ciencies. *Cell*. 1997;89:1–11.

13. Van Dorsten FA, Furter R, Bijkerk M, et al. The *in vitro* kinetics of mitochon-drial and cytosolic creatine kinase determined by saturation transfer ^{31}P NMR. *Biochim Biophys Acta*. 1996;1274:59–66.

14. Furter R, Kaldis P, Furter-Graves EM, et al. Expression of active octameric chicken mitochondrial creatine kinase in *Escherichia coli*. *Biochem J*. 1992; 288:771–775.

15. Gellerich FN, Schlame M, Bohnensack R, Kunz W. Dynamic compartmenta-tion of adenine nucleotides in the mitochondrial intermembrane space of rat heart mitochondria. *Biochim Biophys Acta*. 1987;722:381–391.

16. Kottke M, Adams V, Riesinger I, et al. Mitochondrial boundary membrane contact sites in brain: points of hexokinase and creatine kinase localization, and control of Ca^{2+} transport. *Biochim Biophys Acta*. 1988;935:87–102.

17. Hope MJ, Bally MB, Webb G, et al. Production of large unilamellar vesicles by a rapid extrusion procedure. Characterization of size distribution, trap-ped volume and ability to maintain a membrane potential. *Biochim Biophys Acta*. 1985;812:55–65.

18. Gellerich FN, Kapischke M, Kunz W, et al. The influence of the cytosolic oncotic pressure on the permeability of the mitochondrial outer membrane for ADP: Implications for the kinetic properties of mitochondrial creatine kinase and for ADP channelling into the intermembrane space. *Mol Cell Biochem*. 1994;113/134:85–104.

19. Laterveer FD, Gellerich FN, Nicolay K. Macromolecules increase the chan-nelling of ADP from externally associated hexokinase to the matrix of mito-chondria. *Eur J Biochem*. 1995;232:569–577.

20. Nicolay K, Rojo M, Wallimann T, et al. The role of contact sites between the inner and the outer mitochondrial membrane in energy transfer. *Biochim Biophys Acta*. 1990;1018:229–233.
21. Bittl JA, Ingwall JS. Reaction rates of creatine kinase and ATP synthesis in the isolated rat heart. A ^{31}P NMR magnetization transfer study. *J Biol Chem*. 1985;260:3512–3517.
22. Morrison JF, Cleland WW. Isotope exchange studies of the mechanism of the reaction catalyzed by adenosine triphosphate: creatine phosphotransferase. *J Biol Chem*. 1966;241:673–683.
23. Leenhouts JM, De Gier J, De Kruijff B. A novel property of a mitochondrial presequence. Its ability to induce cardiolipin-specific interbilayer contacts which are dissociated by a transmembrane potential. *FEBS Lett*. 1993;327: 172–176.
24. Veksler VI, Kuznetsov AV, Anflous K, et al. Muscle creatine kinase-deficient mice. II. Cardiac and skeletal muscles exhibit tissue-specific adaptation of the mitochondrial function. *J Biol Chem*. 1995;270:19921–19929.
25. Brdiczka D, Kaldis P, Wallimann T. In vitro complex formation between the octamer of mitochondrial creatine kinase and porin. *J Biol Chem*. 1994; 269:27640–27644.
26. Wilson JE. Hexokinases. In: Beitner EK, ed: *Regulation of Carbohydrate Metabolism*. Boca Raton: CRC Press; 1995:45–85.
27. Laterveer FD, Van der Heijden R, Toonen M, et al. The kinetic consequences of binding of hexokinase-I to the mitochondrial outer membrane. *Biochim Biophys Acta*. 1994;1188:251–259.
28. Gellerich FN, Laterveer FD, Gnaiger E, et al. In: Gnaiger E, Gellerich FN, Wyss M, eds: *Modern Trends in Biothermokinetics*. Innsbruck: Innsbruck University Press; 1994:181–185.
29. Ventura-Clappier R, Kuznetsov AV, D'Albis AS, et al. Muscle creatine kinase-deficient mice. I. Alterations in myofibrillar function. *J Biol Chem*. 1995; 270:19914–19920.
30. Koretsky AP. Insights into cellular metabolism from transgenic mice. *Physiol Rev*. 1995;75:667–688.
31. Koretsky AP, Brosnan MJ, Chen L, et al. NMR detection of creatine kinase expressed in liver of transgenic mice: determination of free ADP levels. *Proc Natl Acad Sci USA*. 1990;87:3112–3116.
32. Brosnan MJ, Chen L, Wheeler CE, et al. Phosphocreatine protects ATP from a fructose load in transgenic mouse liver expressing creatine kinase. *Am J Physiol*. 1991;260:C1191–C1200.

## Chapter 25

Do Changes in the Creatine Kinase System Contribute to Ventricular Dysfunction in the Failing Heart?
Phosphorus Nuclear Magnetic Resonance Spectroscopy Studies

Joanne S. Ingwall, PhD

A longstanding and controversial hypothesis put forth to explain decreased ventricular dysfunction in heart failure is that the failing heart has lower energy reserve needed to fuel the adenosine triphosphatase (ATPase) reactions of the contractile apparatus and ion pumps. Two to three decades ago, this hypothesis was tested by measuring the adenosine triphosphate (ATP) content of the failing heart (for reviews, see references 1 and 2). Because these results showed little or no change in ATP content, this hypothesis fell out of favor. We now know that measuring the ATP content of tissue does not necessarily reflect the energetic state of the heart. New tools including phosphorus nuclear magnetic resonance (^{31}P NMR) spectroscopy now allow us to assess several important thermodynamic and kinetic properties of energy metabolism that cannot be inferred from measurement of ATP content alone. In this chapter we review some of the basic principles of these properties, how they can be studied using ^{31}P NMR spectroscopy, and then apply them to what is currently known about the energetics of the failing heart with special reference to the creatine kinase reaction.

Grant support: NIH SCOR grant on heart failure HL52320

From: Higgins CB, Ingwall JS, Pohost GM, (eds). *Current and Future Applications of Magnetic Resonance in Cardiovascular Disease.* Armonk, NY: Futura Publishing Company, Inc.; © 1998.

A Primer of Bioenergetics

The major reactions responsible for contraction in muscle, namely myofibrillar ATPase and the sarcoplasmic reticular Ca-ATPase, require ATP:

$$MgATP^{-2} + H_2O \rightarrow MgADP^{-1} + Pi^{-2} + H^+.$$

Ventricular tissue contains ~5 μmoles per gram wet weight, which is equivalent to 10 mmol/L (mM) of intracellular water. This amount of ATP is sufficient to maintain ventricular function for only approximately 50 beats. Thus, the cell must continually use and resynthesize ATP to maintain normal ventricular function.

The distinction between the amount or concentration of ATP versus its turnover rate is central to our understanding of bioenergetics. In the normal heart, ATP concentration remains constant but its rate of synthesis and degradation (turnover rate) varies. The energetics of changing cardiac work illustrates this principle. As the workload of the heart increases, oxygen consumption (a good index of ATP synthesis rate) proportionately increases; yet, ATP content is essentially unchanged. Thus ATP turnover rate but not its concentration increases with increasing work. This example also illustrates the important principle that ATP synthesis rate matches ATP utilization rate.

Another important principle essential for our understanding of bioenergetics is that the chemical reactions that use ATP are "driven" by high ratios of ATP to adenosine diphosphate (ADP) but ATP synthesis reactions are inhibited by high ATP/ADP ratios. Inspection of the ATP hydrolysis equation given above shows that the reaction (which is unidirectional) proceeds when the substrate (ATP) concentration is high but slows when the concentrations of the products of ATP hydrolysis (ADP and inorganic phosphate [Pi] are high. There are four major expressions that quantitatively reflect this principle. The first is simply the ATP/ADP ratio. In well-perfused tissue the cytosolic ATP and ADP concentrations are approximately 10 mM and approximately 30 μM, respectively, and this ratio is approximately 300. The second is the adenylate energy charge. It is defined as ATP + 1/2 ADP / ATP + ADP + AMP and distinguishes between utilizable ATP (the numerator) and total adenine nucleotide pool (the denominator). In well-perfused tissue the cytosolic ATP, ADP, and adenosine monophosphate (AMP) concentrations are approximately 10 mM, 30 μM, and 0.1 μM, respectively, and the energy charge is close to 1.

The third expression is the phosphorylation potential, defined as ATP/[ADP $\times$ Pi]. This term is biologically relevant because it takes into account the ability of both end products of ATP hydrolysis, namely Pi and ADP, to inhibit ATPase activity and, at least for ADP, to stimulate ATP synthesis pathways. Under most conditions, the concentrations of ADP and Pi are low, approximately 30 μM and <1 mM, respectively, and the phosphorylation potential is approximately 300 mM^{-1}. When ATP is hydrolyzed, the phosphorylation potential decreases in proportion to the increases in both ADP and Pi. For example, a doubling of ADP and Pi would decrease the phosphorylation potential from approximately 300 mM^{-1} to approximately 80 mM^{-1}. In this way the phosphorylation potential is a sensitive marker of the energy state of the cell. It is the critical component of the thermodynamic quantity representing the free energy of ATP hydrolysis.

The fourth expression, the free energy of ATP hydrolysis, ΔG, defines the chemical driving force for all ATP utilizing reactions in the cell. It is calculated from the constant value for ATP hydrolysis under standard conditions, ΔG^0, corrected for the actual concentrations of ATP, ADP, and Pi in the cytosol. The expression is

$$\Delta G = \Delta G^0 - RT \ln [ATP]/[ADP][Pi]$$

where ΔG^0 is the standard free energy change of ATP hydrolysis (-30.5 kJ/mol under standard conditions of molarity, temperature, pH and Mg^{2+}), R is the gas constant (8.3 J/mol·K) and T is the absolute temperature in Kelvin. Note that the argument of the ln term is the phosphorylation potential. The value of ΔG for pyruvate-perfused rat heart with a typical rate-pressure product of 28,000 mm Hg sec^{-1} is -69.9 ± 2.0 kJ/mole; for a glucose-perfused heart, which has higher Pi concentration, ΔG becomes less negative, -57.7 ± 0.6 kJ/mol. The less negative value means that the glucose-only perfused heart has a lower driving force for ATP utilizing reactions. Because it is often confusing to describe changes for a negative number, it is convenient to describe changes in ΔG in terms of its absolute value.

Given the critical need to maintain both a constant and high level of ATP and the ATP/[ADP][Pi] ratio, it is not surprising that the cell uses many reactions and pathways to synthesize ATP and to keep ADP and Pi low. The remarkable feature of intermediary metabolism is that a constant ATP concentration is maintained by the integration of multiple pathways. The subject of this chapter is the enzyme which transfers the phosphoryl group to and from ATP most rapidly, namely the creatine kinase reaction.

The Creatine Kinase Reaction

Creatine kinase catalyzes the transfer of the phosphoryl group between phosphocreatine (PCr) and ATP:

$$PCr^{-2} + MgADP^{-1} + H^+ \leftrightarrow creatine + MgATP^{-2}.$$

The reaction consumes neither oxygen nor carbon-based substrates. In heart, the PCr concentration is twice the ATP concentration. The overall equilibrium position is far to the right, Keq ~144 at pH 7.

Creatine kinase is highly abundant in excitable tissues. It exists as a family of five isoenzymes: BB, MB, MM, and the ubiquitous and sarcomeric mitochondrial isoforms. Discoveries of the localization of the mitochondrial creatine kinase isoenzymes on the inner mitochondrial membrane[3] and some of the MM isoenzyme in the M-band of the myofibril[4] have led to the hypothesis that the creatine-PCr "shuttles" chemical energy between sites of ATP production (mitochondria) and sites of ATP utilization (myofibrils and ion transport across membranes) (see reference 5 for a review).

^{31}P NMR spectra of hearts is uniquely well suited to provide information about the creatine kinase reaction *in vivo*. Standard spectra such as shown in Figure 1 provides information about the amounts of ATP, PCr as well as Pi in the heart and intracellular pH. If one also knows the total creatine content of the tissue, one can calculate the free ADP concentration in the cytosol from the creatine kinase equilibrium expression:

$$[ADP] = [ATP] \, [creatine]/[PCr] \, [H^+] \, Keq.$$

This information is sufficient to calculate all the expressions described above defining the energetic state of the heart. In this way, creatine kinase is an *in vivo* reporter of the bioenergetic state of the heart.

Furthermore, using the NMR technique of magnetization transfer, the unidirectional velocity of the creatine kinase reaction can be measured *in vivo*. Generally this measurement is performed in the direction of phosphoryl transfer from PCr to ADP. Its application to the heart has been described in detail.[6] The opportunity to measure the reaction velocity of a single protein (or protein family in this case) in the intact beating heart is unique. This approach allows us to understand how this enzyme works *in vivo* and, under some conditions, to compare how it works *in vivo* versus in solution. We have learned the following from such measurements: (1) ATP synthesis via creatine kinase is 10 times faster than net ATP synthesis rate estimated from the physiological index of oxygen consumption.[7] Because its reaction velocity is high, creatine kinase effectively functions to resupply ATP during high demand conditions, to keep [ADP] and [Pi] low, thereby maintaining a high driving force for all ATPase reactions, and to buffer intracellular hydrogen ion concentration; (2) the ratio of measured creatine kinase reaction velocity in the beating heart to maximal capacity of the reaction, known as V_{max}, is approximately -0.1.[7] This means that most of the enzyme activity (capacity) is not used under normal workload conditions. It is not known whether enzyme activity can be recruited

A) Non-Failing Heart - Untreated

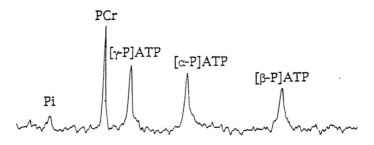

B) Failing Heart - Untreated

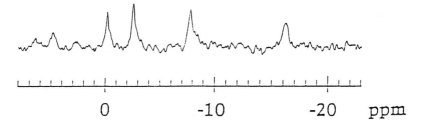

0   -10   -20   ppm

FIGURE 1. Representative plots of ^{31}P nuclear magnetic resonance spectra from **(A)** an untreated nonfailing hamster heart, and **(B)** an untreated failing hamster heart. The major resonances are assigned (from left to right) as inorganic phosphate (Pi), phosphocreatine (PCr), and γ-, α-, and β-phosphates of ATP. Relative ATP contents for the intact hearts were determined by integrating [β-P]ATP peak resonance areas. The [β-P]ATP areas for the untreated failing heart are, on average, 23% lower than for the nonfailing hamster heart. (Redrawn from Reference 10.)

for use under times of high energy demand. (3) Comparison of measured and predicted (from known solution kinetics) reaction velocities are usually in good agreement. However, lack of agreement in hypoxia and ischemia, when the reaction velocity measured *in vivo* is lower than predicted from the rate equation,[8,9] and when failing aged hearts were supplied with angiotensin-converting enzymes (ACE) inhibitors,[10] when velocity was higher than predicted from the rate equation, show that the enzyme is regulated *in vivo* by mechanisms in addition to substrate control. These are as yet undefined.

The Creatine Kinase System in Failing Myocardium

The properties of the creatine kinase reaction that can be learned using biopsy specimens of the human heart are limited to measurement of its tissue activity and the content of its substrates. Tissue creatine kinase activity, or V_{max}, represents the maximum capacity of the reaction. Because neither ATP nor PCr are well preserved in biopsy specimens from the human heart, we usually measure only total creatine content. Even with this limited information, we and others have obtained evidence that suggests that the capacity for ATP resynthesis via the creatine kinase reaction is compromised in the failing myocardium. Tissue activity of creatine kinase was 30% to 50% lower[11,12] and the tissue content of the guanidino substrate for the reaction, ie, the sum of free creatine and PCr, was 60% lower.[11] Consistent with the decrease in total creatine content, ^{31}P NMR spectroscopy studies of the failing human myocardium by several groups[13-15] have shown that PCr is decreased compared to nonfailing myocardium. These reports describe lower ratios of PCr to ATP resonance areas in the ^{31}P NMR spectrum. If (as occurs in at least some animal models of severe failure) ATP content is also lower in failing human myocardium, then the decrease in PCr content would be even greater than reported by the ratio of PCr/ATP.

The changes in V_{max} and guanidino pool observed in human heart failure are faithfully reproduced in animal models of heart failure. These results have been recently reviewed.[1] One of the major advantages of studying small animal models of heart failure is that we can use ^{31}P NMR spectroscopy to measure the turnover rate of the phosphoryl group in the intact beating heart while simultaneously measuring contractile performance. We and our colleagues have observed decreased creatine kinase reaction velocity in several animal models of heart failure, each with a different etiology: the 18-month-old failing spontaneously hypertensive rat heart,[16] the 10-month-old failing hamster heart,[10] the rat heart 8 weeks after myocardial infarction[17] and the furazolidone-treated turkey poult.[18] Consistent with depressed cardiac performance in congestive heart failure in humans and in other animal models of failure, isovolumic contractile performance measured as the rate pressure product in hearts isolated from all of these failing animals was lower (typically 50% to 70% lower) than for hearts isolated from age-matched nonfailing animals perfused under the same conditions of load and coronary flow. Thus in concert with the decrease in contractile performance, the tissue content of PCr, the capacity for ATP synthesis via the creatine kinase reaction measured as tissue enzyme activity

(V_{max}) and the rate of phosphoryl transfer measured as creatine kinase reaction velocity *in vivo* are all lower in the severely failing mammalian myocardium.

From these measurements, we conclude that the creatine kinase phenotype in failing myocardium is characterized by decreases in both total creatine kinase activity (V_{max}) and the guanidino pool. These decreases are independent of species and etiology, strongly suggesting that this is a property of failing myocardium. We also conclude that decreased V_{max} and PCr content combine to limit the velocity of the creatine kinase reaction. Moreover, decreased creatine kinase reaction velocity parallels decreases in ventricular performance.

Significance of Changes in the Creatine Kinase Reaction in Heart Failure

The critical questions now become: does decreased phosphoryl transfer via the creatine kinase reaction matter? Does it compromise the energetic state of the heart? Does decreased creatine kinase reaction velocity lead to ventricular dysfunction? What is cause and what is consequence?

To address these questions, we need to develop strategies to perturb the *in vivo* creatine kinase reaction selectively and then define the consequences. This must be done using animal models. There are several approaches to this problem. The first is to acutely and selectively inhibit the creatine kinase reaction in the normal heart and measure parameters of bioenergetics and of contractile performance. There are at least three ways known to chemically attack the labile sulfhydryl groups at or near the active site of creatine kinase in the intact heart and thereby alter enzyme velocity: (1) supplying a small amount of iodoacetamide[19]; (2) supplying an exogenous nitric oxide (NO) donor[20]; and (3) supplying reactive oxygen species[21] (this may overlap with #2). The second approach is to replace the creatine pool with a poorly hydrolyzable guanidino substrate. Several creatine analogs have been used in this way, including β-guanidinoproprionic acid and β-guanidinobutyric acid.[22,23] Replacing the creatine pool is accomplished by supplying the new substrate in the diet for several weeks. During this time adaptation to the new steady state may, and does, occur. A third strategy is to bioengineer mice with the genes for one or more of the creatine kinase isoenzymes ablated. Be Weiringa of the Netherlands has succeeded in creating mice with the genes for M-CK and/or mitochondrial CK ablated.[24] This approach also allows for substantial time for adaptations in the ATP-synthesizing and utilizing pathways to occur.

We and others have now used each of these experimental tools. Our objective has been to define the relation between the new energetic state created by decreasing or ablating creatine kinase reaction velocity and contractile performance of the heart. Because one definition of the failing heart is the inability in acutely increase its workload, ie, recruit its contractile reserve, our focus has been on defining the relation between the creatine kinase reaction velocity and contractile reserve. We suggest that a useful term describing the biochemical analogue to contractile reserve is energy reserve. Here we briefly describe some recent results from our laboratory using acute inhibition of creatine kinase activity as a way of perturbing, as selectively as possible, this energy reserve system and assessing its consequences using a combination of ^{31}P NMR spectroscopy and physiology.

Does Decreasing Creatine Kinase Activity Change the Bioenergetic State of the Heart?

Supplying the intact rat heart with small amounts (up to 120 μmol) of the sulfhydryl group modifier iodoacetamide resulted in acute inhibition of creatine kinase activity to as little as <1% of control. Neither the indices of respiration measured in mitochondria isolated from these hearts nor rates of glycolytic flux measured in the intact heart using radiolabeled glucose decreased with supplying iodoacetamide slowly and in low amounts.[19] Neither were the adenylate kinase and myofibrillar ATPase activities affected. In terms of physiological measures of ATP supply and utilization, normal baseline performance assessed as isovolumic contractile performance and normal oxygen consumption-rate pressure product relations were maintained. Thus, at least in terms of the major ATP synthesizing reactions and the major ATPase of the cell, inhibition appears to be specific.

^{31}P NMR spectra of these hearts at baseline levels of cardiac performance showed that inhibiting creatine kinase to <1% of control decreased [PCr] by approximately 30% with a concomitant increase in calculated free [ADP] (from approximately 60 to 110 μM).[25] [ATP], [Pi,] the total creatine pool and the intracellular pH were all unchanged. By varying the amount of iodoacetamide supplied to the heart, graded inhibition could be achieved and graded decreases in [PCr] and increases in free [ADP] were observed.[25] The four indices of the energetic state of the heart can be calculated from this information. The ATP/ADP ratio decreased from approximately 200 in glucose-supplied uninhibited hearts to approximately 85 in hearts with inhibited creatine kinase. The adenylate energy charge decreased imperceptibly from 0.997 to 0.994. The phosphorylation potential decreased from approximately 36

to approximately 17 mM^{-1}. The free energy of ATP hydrolysis decreased slightly from -58.5 to -56.5 kJ/mol. Thus, those indices that emphasize the contribution of increased [ADP] changed the most. These results show that the energetic state of the heart was changed by acutely inhibiting creatine kinase, but not enough to alter baseline cardiac performance.

Does Decreased Creatine Kinase Activity Compromise the Contractile Reserve of the Heart?

In contrast to relatively modest changes in ^{31}P NMR measured metabolites in creatine kinase inhibited hearts at normal levels of work, all of the metabolites changed with inotropic challenge, ie, when the heart was challenged to recruit its energy reserve to support its contractile reserve.[19,25] When hearts with <1% remaining creatine kinase activity were abruptly exposed to buffer containing high concentrations of Ca^{2+}, [ATP] fell to approximately 8 mM, PCr fell even further from approximately 11 mM to approximately 8 mM, Pi increased to approximately 11 mM and calculated free [ADP] increased to approximately 140 μM. In control (uninhibited) hearts, the changes were less dramatic: [ATP] did not change, PCr fell from 16 to 12 mM and Pi increased by approximately 4 μM and free [ADP] increased from approximately 60 to approximately 110 μM. The changes in creatine kinase-inhibited hearts were remarkable in two respects. First, although the changes in PCr and Pi were expected with this challenge, they occurred *even though* the increase in isovolumic contractile performance elicited by high [Ca^{2+}] was less than half that observed for normal hearts. Second, [ATP] actually decreased, showing that the remaining intact ATP synthesis pathways were not adequate to resupply ATP at high workloads. These results are shown in Figure 2, where the increases in rate-pressure product are plotted against the absolute value of the free energy of ATP hydrolysis for normal hearts and for hearts with <1% remaining creatine kinase activity. These results show that acutely decreasing energy reserve decreases contractile reserve of the heart.

Similar results have been obtained using other strategies to chronically reduce creatine kinase reaction velocity. In rat hearts in which the myocardial PCr pool was replaced with a poorly hydrolyzable guanidino analog, β-guanidinopropionic, PCr content, creatine kinase reaction velocity and heart function all decreased under high workload conditions.[18,22,23,26]

Finally depleting M creatine kinase by transgenic technology reduced the ability of skeletal muscle to sustain burst work.[24] Each of these experiments shows that decreasing energy reserve limits the abil-

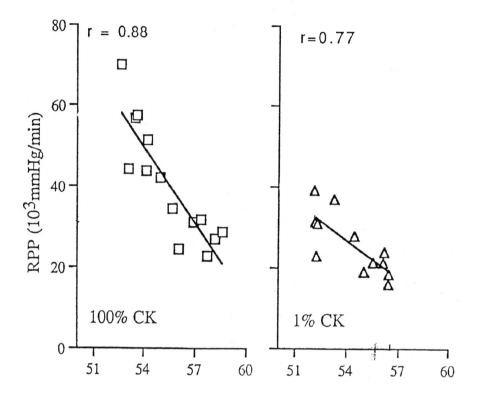

Free Energy Release from ATP Hydrolysis (kJ/mol)

FIGURE 2. Relation of free energy release from ATP hydrolysis (ΔG~P on the x-axis) and isovolumic contractile performance (RPP) for a control heart and a heart with <1% creatine kinase (CK) activity. Linear regressions were performed within data range of each group. Regression equations are y = −6.35x + 387 (r = 0.88) and y = 3.18x + 198 (r = 0.77) for hearts with 100 and 1% CK activity, respectively, where x is ΔG~P and y is RPP. (Redrawn from Reference 25.)

ity of striated muscle to increase contractile performance. Moreover, the perturbations which result in chronic impairment of creatine kinase activity, such as the M creatine kinase knockout, can elicit compensatory changes in other pathways for ATP synthesis. Most notable, glycolytic capacity and the fractional cell volume of mitochondria increased in striated muscle of the M creatine kinase knockout mouse.

These results illustrate the important principle that ATP synthesis occurs by the integration of all ATP synthesizing pathways. When one pathway is diminished or eliminated (in this case the creatine kinase reaction), compensatory increases occur in the others. The biochemical remodeling of the myocyte also emphasizes the importance of the creatine kinase system for phosphoryl transfer. Taken together, and of great importance for understanding the bioenergetics of heart failure, these results also show that reducing energy reserve of the heart by selectively inhibiting creatine kinase activity leads to decreased contractile reserve.

Acknowledgment

I would like to acknowledge my many colleagues who have contributed to this body of work over the last 20 years, especially Paul Allen, John Bittl, Jan Friedrich, Judy Gwathmey, Baron Hamman, Martha Kramer, Luigi Nascimben, Ilana Reis, and Rong Tian.

References

1. Ingwall JS. Is cardiac failure a consequence of decreased energy reserve? *Circulation.* 1993;87(suppl VII):VII-58–VII-62.
2. Scheuer J. Metabolic factors in myocardial failure. *Circulation.* 1993;87(suppl VII):VII-55–VII-57.
3. Jacobus WE, Lehninger AL. Creatine kinase of rat heart mitochondria. *J Biol Chem.* 1973;248:4803–4810.
4. Wallimann T, Schlosser T, Eppenberger HM. Function of M-line-bound creatine kinase as intramyofibrillar ATP regenerator at the receiving end of the phosphorylcreatine shuttle in muscle. *J Biol Chem.* 1984;259:5238–5246.
5. Wallimann T, Wyss M, Brdiczka D, et al. Intracellular compartmentation, structure and function of creatine kinase isozymes in tissue with high and fluctuating energy demands: the 'phosphocreatine circuit' for cellular energy homeostasis. *Biochem J.* 1992;281:21–40.
6. Friedrich J, Nascimben L, Liao R, et al. Phosphocreatine T_1 measurements with and without exchange in the heart. *Magn Reson Med.* 1993;30:45–50.
7. Bittl JA, Ingwall JS. Reaction rates of creatine kinase and ATP synthesis in the isolated rat heart. *J Biol Chem.* 1985;260:3512–3517.
8. Bittl JA, Balschi JA, Ingwall JS. Contractile failure and high-energyphosphate turnover during hypoxia: ^{31}P-NMR surface coil studies in living rat. *Circ Res.* 1987;60:871–878.
9. Ingwall JS, Kobayashi K, Bittl JA. *In vivo* enzymology of the creatine kinase reaction in the isolated rat heart: ^{31}P magnetization transfer studies. In: Smirnoff VN, Katz A, eds. *Proceedings of the 6th Joint USA-USSR Symposium on Myocardial Metabolism.* New York, NY: Gordon and Breach; 1987:3–48.
10. Nasimben L, Friedrich J, Liao R, et al. Enalapril treatment increases cardiac performance and energy reserve via the creatine kinase reaction in myocardium of syrian hamsters with advanced heart failure. *Circulation.* 1995;91:1824–1833.
11. Nascimben L, Ingwall JS, Pauletto P, et al. Creatine kinase system in failing and nonfailing human myocardium. *Circulation.* In press.

12. Sylven C, Lin L, Jansson E, et al. Ventricular adenine nucleotide translocator mRNA is upregulated in dialted cardiomyopathy. *Cardiovasc Res.* 1993;27: 1295–1299.
13. Conway MA, Allis J, Ouwerkerk R, et al. Detection of low phosphocreatine to ATP ratio in failing hypertrophied human myocardium by ^{31}P magnetic resonance spectroscopy. *Lancet* 1991;338:973–976.
14 Hardy CJ, Weiss RG, Bottomley PA, et al. Altered myocardial high-energy phosphate metabolites in patients with dialated cardiomyopathy. *Am Heart J.* 1991;122:795–801.
15. Neubauer S, Krahe T, Schnidler R, et al. [31]P magnetic resonance spectroscopy in dialated cardiomyopathy and coronary artery disease: altered high-energy phosphate metabolism in heart failure. *Circulation.* 1992;86: 1810–1818.
16. Bittle JA, Ingwall JS. Intracellular high-energy phosphate transfer in normal and hypertrophied myocardium. *Circulation.* 1987;75(suppl I):I-96. Abstract.
17. Neubauer S, Horn M, Naumann A, et al. Impairment of energy metabolism in intact residual myocardium of rat hearts with chronic myocardial infarction. *J Clin Invest.* 1995;95:1092–1100.
18. Liao R, Nascimben L, Friedrich J, et al. Decreased energy reserve in an animal model of dialted cardiomyopathy: Relationship to contractile performance. *Circ Res.* 1996;78:893–902.
19. Hamman BL, Bittl JA, Jacobus WE, et al. Inhibition of creatine kinase reaction decreases the contractile reserve of the isolated rat heart. *Am J Physiol.* 1995;269:H1030–1036.
20. Gross WL, Bak MI, Ingwall JS, et al. Nitric oxide inhibits creatine kinase and regulates rat heart contractile reserve. *Proc Natl Acad Sci.* 1996;93:5604–5609.
21. Mekhfi H, Veksler V, Mateo P, et al. Creatine kinase is the main target of reactive oxygen species in cardiac myofibrils. *Circ Res.* 1996;78:1016–1027.
22. Zweier JL, Jacobus WE, Korecky B, et al. Bioenergetic consequences of cardiac phosphocreatine depletion induced by creatine analogue feeding. *J Biol Chem.* 1991;266:20296–20304.
23. Kapelko VI, Kuprianov VV, Novikova NA et al. The cardiac contractile failure induced by chronic creatine and phosphocreatine deficiency. *J Mol Cell Cardiol.* 1988;20:465–479.
24. Van Deursen J, Heerschap A, Oerlemans F, et al. Skeletal muscles of mice deficient in muscle creatine kinase lack burst activity. *Cell.* 1993;74:621–631.
25. Tian R, Ingwall JS. Energetic basis for reduced contractile reserve in isolated rat hearts. *Am J Physiol.* 1996;270:H1207–1216.
26. Shoubridge EA, Jeffry FMH, Keogh JM, et al. CK kinetics, ATP turnover and cardiac performance in hearts depleted of creatine with the substrate analog β-guanidinopropionic acid. *Biochim Biophys Acta.* 1985;847:25–32.

## Chapter 26

Phosphorus Nuclear Magnetic Resonance Spectroscopy in the Hypertrophied Left Ventricle

Robert J. Bache, MD, Jianyi Zhang, MD, PhD, Arthur H.L. From, MD, Kamil Ugurbil, PhD

Left ventricular pressure overload initially leads to an increase in systolic wall stress followed by the development of myocardial hypertrophy. As hypertrophy occurs, systolic wall stress decreases in proportion to the increased wall thickness so that systolic wall stress returns to near-normal levels.[1] Although myocardial hypertrophy appears to be an appropriate response to an increased systolic load, both clinical and experimental data indicate that the hypertrophied left ventricle does not behave normally. Thus, patients with left ventricular hypertrophy secondary to pressure overload can experience typical exertional angina pectoris despite angiographically normal epicardial coronary arteries.[2] Patients with pressure overload left ventricular hypertrophy commonly develop electrocardiograph repolarization changes either at rest or during exercise that are similar to those seen with subendocardial ischemia.[3] Experimental studies of left ventricular pressure overload have demonstrated that a period of apparently stable compensated hypertrophy can be followed by progressive myocardial dysfunction.[4] These findings have been taken as evidence that the hypertrophied left ventricle has increased vulnerability to abnormalities of perfusion or energy metabolism.

This study was supported by US Public Health Service Grants HL21872, HL32427 and HL50470 from the National Heart, Lung and Blood Institute, and from the Department of Veterans Affairs Medical Research funds.

From: Higgins CB, Ingwall JS, Pohost GM, (eds). *Current and Future Applications of Magnetic Resonance in Cardiovascular Disease.* Armonk, NY: Futura Publishing Company, Inc.; © 1998.

Experimental Models

High-energy phosphate metabolism can be studied in large animal models of left ventricular hypertrophy (LVH) *in vivo* using phosphorus nuclear magnetic resonance (^{31}P NMR) spectroscopy.[5] Severe LVH can be produced in dogs by banding the ascending aorta at approximately 8 weeks of age.[6] During the surgical procedure the aortic band is tightened to produce a peak systolic pressure gradient of 20 to 25 mm Hg. As the animals subsequently undergo normal body growth in the face of a fixed degree of aortic narrowing, the systolic pressure gradient increases to approximately 100 mm Hg at adulthood. By initially applying a mild degree of stenosis and allowing the pressure overload to increase gradually, myocardial injury (which has been reported with acute imposition of severe pressure overload) is avoided. The gradually increasing aortic stenosis does not result in growth retardation and typically results in severe hypertrophy with a near doubling of left ventricular mass.[6] Ascending aortic banding can also be performed in adult animals, but a peak systolic gradient of no greater than 50 mm Hg is generally tolerated acutely. When this is done a lesser degree of hypertrophy occurs, typically with a 30% to 50% increase in left ventricular mass.[7]

Phosphorus Nuclear Magnetic Resonance Spectroscopy

^{31}P NMR spectroscopy was performed in intubated, open-chest animals anesthetized with α-chloralose.[5] Studies were carried out in a 4.7-T 40-cm bore magnet interfaced with an SIS Corporation console. Radiofrequency (RF) transmission and signal detection were performed using 28- and 35-mm diameter surface coils for normal and LVH hearts, respectively. The coil was cemented to a sheet of silicone rubber 0.7 mm in thickness; a capillary containing 15 μL of 3M phosphonoacetic acid was placed at the coil center to serve as a reference. The proton signal from water detected with the surface coil was used to homogenize the magnetic field and to adjust the position of the animal in the magnet so that the coil was at or near the magnet and gradient isocenters. The left ventricular pressure signal was used to gate NMR data acquisition to the cardiac cycle, and respiratory gating was achieved by triggering the ventilator to the cardiac cycle between data acquisitions.[8] Spectra were recorded in late diastole with a pulse repetition time of 6 to 7 seconds. This repetition time allowed full relaxation of adenosine triphosphate (ATP) and inorganic phosphate (Pi) and approximately

95% relaxation of phosphocreatine (PCr). The PCr resonance was corrected for this minor saturation.

Signal origin was restricted to an ISIS column coaxial with the surface coil and perpendicular to the left ventricular wall as previously described; column dimensions were 18 mm × 18 mm in normal hearts and 23 mm × 23 mm in LVH hearts.[5] Within this column the signal was further localized to 5 voxels across the left ventricular wall from epicardium to endocardium using the B_1 gradient centered about 135°, 120°, 90°, 60°, and 45° phase angles. The details of the adiabatic inversion pulses, the plane rotation adiabatic BIR-4 pulse, Fourier coefficients, and the multiplication factors used to construct the voxels have been previously reported.[9] When the B_1 gradient is used for localization along the coil axis, an increase in phase angle shifts the voxel further from the surface coil and deeper into the left ventricular muscle. Because of the nonlinear nature of the B_1 gradient, voxel width is largest for the 45° (deepest) voxel; this voxel is centered approximately 1 radius distance from the coil. Despite the nonuniform voxel volume, the detected signal per unit spins is nearly uniform between voxels because the decreasing sensitivity with increasing distance from the coil compensates for the increasing voxel volume. This allows voxel intensities to be compared directly, except for the innermost (subendocardial) voxel where metabolite content may be underestimated because of a partial volume effect, because part of this voxel is occupied by blood in the left ventricular chamber. For each measurement 96 scans were accumulated in 10 minutes to construct a spatially localized spectra set. At the conclusion of study, a myocardial biopsy was obtained for measurement of ATP content with high-performance liquid chromatography to allow calibration of the spectra. This procedure is based on the finding that chemically measured ATP was essentially identical with ATP determined with ^{31}P NMR spectroscopy in normoxic perfused rat hearts.[10]

Severe Left Ventricular Hypertrophy

Animals with severe LVH secondary to chronic pressure overload demonstrated prominent abnormalities of myocardial high-energy phosphates (HEP). Myocardial ATP content was 23.9 ± 0.84 μmol/g dry weight in normal hearts. ATP values were normal in animals with mild LVH,[10] but were decreased by 42% in animals with severe LVH.[5] Myocardial ATP content was uniform across the wall of the left ventricle from epicardium to endocardium both in normal animals and in animals with hypertrophy. The myocardial PCr/ATP ratio demonstrated significant transmural nonuniformity, with values in the suben-

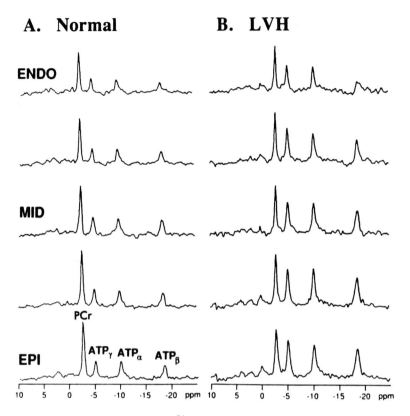

FIGURE 1. Transmurally localized ^{31}P NMR spectra from a normal heart **(A)** and a heart with severe LVH **(B)** produced by banding the ascending aorta. Each transmural data set consists of a stack of 5 spectra corresponding to voxels centered around phase angles of 145°, 120°, 90°, 60°, and 45°. The 145° voxel and the 45° voxel are the innermost and outermost voxels relative to the surface coil. ENDO indicates subendocardial voxel; MID, midwall voxel; EPI, subepicardial voxel. Spectra are scaled to optimize visualization of the resonance peaks so that only the PCr/ATP ratios can be compared between spectra. (Reproduced with permission from Reference 5.)

docardium significantly lower than in the subepicardium. Myocardial PCr/ATP values were not altered in animals with mild LVH.[11] In contrast, in animals with severe hypertrophy myocardial PCr/ATP ratios were significantly decreased in all transmural layers with a tendency for greatest reduction in the subendocardium (Figure 1). Mean PCr was 58% less in animals with severe LVH than in normal animals.[5] The decrease in PCr was associated with a significant reduction of myocardial total creatine from 116 ± 3 μmol/g dry weight in normal hearts to 90 ± 5 μmol/g dry weight in animals with severe LVH. Despite the

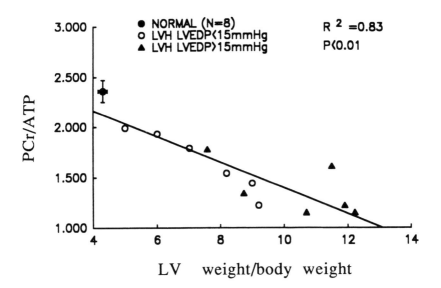

FIGURE 2. Relative severity of LVH expressed as the ratio of left ventricular weight/body weight plotted against PCr/ATP ratios. Filled circle with brackets from normal hearts; open circles from LVH animals with end-diastolic pressures less than 15 mm Hg; filled triangles from LVH hearts with left ventricular end-diastolic pressures greater than 15 mm Hg. (Reproduced with permission from Reference 5.)

decreased PCr/ATP ratio in severely hypertrophied hearts, inorganic phosphate was not detected during basal conditions. The abnormality of the PCr/ATP ratio was directly related to the degree of hypertrophy, so that the most severely hypertrophied hearts had the most marked reduction of the PCr/ATP ratio (Figure 2). The cause of the lower ATP and PCr levels in the severely hypertrophied hearts is unclear. ATP synthetic capacity appears to be adequate, since the hypertrophied hearts are able to respond with increases of contractile activity during moderate stress produced by pacing or inotropic stimulation without further reduction of ATP (at least in the subepicardium). It is possible, however, that repetitive episodes of stress induced ischemia could result in decreased myocardial ATP content by causing loss of adenine nucleotide precursors which typically require several days for *de novo* resynthesis.

Using the measured values of ATP, PCr, and creatine (as well as pH and magnesium that can be estimated from the ^{31}P spectra), it is possible to calculate the myocardial free adenosine diphosphate (ADP) concentration using the creatine kinase equilibrium.[12] Using data obtained during basal conditions this calculation yields values for free

ADP in the severely hypertrophied hearts which are approximately 80% greater than normal.[5] In the intact heart ATP synthesis is kinetically regulated by its primary substrates which include oxygen, nicotinamide adenine dinucleotide phosphate (NADH), ADP, and inorganic phosphate.[3] Thus, the increased ADP levels could be the result of inadequate delivery of oxygen secondary to deficiencies of perfusion or diffusion in severely hypertrophied myocardium. Similarly, decreased NADH generation secondary to inadequate exogenous substrate or disordered intermediary metabolism would require that ADP levels rise to support ATP synthesis. A reduction of the magnitude of the mitochondrial proton gradient or altered properties of the mitochondrial H^+ adenosine triphosphatase (ATPase) so that the V_{max} or K_m values with respect to ADP are increased would have a similar effect. All of these alterations have in common the need to increase free ADP to support a given rate of ATP synthesis.

To determine whether high-energy phosphate abnormalities in hypertrophied myocardium are the result of abnormal perfusion, myocardial blood flow was measured using the radioactive microsphere technique. Microspheres, 15 μm in diameter, labeled with gamma-emitting radionuclides were injected into the left atrium. The microspheres are uniformly mixed during passage through the left ventricle and distributed in proportion to blood flow, so that tissue radioactivity can be used to compute flow rates. To determine if the decreased PCr/ATP ratio (increased free ADP) in the severely hypertrophied left ventricle resulted from hypoperfusion, coronary blood flow was increased without changing the cardiac workload by administration of adenosine (1 mg/kg per minute intravenously), which acts as a selective coronary vasodilator.[5] Although minimum coronary resistance is impaired in severely hypertrophied hearts, coronary perfusion pressure is increased in this model of LVH because the coronary arteries arise proximal to the constricting aortic band.[14] Adenosine caused a threefold increase in myocardial blood flow in the severely hypertrophied left ventricles; blood flow increased in all transmural layers across the wall of the ventricle. Adenosine caused no change in high energy phosphate content in normal or mildly hypertrophied ventricles. Similarly, the depressed ATP and PCr values, and the abnormally increased free ADP were not corrected by increasing coronary blood flow in the hearts with severe LVH.[5] Failure of hyperperfusion to increase the ATP levels was not surprising, because synthesis of ATP precursor is very slow, often requiring several days.[15] However, this is not the case with regard to PCr, because substantial amounts of free creatine are available in the myocardium. The enzyme that generates PCr, creatine kinase, is in equilibrium and consequently responds passively to the concentrations of its reactants.[12] In normoxic myocardium the rate-limiting reactant appears to be ADP, since ATP levels are high relative to the K_m value with respect to creatine kinase.[16] Although a primary alteration of the properties of creatine kinase in severely hypertrophied myocardium cannot be excluded, the failure of PCr to rise despite a marked increase in coronary blood flow likely resulted from persistently high levels of ADP. Failure of hyperperfusion to correct the elevated ADP values excludes the possibility that oxygen delivery by blood flowing through the coronary capillaries is limiting. However, the data do not exclude limitation of oxygen diffusion to the mitochondria which could result from the increased intercapillary diffusion distance in the hypertrophied myocardium.[17] Limitation of carbon substrate delivery to the myocyte seems excluded by failure of hyperperfusion to decrease the free ADP concentration. The findings demonstrate that the high-energy phosphate alterations in the severely hypertrophied hearts cannot be ascribed to persistent coronary hypoperfusion.

Myocardial Response to Stress

In the pressure overloaded hypertrophied left ventricle, treadmill exercise or pacing-induced tachycardia can result in an abnormal transmural distribution of perfusion with a decrease in the subendocardial/subepicardial blood flow ratio below unity.[6] In addition, exercise causes an exaggerated increase in oxygen demands in the pressure overloaded hypertrophied left ventricle, likely because of the exaggerated increase in left ventricular systolic pressure that occurs during exercise.[18] Both insufficient coronary blood flow and excessive increases in metabolic demands could contribute to the development of myocardial ischemia during stress in the hypertrophied heart. The response of myocardial high-energy phosphate content to increases of metabolic demands produced by atrial pacing and dobutamine was examined using ^{31}P NMR in animals with LVH produced by banding of the ascending aorta.[11] In normal hearts atrial pacing at 200 and 240 beats per minute resulted in increases of myocardial blood flow in proportion to the increased oxygen demands produced by the tachycardia; the increase in blood flow was uniform across the left ventricular wall. In animals with mild LVH (left ventricular/body weight = 5.7 ± 0.2 g/kg as compared with 4.3 ± 0.1 g/kg in normal animals), pacing produced a variable response; in all animals subepicardial blood flow increased during pacing, but in some animals subendocardial flow failed to increase or even decreased despite the increased contractile work caused by pacing. Myocardial ATP and PCr did not change in the normal hearts or in the subepicardium of the hypertrophied hearts during pacing as fast as 240 beats per minute. However, in hypertro-

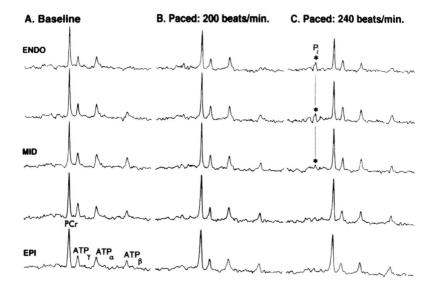

FIGURE 3. Transmural responses of phosphorylated metabolites detected by ^{31}P-NMR spectroscopy during sinus rhythm **(A)**, pacing at 200 **(B)**, and 240 beats per minute **(C)** in an animal with left ventricular hypertrophy that developed subendocardial underperfusion during pacing. *Pi indicates inorganic phosphate. (Reproduced with permission from Reference 11.)

phied hearts in which the subendocardial/subepicardial blood flow ratio decreased during pacing (as evidence of relative subendocardial underperfusion), ^{31}P NMR spectra demonstrated loss of PCr with accumulation of inorganic phosphate in the subendocardium (Figure 3). The response of subendocardial PCr during pacing at 240 beats per minute was directly related to perfusion, so that decreases in subendocardial blood flow were associated with loss of subendocardial PCr. The loss of PCr and accumulation of Pi in the subendocardium of the hypertrophied left ventricles during pacing is similar to changes that occur during subendocardial ischemia produced by stress in the presence of a proximal coronary artery stenosis.[19] Thus, the findings suggest that in the hypertrophied left ventricle tachycardia can cause redistribution of blood flow away from the subendocardium, thereby resulting in subendocardial ischemia. This abnormality is the result of increased extravascular forces during tachycardia in the hypertrophied heart (increased left ventricular filling pressure and delayed relaxation), because relative subendocardial underperfusion persists even during maximum coronary vasodilation with adenosine.[20] The development of subendocardial ischemia during tachycardia would be expected to further impair myocardial relaxation and cause increased ventricular stiffness, thereby further impeding subendocardial blood flow and worsening the degree of ischemia.[21]

Dobutamine has been commonly used to mimic the effects of exercise on the heart. Unlike pacing, dobutamine results in prominent increases of myocardial contractility (as well as heart rate). Although the positive inotropic effect causes a greater increase in myocardial metabolic demands than pacing, the increased contractility increases the velocity of both contraction and relaxation, thereby shortening the duration of systole and augmenting the diastolic perfusion period. The resultant decrease in extravascular compressive forces which impede coronary blood flow may be especially important in the hypertrophied heart where impaired relaxation can encroach on the diastolic perfusion period, especially at high heart rates. Dobutamine causes both metabolic coronary vasodilation as a result of the increased myocardial oxygen consumption which it produces as well as vasodilation secondary to stimulation of coronary β-adrenoceptors.[22] In normal hearts dobutamine in doses of 15 and 30 $\mu g/kg$ per minute resulted in increases in myocardial oxygen consumption and coronary blood flow with no change in the transmural distribution of perfusion.[11] Dobutamine caused a decrease of myocardial PCr that was more marked in hypertrophied than in normal hearts. Unlike pacing, the decrease of PCr during dobutamine infusion was transmurally uniform or more prominent in the subepicardium (Figure 4). Dobutamine also caused an increase in inorganic phosphate which was more marked in hypertrophied than in normal hearts. The changes in PCr and Pi could have resulted from inadequate perfusion with an insufficient oxygen supply during the high work state achieved during dobutamine infusion, or from a need to raise inorganic phosphate and ADP to support the increased work state even in the presence of sufficient oxygen delivery. To determine whether the high-energy phosphate changes resulted from insufficient perfusion, blood flow was increased by administration of adenosine during dobutamine infusion. Adenosine caused an approximately 50% further increase in coronary flow, but the decreased PCr and increased Pi produced by dobutamine were not corrected.[11] The finding that increasing blood flow did not correct the alterations in PCr and Pi during dobutamine indicates that these changes were not the result of inadequate myocardial perfusion. However, it is possible that the increased intercapillary diffusion distance in the hypertrophied heart could limit delivery of oxygen and carbon substrate, resulting in the changes in PCr and inorganic phosphate during dobutamine infusion.[17]

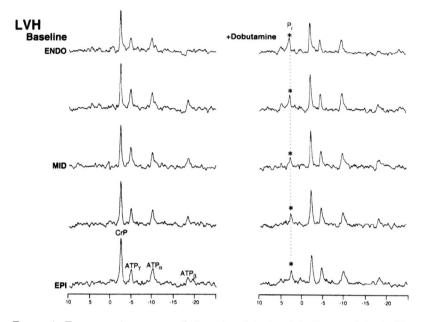

FIGURE 4. Transmural response of phosphorylated metabolites as detected by
^{31}P-NMR spectroscopy during basal conditions and during infusion of dobutamine, 30 μg/kg per minute in an animal with left ventricular hypertrophy. Note
the appearance of inorganic phosphate (Pi) in all transmural layers that was
accompanied by a decrease in PCr resonance during dobutamine administration. (Reproduced with permission from Reference 11.)

2-Deoxyglucose Uptake in the Hypertrophied Heart

Myocardial hypertrophy resulting from pressure or volume overload has been demonstrated to result in defective long chain fatty acid
metabolism in perfused guinea pig and rat hearts.[23,24] Conversely, concentrations of several glycolytic enzymes are increased in hypertrophied myocardium,[23,25] and glucose uptake assessed with dual-tracer
autoradiography has been found to be greater in left ventricles of hypertensive rats than normotensive rats.[26] ^{31}P NMR spectroscopy has
potential to assess alterations in glucose uptake by the heart because
of the ability to detect 2-deoxyglucose 6-phosphate (2DGP). 2-Deoxy-
glucose (2DG) is a glucose analogue that is transported by the sarcolem-
mal glucose transporter and phosphorylated in the C-6 position by
hexokinase to yield 2DGP.[27] 2DG uptake is subject to insulin control
and is increased as blood levels of competing oxidative substrates such
as fatty acids and lactate are decreased. The clearance of 2DGP from
the myocardium is extremely slow, because it cannot undergo further

glycolytic metabolism and is only slowly dephosphorylated by 6-phosphoglucose phosphatase. These considerations suggest that ^{31}P NMR detection of 2DGP accumulation in the myocardium would have potential for assessing the fractional rate of glucose uptake by the heart.

The feasibility of assessing myocardial hexose uptake *in vivo* by measuring 2DGP accumulation with ^{31}P NMR spectroscopy was assessed in dogs with LVH produced by ascending aortic banding.[28] At the time of study, animals had severe LVH with a 90% average increase in the left ventricular/body weight ratio. Animals were anesthetized with sodium pentobarbital and studied in the open-chest state with a surface coil sutured to the epicardial surface of the anterior left ventricular wall. After baseline ^{31}P NMR spectra had been obtained, 2DG was infused into the left anterior descending coronary artery at a rate of 15 μmol/kg body weight per minute while transmurally differentiated spectra were acquired at 15-minute intervals. Infusion of 2DG caused no change in systemic hemodynamic variables or myocardial blood flow. Arterial levels of free fatty acids, glucose and insulin were similar in normal and hypertrophied hearts, and were not changed by infusion of 2DG. Arterial lactate and norepinephrine levels were higher in animals with LVH than in normal animals, but these values were not significantly altered by infusion of 2DG. Normal hearts demonstrated no change in phosphorus spectra during a one hour infusion of 2DG and no detectable 2DGP accumulation. Time-dependent 2DGP accumulation was observed in 7 of 8 animals with LVH. As shown in the representative spectra from one animal with LVH in Figure 5, 2DGP accumulation was most marked in the subendocardium of hypertrophied hearts. After 1 hour of 2DG infusion, total 2DGP accumulation was directly related to the left ventricular weight/body weight ratio, indicating that 2DG uptake was greatest in hearts with the most severe hypertrophy (Figure 6). Increased accumulation of 2DGP in animals with LVH was not the result of the increased left ventricular systolic pressure in this group, because acute aortic constriction to produce similar levels of left ventricular systolic pressure in a group of normal dogs did not result in accumulation of 2DGP.

The findings in these animals indicate that myocardial 2DGP accumulation can be detected in the pressure overloaded hypertrophied left ventricle *in vivo* using ^{31}P NMR spectroscopy. Failure to observe 2DGP accumulation in normal hearts was likely related to the relative insensitivity of the NMR technique. The threshold for consistently resolvable phosphate metabolite is 2–4 μmol/g dry weight; in contrast, positron emission tomography using ^{18}F-fluorodeoxyglucose is at least three orders of magnitude more sensitive than this.[29] Furthermore, the relatively large concentrations of 2DG which must be used to provide sufficient sensitivity for detection of 2DGP accumulation by ^{31}P NMR

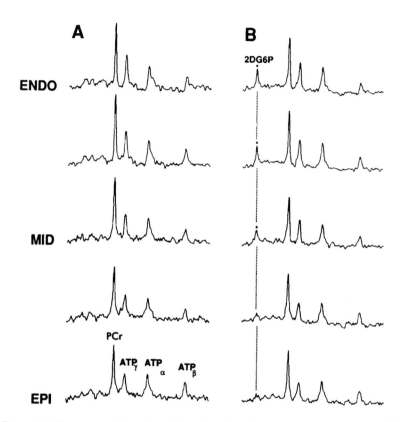

FIGURE 5. Transmurally localized phosphorylated metabolites detected by ³¹P NMR spectroscopy in an animal with left ventricular hypertrophy during control conditions **(A)** and at 45 minutes of intracoronary infusion of 2-deoxyglucose (15 μmol/kg per minute). **(B)** 2DGP identifies the 2-deoxyglucose-6-phosphate resonance. ENDO, subendocardium; MID, midwall; EPI, subepicardium; CP, phosphocreatine. (Reproduced with permission from Reference 28.)

spectroscopy would likely interfere with glucose metabolism because of competitive inhibition of glucose uptake and metabolism by 2DG. Nevertheless, the finding of increased 2DGP accumulation in these canine hearts with LVH *in vivo* is in agreement with previous *in vitro* studies in rodent hearts that have documented increased glucose utilization by hypertrophied myocardium, and demonstrate that the increase in 2DG uptake is related to the severity of LVH. The more prominent 2DGP accumulation in the subendocardium is in agreement with reports that subendocardial glucose uptake exceeds subepicardial uptake in both normal and hypertensive rat left ventricle.[26,30] The findings suggest increased dependence on glucose metabolism, especially in

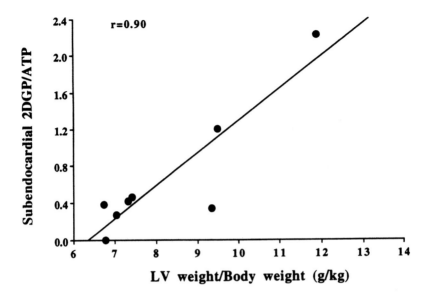

FIGURE 6. Subendocardial 2-deoxyglucose-6-phosphate (2DGP), expressed relative to ATP, plotted against the relative severity of left ventricular (LV) hypertrophy, expressed as the ratio of LV weight/body weight in 8 animals with left ventricular hypertrophy. (Reprinted with permission from Reference 28.)

subendocardium of the chronically pressure-overloaded hypertrophied left ventricle.

References

1. Hood WP, Rackley CE, Rolette E. Wall stress in the normal and hypertrophied left ventricle. *Am J Cardiol.* 1968;22:550–558.
2. Goodwin JR. Hypertrophic disease of the myocardium. *Prog Cardiovasc Dis.* 1973;16:199–238.
3. Wrobewski EM, Pearl FJ, Hammer WJ, et al. False-positive stress test due to undetected left ventricular hypertrophy. *Am J Epidemiol.* 1982;115:412–417.
4. Meerson FZ. The myocardium in hyperfusion, hypertrophy and heart failure. *Circ Res.* 1969;25:111–118.
5. Zhang J, Merkle H, Hendrich K, et al. Bioenergetic abnormalities associated with severe left ventricular hypertrophy. *J Clin Invest.* 1993;92:993–1003.
6. Bache RJ, Vrobel TR, Ring WS. Regional myocardial blood flow during exercise in dogs with chronic left ventricular hypertrophy. *Circ Res.* 1981;49:742–750.
7. Bache RJ, Dai XZ, Alyono D, et al. Myocardial blood flow during exercise in dogs with left ventricular hypertrophy produced by aortic banding and perinephritic hypertension. *Circulation.* 1987;76:835–842.
8. Robitaille P, Markle H, Sublett E, et al. Spectroscopic imaging and spatial

localization using adiabatic pulses and applications to detect transmural metabolite distribution in the canine heart. *Magn Reson Med.* 1989;10:14–37.

9. Hendrich K, Liu H, Merkle H, et al. B_1 voxel-shifting of phase-modulated spectroscopic localization techniques. *J Magn Reson.* 1992;97:486–497.

10. Humphrey SM, Garlick PB. NMR-visible ATP and PI in normoxic and reperfused rat hearts: a quantitative study. *Am J Physiol.* 1991;260 (Heart Circ Physiol 29):H6–H12.

11. Bache RJ, Zhang J, Path G, et al. High-energy phosphate responses to tachycardia and inotropic stimulation in left ventricular hypertrophy. *Am J Physiol.* 1994;266 (Heart Circ Physiol 35):H1959–H1970.

12. Wyss M, Smeitink J, Wevers RA, Wallimann T. Mitochondrial creatine kinase: A key enzyme of aerobic energy metabolism. *Biochim Biophysica Acta.* 1992;1102:119–166.

13. From AHL, Zimmer SD, Mirchurski SP, et al. Regulation of the oxidative phosphorylation rate in the intact cell. *Biochemistry.* 1990;29:3731–3743.

14. Mueller TM, Marcus ML, Kerber RE, et al. Effect of renal hypertension and left ventricular hypertrophy on the coronary circulation in dogs. *Circ Res.* 1978;42:543–551.

15. Manfredi JP, Holmes EW. Purine salvage pathways in myocardium. *Ann Rev Physiol.* 1985;47:691–705.

16. Ugurbil K, Petein M, Maidan R, et al. Measurement of an individual rate constant in the presence of multiple exchanges; application to myocardial creatine kinase reaction. *Biochemistry.* 1986;25:100–107.

17. Breisch EA, White FC, Bloor CM. Myocardial characteristics of pressure overload hypertrophy. A structural and functional study. *Lab Invest.* 1984; 51:333–342.

18. Bache RJ, Dai XZ. Myocardial oxygen consumption during exercise in the presence of left ventricular hypertrophy secondary to supravalvular aortic stenosis. *J Am Coll Cardiol.* 1990;15:1157–1164.

19. Path G, Robitaille P, Merkle H, et al. The correlation between transmural high energy phosphate levels and myocardial blood flow in the presence of graded coronary stenosis. *Circ Res.* 1990;67:660–673.

20. Bache RJ, Cobb FR. Effect of maximum coronary vasodilation on transmural myocardial perfusion during tachycardia in the awake dog. *Circ Res.* 1977; 41:648–656.

21. Apstein CS, Mueller M, Hood WB Jr. Ventricular contracture and compliance changes with global ischemia and reperfusion and their effect on coronary resistance in the rat. *Circ Res.* 1977;41:206–217.

22. Ruffolo RR, Yaden EL. Vascular effects of the stereoisomers of dobutamine. *J Pharmacol Exp Ther.* 1983;224:46–50.

23. Wittels B, Spann JF Jr. Defective lipid metabolism in the failing heart. *J Clin Invest.* 1968;47:1787–1794.

24. El Alaqui-Talibi Z, Landormy S, Loireau A, Moravec J. Fatty acid oxidation and mechanical performance of volume-overloaded rat hearts. *Am J Physiol.* 1992;262:H1068–H1074.

25. Bishop SP, Altschuld RA. Increased glycolytic metabolism in cardiac hypertrophy and congestive failure. *Am J Physiol.* 1970;218:153–159.

26. Yonekura Y, Brill AB, Som P, et al. Regional myocardial substrate uptake in hypertensive rats: A quantitative autoradiographic measurement. *Science.* 1985;227:1494–1496.

27. Sokoloff L. The radioactive deoxyglucose method: theory, procedure, and applications for the measurement of local glucose utilization in the central nervous system. *Adv Neurochem.* 1982;4:1–82.

28. Zhang J, Duncker DJ, Ya X, et al. Effect of left ventricular hypertrophy secondary to chronic pressure overload on Transmural myocardial 2-deoxyglucose uptake. *Circulation.* 1995;92:1274–1283.
29. Ratib O, Phelps ME, Huang SC, et al. Positron tomography with deoxyglucose for estimating local myocardial glucose metabolism. *J Nucl Med.* 1982; 23:577–586.
30. Takalla TES, Hassinen IE. Effect of mechanical workload on the transmural distribution of glucose uptake in the isolated perfused rat heart studied by regional deoxyglucose trapping. *Circ Res.* 1981;49:62–69.

## Chapter 27

Energy Metabolism of the Right Ventricle

Gregory G. Schwartz, MD, PhD,
Clifford R. Greyson, MD, Barry M. Massie, MD,
Michael W. Weiner, MD,
and Judith A. Wisneski, MD

While differences in structure, function, and perfusion between the right and left ventricles (RV and LV) are well appreciated, differences in energy metabolism have received relatively little investigative attention. In this chapter, we explore the similarities and differences in normal RV versus LV energy metabolism, the potential advantages of the RV as model for studying the regulation of myocardial energy metabolism, and the potential implications of these similarities and differences in the pathophysiology of common conditions affecting the RV.

Energy Consumption of Right Ventricle versus Left Ventricle Myocardium

The rate of energy consumption by the RV is lower than that of the LV (Table 1). The RV normally develops much lower systolic pressure than the LV because of the lower resistance of the pulmonary circulation, compared with the systemic. Consequently, RV stroke work (defined as the integral of the instantaneous product of RV pressure and pulmonary artery flow over the ejection period) is normally approximately 25% of simultaneous LV stroke work.[1] As expected, the

Supported by NIH grants HL02155 and HL49944 and the Department of Veterans Affairs Medical Research Service.

From: Higgins CB, Ingwall JS, Pohost GM, (eds). *Current and Future Applications of Magnetic Resonance in Cardiovascular Disease.* Armonk, NY: Futura Publishing Company, Inc.; © 1998.

TABLE 1

Significant Differences in Structure, Function, and Metabolism Between Right and Left Ventricles

Characteristic	Right ventricle	Left ventricle	Species	Reference
Free wall thickness (mm)	3–4	8–12	human, dog, pig	15,19
Typical developed pressure (mm Hg)	25	120	human, dog, pig	15
Resting blood flow (mL/g/min)	0.5–0.7	0.8–0.10	dog	4,19
Resting MVO$_2$ (μmol/g/min)	3–4	5–6	pig	3
Coronary venous O$_2$ content (μmol/mL)	2.5–3.0	1.0–2.0	pig	3,5
Coronary arteriovenous oxygen extraction (μmol/mL)	4	5–6	pig	3,5
Mitochondrial/myofibrillar volume ratio (%)	31	34	pig	7
Max. rate of pyruvate oxidation (state 3 O$_2$ consumption, nmol/min/mg protein)	4.5	8	rat	9
Lactate dehydrogenase activity (μmol/s/g dry wt)	32	39	human	11
Myosin isoform distribution (V$_1$/V$_3$ ratio)	1.9	1.4	rat	12

smaller stroke work of the RV is accompanied by a lower rate of myocardial oxygen consumption (MVO$_2$) in the RV free wall, compared with the LV. However, the difference in MVO$_2$ is not as great as that in stroke work: In most studies, RV free wall MVO$_2$ is approximately 70% of simultaneous LV MVO$_2$.[2] MVO$_2$ of the interventricular septum is intermediate between the free walls of the two ventricles.[4] Selective sampling of coronary venous blood from RV and LV veins reveals that MVO$_2$ in RV free wall of the anesthesized pig averages 3.6 μmol$\cdot$g^{-1} $\cdot$min^{-1}, compared with 5.1 μmol$\cdot$g$^{-1}\cdot$min^{-1} in the LV free wall under baseline conditions.[5] The most likely explanation for the relatively modest difference in MVO$_2$ between RV and LV free walls is that the thin RV free wall is subjected to higher wall tension *per unit intracavitary pressure* than the thicker LV wall.

The lower MVO$_2$ of the RV free wall is the result of both to lower coronary flow[2,4] and lower transcoronary oxygen (O$_2$) extraction. For instance, transcoronary O$_2$ extraction by the RV averages 60%, and LV extraction averages 79% under baseline conditions in the anesthetized pig.[3,5] Under conditions of near-maximal hemodynamic stress (eg, pressure overload and/or inotropic sitmulation) increases in RV free wall MVO_2 to greater than 3 times baseline have been documented.[2] Because maximal myocardial blood flow during pharmacological vasodilation is similar in both ventricles,[6] the RV posesses greater flow and O_2 extraction reserve than the LV.

Energy Generation by Right Ventricle versus Left Ventricle Myocardium

Most, but not all studies indicate that the energy generating capacity of RV myocardium is lower than that of LV. Morphometric studies in both pigs and dogs reveal a slightly lower mitochondrial density in RV myocardium, compared with LV.[7,8] In the rat heart, maximal rates of oxidation of various carbon substrates *in vitro* are 20% to 50% lower for RV homogenates, compared with LV homogenates.[9] Limited available data indicate that differences in the activities of enzymes of glycolytic and oxidative metabolism or energy transfer between the two ventricles are modest. In normal rats, the activities of citrate synthase, isocitrate dehydrogenase, cytochrome c oxidase, and creatine kinase are not significantly different in RV versus LV,[9,10] but the activity of lactate dehydrogenase has been found to be lower in RV free wall of rat[10] and human hearts.[11]

Differences in Composition and Function of Contractile Proteins

In rat heart, expression of V_1 myosin isoform (containing α heavy chains) exceeds that of V_3 (containing β heavy chains), with the greatest expression of V_1 in the RV.[12] The V_1 isoform of myosin is characterized by a higher calcium-stimulated adenosine triphosphatase (ATPase) activity than the V_3 isoform resulting in a higher rate of cross-bridge cycling, higher velocity of shortening, and shorter time of crossbridge interaction. Conversely, V_3 is characterized by slower cross-bridge cycling and greater time of crossbridge interaction. These differences in myosin isoform expression may be adaptive to the usual role of the RV as a volume-adaptive, low-pressure pump, and the role of the LV as a pressure-adaptive, high-pressure pump. Although the expression of V_3 predominates in both ventricles of the human heart, immunofluorescent microscopy using monoclonal antibodies to α and β heavy chains demonstrates a greater proportion of α-staining cells in human RV than in LV.[13] Myofilament calcium sensitivity may also differ between the two ventricles. RV myocardium of normal (WKY) rats displays lower calcium sensitivity (pCa_{50} and maximal calcium-activated force) than LV myocardium, but the differences are diminished in the setting of RV hypertrophy.[1]

Advantages of the Right Ventricle as a Model to Study the Energetic Response to Increased Cardiac Workload

Large and rapid changes in cardiac workload imposed by physical activity and neurohormonal influences result in parallel changes in the rate of energy utilization (adenosine triphosphate [ATP] hydrolysis). Myocardial energy use during maximal exercise or pharmacological stress may rise to 4 to 5 times resting levels.[15] Accordingly, the rate of ATP production must be subject to rapid regulation over a wide dynamic range. Because of the limited capacity of the heart to synthesize ATP by anaerobic glycolysis, the rate of ATP synthesis by oxidative phosphorylation must remain closely coupled to the changing rate of ATP hydrolysis. The control mechanisms involved in balancing ATP synthesis and hydrolysis have been the subject of considerable investigation over many years. Workload-dependent increases in the concentrations of ATP hydrolysis products (adenosine diphosphate [ADP] and inorganic phosphate), changes in mitochondrial redox potential (increased mitochondrial $NADH/NAD^+$ ratio), and calcium-mediated activation of enzymes of the tricarboxylic acid cycle and/or electron transport have been proposed as potential mechanisms for the stimulation of oxidative phosphorylation in response to increased cardiac energy demand.[16,17]

Most studies investigating the potential mechanisms of energetic regulation in response to increased cardiac workload have been performed in the LV of isolated or intact hearts. However, data from studies in both pigs and dogs indicate that when workload is increased to high levels, relative ("demand") myocardial ischemia may develop in the LV, even in the absence of coronary stenosis or functional abnormalities of the coronary circulation.[5,15] At high LV workloads, the metabolic consequences of myocardial ischemia (including decreased concentration of phosphocreatine, increased concentrations of ATP hydrolysis products, and increased $NADH/NAD^+$) may therefore be difficult to distinguish from physiological regulatory changes in energy metabolism. For example, when MVO_2 of the porcine LV was increased to 2 to

3 times baseline by dobutamine infusion without or with simultaneous aortic constriction, subendocardial/subepicardial blood flow ratio diminished while the ratio of phosphocreatine/ATP concentration (determined by phophorus nuclear magnetic resonance [^{31}P NMR]) decreased and myocardial lactate release (quantified by an isotopic tracer technique) increased[5] (Figure 1).

As a model for the study of the regulation of oxidative phosphorylation, the RV has the particular advantage of being less susceptible to demand ischemia than the LV under most conditions. Because of its lower intracavitary (and presumably, intramyocardial) pressure during systole, perfusion of RV myocardium normally occurs throughout the cardiac cycle, in contrast to the predominantly diastolic perfusion of the LV.[19] As a consequence, the RV is less susceptible to demand ischemia when tachycardia shortens the duration of diastole. In addition, the lower extraction of O_2 from right coronary, compared with left coronary arterial blood under resting conditions provides the RV with additional O_2 extraction reserve as metabolic demand increases. Unlike the LV, experimental demonstration of demand ischemia of the RV free wall is limited to situations where RV afterload is increased to the point that cardiac output and systemic arterial pressure fall. Under these circumstances, reductions in RV subendocardial perfusion and phosphocreatine concentration have been documented, with reversal upon an increase in coronary perfusion pressure.[20,21] However, acute RV pressure overload can be produced without RV hypoperfusion if pulmonary artery constriction is carefully adjusted to increase RV systolic pressure without causing a fall in coronary perfusion pressure.[22]

Assessment of Right Ventricular Energy Metabolism Using ^{31}Phosphorus Nuclear Magnetic Resonance Spectroscopy

^{31}P NMR spectroscopy has proven to be a technique of great value in the study of myocardial energy metabolism because of its ability to provide repetitive, nondestructive measurements of key phosphorus energy metabolites. The first ^{31}P NMR spectra from the RV were obtained with an intravascular catheter coil inserted via the external jugular vein of dogs to the RV apex.[23] The NMR signal detected by this technique is presumed to arise primarily from the interventricular septum, whose mass is much greater than the thin apical portion of the RV free wall.

The thinness of the RV free wall presents a technical challenge to the application of NMR spectroscopy to study RV energy metabolism.

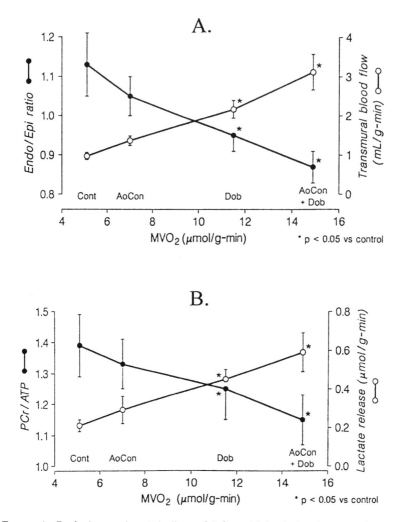

FIGURE 1. Perfusion and metabolism of *left* ventricle during increased metabolic demand (MVO$_2$) imposed by aortic constriction (AoCon), intravenous dobutamine infusion (Dob) and the combination of the two interventions (AoCon+Dob) in 10 pigs. **A:** Mean transmural blood flow and subendocardial/subepicardial blood flow ratio. **B:** Subendocardially weighted PCr/ATP ratio (by ^{31}P NMR) and lactate release (by isotope dilution technique). At high workloads, a significant decrease in endo/epi blood flow ratio and PCr/ATP ratio and a significant increase in lactate release are observed, consistent with the development of relative myocardial ischemia in the LV subendocardium (demand ischemia). At high LV workloads, ischemic metabolic changes may therefore be difficult to distinguish from physiologic regulatory changes in energy metabolism. (Reproduced with permission from Reference 5.)

In normal pigs and humans, the thickness of the RV free wall is 3 to 4 mm, about 40% of the thickness of the LV free wall.[24,25] Thus, *in vivo* spectroscopy of the RV free wall necessitates pulse sequences that provide precise localization and/or a surface coil designed to provide a sufficient signal from the thin volume of RV lying directly beneath it, while excluding signal from a deeper, but much larger volume of intracavitary blood.

Based on a design originally intended for spectroscopy of skin,[26] our laboratory has developed a 3.5 × 1.0 × 0.3 cm elliptical surface coil using a two-turn crossover design (Figure 2). This design provides high sensitivity within a few millimeters of the central portion of the coil, but sharply decremental sensitivity with increasing distance from

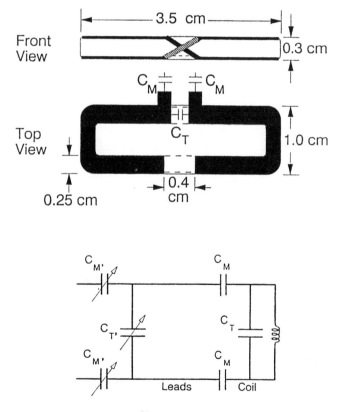

FIGURE 2. Schematic drawing of ^{31}P NMR surface coil designed for use on the porcine RV free wall at 2 T. Fixed match capacitance (C_M), 51 pF; fixed tune capacitance (C_T), 200 pF; variable match capacitance (C_M), 1–30 pF; variable tune capacitance (C_T), 1–30 pF. (Reproduced with permission from Reference 24.)

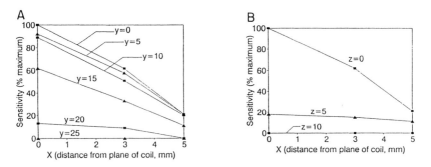

FIGURE 3. Sensitivity profile of RV free wall surface coil shown in Figure 2. Coil lies in *y-z* plane with long axis parallel to *y* and short axis parallel to *z* and B_0 field. Coil long axis spans -17.5 mm$<y<17.5$ mm; coil short axis spans -5 mm$<x<5$ mm. Values of *x* indicate distance from plane of coil. *In vivo*, RV free wall would extend from $x=0$ (plane of coil) to $x\approx3-4$ mm. RV chamber blood would be present at $x>3-4$ mm. **A:** Sensitivity versus x at various values of y (in mm), with $z=0$. **B:** Sensitivity versus x at various values of z (in mm), with $y=0$. Note that coil sensitivity declines sharply at $x=5$ mm, thereby minimizing signal from RV chamber blood in vivo. Coil sensitivity also declines rapidly at values of y and z that exceed coil dimensions, thereby minimizing signal from laterally adjacent regions in vivo. (Reproduced with permission from Reference 24.)

the plane of the coil (Figure 3).[24] We have used this coil to investigate energy metabolism of the RV free wall in open-chest, anesthetized pigs. At a B_0 field strength of 2 T, ^{31}P spectra were obtained from 800 acquisitions at a repetition time of 1.8 seconds. Signal-to-noise for phosphocreatine (PCr) averaged 13:1. The concentration ratio of PCr to ATP in porcine RV under baseline hemodynamic conditions (1.7–2.3) was similar to that determined by direct biochemical analysis of canine[20] and porcine[27] RV, and by direct biochemical analysis[28] or ^{31}P NMR[29,30] in canine, ovine, or porcine LV.

Relation Among Oxygen Consumption, High-Energy Phosphates, and Carbon Substrate Uptake in Right Ventricles: Implications for the Regulation of Oxidative Phosphorylation

We addressed the question of whether increased RV workload and MVO_2 are accompanied by decreased PCr/ATP (implying increased free ADP).[3] To this end, RV free wall blood flow, MVO_2, and carbon substrate uptake were measured in the myocardium directly beneath the ^{31}P surface coil. Regional blood flow was measured with radioactive

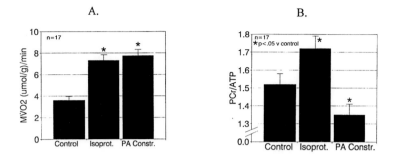

FIGURE 4. **A:** Oxygen consumption (MVO_2) of RV free wall under control conditions (mean RV systolic pressure 34 mm Hg), with isoproterenol stimulation (0.15 μg/kg/min IV), and pulmonary artery (PA) constriction (mean RV systolic pressure 63 mm Hg). Note that both isoproterenol and PA constriction produced nearly equal increases in MVO_2. **B:** Ratio of phosphocreatine (PCr) to ATP in RV free wall, determined by ^{31}P NMR without correction for partial saturation. Note that PCr/ATP rose with isoproterenol, but fell with PA constriction.* P<.05 vs. control. (Reproduced with permission from Reference 3.)

microspheres, and oxygen and substrate uptake were determined from paired arterial and RV coronary venous blood samples. The metabolic responses to two interventions that increased RV workload were compared: acute RV pressure overload imposed by pulmonary artery (PA) constriction versus inotropic and chronotropic stimulation with intravenous isoproterenol.[3] The two interventions produced nearly equal increases in RV MVO_2, to approximately twice baseline (Figure 4A). PA constriction caused a significant fall in PCr/ATP (from a mean baseline value of 1.52 to 1.35, not corrected for partial saturation), implying an increase in free ADP concentration. However, isoproterenol stimulation caused an unexpected and significant *increase* in PCr/ATP, to a mean value of 1.72 (Figure 4B), implying a *decrease* in free ADP concentration. RV free wall blood flow and lactate consumption increased from baseline by similar extents during both interventions, implying that the fall in PCr/ATP during PA constriction was not due to relative RV ischemia. Considering the observed changes in PCr/ATP, changes in free Mg^{2+} estimated from the chemical shift difference between α- and β-ATP peaks, and assuming literature values for ^{31}P longitudinal relaxation times and total myocardial creatine concentration, the creatine kinase equilibrium predicts that RV free ADP concentration averaged 48 nmol/g wet weight at baseline, increasing to a mean of 59 nmol/g wet weight during PA constriction, but decreasing to a mean of 24 nmol/g wet weight during isoproterenol.[3] Thus, despite nearly equal MVO_2 during PA constriction and isoproterenol, there was a 2.5-fold difference in estimated free ADP concentration. While increased

ADP may have contributed to the stimulation of oxidative phosphorylation during PA constriction, other factors must have stimulated this process during isoproterenol in the face of decreased free ADP.

The answer to this seeming dichotomy may lie in the differing patterns of carbon substrate uptake during the two interventions. Both glucose and free fatty acid (FFA) uptake were much higher during isoproterenol, compared with PA constriction. During PA constriction, glucose and FFA uptake increased to mean levels of 1.5 and 1.2 times baseline, but these increases were less than proportionate to the mean increase in MVO_2 to 2.2 times baseline. In contrast, isoproterenol-induced increases in glucose and FFA uptake were greater than proportionate to the rise in MVO_2: glucose and FFA uptake increased to means of 2.5 and 4.6 times baseline, respectively, while MVO_2 increased to a mean of 2.0 times baseline. The higher glucose uptake during isoproterenol may be related to an ninefold increase in plasma insulin concentration from a mean baseline level of 5.5 $\mu U/mL$ to 46 $\mu U/mL$ during isoproterenol. In addition, there is evidence that catecholamine stimulation can cause translocation of glucose transporter proteins to the plasma membrane of cardiac myocytes.[31] The higher FFA uptake during isoproterenol is most likely related to catecholamine-induced peripheral lipolysis, resulting in a rise in arterial FFA concentration to approximately twice baseline. PA constriction, on the other hand, caused no increase in circulating FFA concentration, and therefore a much smaller increase in FFA uptake from baseline.

The relation between MVO_2 and exogenous carbon substrate uptake can be further quantified by calculating an oxygen extraction ratio (OER) for each substrate. A stoichiometric equivalence exists between substrate oxidation and oxygen consumption.[32] For each mole of lactate oxidized, 3 mol of O_2 are consumed; for each mole of glucose oxidized, 6 mol of O_2 are consumed; and for each mole of FFA, approximately 23.5 mol of O_2 are consumed. In the steady-state, one would expect that MVO_2 could be fully accounted for by the uptake of exogenous substrates (ie, if the sum of OERs for exogenous substrates = 1.0, there is no net accumulation or depletion of endogenous substrates such as myocardial glycogen and triglycerides). In fact, this was the case under baseline conditions in the porcine RV, with the sum of OERs for lactate, glucose, and FFA averaging 0.98. However, a significant divergence in the sum of OERs was apparent in comparing PA constriction (mean sum of OERs = 0.63) to isoproterenol stimulation (mean sum of OERs = 1.36). Thus, uptake of exogenous lactate, glucose and FFA could account for only 63% of measured MVO_2 during PA constriction, but exceeded the amount required to account for MVO_2 by 36% during isoproterenol. While such imbalances between exogenous substrate uptake and MVO_2 cannot be maintained indefinitely, these measurements were made in a quasi-steady state, after approximately 45 minutes under each condition.

Do the differences in carbon substrate uptake during these two interventions help explain the divergent changes in the PCr/ATP ratio measured by ^{31}P NMR? The answer may lie in the multifactorial control of oxidative phosphorylation, with positive regulation by ATP hydrolysis products (ADP, inorganic phosphate), mitochondrial NADH concentration, and/or mitochondrial calcium concentration.[16]

When ATP use was increased by PA constriction, the uptake of exogenous substrate by the RV was insufficient to account for the increased flux of reducing equivalents through the electron transport chain (based on measured MVO_2). With a relative deficit of exogenous substrate uptake, the mitochondrial redox potential ($NADH/NAD^+$ ratio) may have been too low (oxidized) to adequately stimulate the rate of oxidative phosphorylation. This may have caused ADP and inorganic phosphate concentrations to rise until these metabolites achieved levels sufficient to provide an alternative stimulus to respiration.

Conversely, the estimated 50% decline in free ADP concentration during isoproterenol stimulation would be expected to exert *negative* feedback on the rate of oxidative phosphorylation; yet this rate *increased* by twofold over baseline (based on the increase in MVO_2). Another factor must have exerted a stimulatory influence on the rate of oxidative phosphorylation. Most likely, this factor was a more reduced mitochondrial redox potential (increased $NADH/NAD^+$ ratio) due to the robust uptake of exogenous substrates, particularly FFA. Scholz et al[33] showed that addition of lactate or pyruvate to glucose in the perfusate of isolate rabbit hearts caused an increase in epicardial NADH fluorescence. Similarly, Hassinen et al[34] showed that addition of hexanoate to the perfusate of isolated rat hearts caused a dose-dependent increase in NADH fluorescence accompanied by increasing phosphorylation potential (PCr/inorganic phosphate ratio). Starnes et al[35] found that perfusion of rat hearts with palmitate increased PCr/ATP by 10% and $NADH/NAD^+$ by 39%, compared with glucose perfusion. Alternatively, isoproterenol may increase the mitochondrial $NADH/NAD^+$ ratio by increasing intracellular calcium, with consequent stimulation of calcium-sensitive dehydrogenases (eg, pyruvate, isocitrate and α-ketoglutarate dehydrogenase) whose action results in the formation of NADH.

We tested the hypothesis that greater use of FFA by RV myocardium increases mitochondrial NADH and decreases free [ADP], the latter reflected by a rise in PCr/ATP measured by ^{31}P NMR. To test the hypothesis, we stimulated MVO_2 with isoproterenol while FFA metabolism was blocked by the carnitine palmitoyltransferase I inhibitor, oxfenicine.[36] In the presence of oxfenicine, RV FFA uptake did not increase with isoproterenol, despite a large increase in the circulating FFA concentration. The RV PCr/ATP ratio *decreased* from baseline during isoproterenol stimulation with oxfenicine, compared to a significant *increase* from baseline during isoproterenol without oxfenicine. Consistent with these data are recent results by Balschi et al[37] demonstrating that PCr/ATP in canine LV declines during phenylephrine stimulation of workload in the presence of oxfenicine, but not in the absence of oxfenicine. The data of these studies support the hypothesis that high FFA uptake and metabolism are responsible for maintaining or increasing the PCr/ATP ratio during increased myocardial workstates.

Energetic Response to Acute Right Ventricle Pressure Overload

Acute RV pressure overload occurs in the clinical settings such as massive pulmonary embolism, hypoxic pulmonary vasoconstriction, prolonged cardiopulmonary bypass, and after cardiac transplantation when the donor heart is commonly faced with high resistance in the recipient's pulmonary circulation. Because RV failure is an important determinant of morbidity and mortality in these conditions, an understanding of the mechanism of RV failure in these situations is important.

In anesthetized, open-chest pigs,[22] the PA was gradually and progressively constricted to produce an increase in RV systolic pressure to approximately 45 mm Hg from a baseline of approximately 30 mm Hg. With this degree of RV pressure overload, systemic arterial pressure was unchanged, RV free wall blood flow increased transmurally, contractile function was maintained, and persistent RV coronary vasodilator reserve could be demonstrated by infusion of intravenous adenosine. Thus, it is highly unlikely that this degree of PA constriction caused RV free wall ischemia. Nonetheless, PCr/ATP in the RV free wall decreased significantly. Further constriction of the PA (to achieve maximum RV systolic pressure before systemic pressure began to fall) produced a further decrease in the PCr/ATP ratio along with significant RV dilatation. During this more severe level of PA constriction, RV free wall blood flow was increased by raising the coronary perfusion pressure with simultaneous aortic constriction. Despite increased RV perfusion, the PCr/ATP ratio did not recover. Upon release of the PA constriction, the reduction in PCr/ATP was fully reversible, but the RV remained significantly dilated even though preload and afterload were no higher than baseline. These findings suggest that increased RV workload imposed by acute pressure overload is accompanied by a nonischemic increase in the concentration of free ADP that may serve to stimulate the rate of oxidative phosphorylation. Furthermore, the results of this study indicate the onset of RV contractile dysfunction in acute pressure overload coincides with the exhaustion of coronary vasodilator reserve, rather than with the initial decline in high-energy phosphate concentration.

Energy Metabolism in Right Ventricular Ischemia

Right ventricular ischemia and infarction may occur in the clinical setting of inferior myocardial infarction due to thrombotic occlusion of the right coronary artery. While most survivors of RV infarction regain RV systolic function and do not suffer from chronic RV failure, clinically significant RV dysfunction and failure is common in the early phase of RV infarction and may contribute substantially to morbidity and mortality.[38] Such RV dysfunction is usually treated with volume loading, and if necessary, inotropic stimulation. However, inotropic stimulation of ischemic myocardium has the potential to worsen myocardial energy demand/oxygen supply imbalance, with resultant depletion of myocardial high energy phosphates and increased tissue acidosis from accelerated anaerobic metabolism.[39] We investigated the metabolic consequences of prolonged, moderate ischemia in the porcine RV, and the response of the RV to inotropic stimulation with dobutamine (Figure 5).[27] When RV free wall blood flow was reduced by approximately 45% for 100 minutes by constricting the proximal right coronary artery, regional systolic shortening declined by 75%, accompanied by net lactate release and coronary venous acidosis. Surprisingly, however, there were no significant changes in RV PCr or ATP concentrations determined either by direct biochemical analysis or by ^{31}P NMR. Furthermore, when the heart was stimulated with dobutamine during continued RV ischemia, systolic function of the ischemic RV free wall did not improve, while global measures of RV function increased due to stimulation of non-ischemic regions of the heart. In the ischemic region, dobutamine stimulation had no deleterious effects on any measured parameter of energy metabolism, including high-energy phosphate concentrations, lactate release, or coronary venous pH. Thus, the RV exhibits metabolic adaptation to prolonged, moderate ischemia by maintaining high energy phosphate levels despite reduced blood flow, contractile function, and accelerated anaerobic metabolism. These results are similar to those obtained in the moderately ischemic LV by Arai et al.[40] Furthermore, inotropic stimulation with dobutamine enhances global RV function by stimulation of nonischemic regions of myocardium, but does not reduce high-energy phosphate or increase tissue acidosis or lactate release from the ischemic zone.

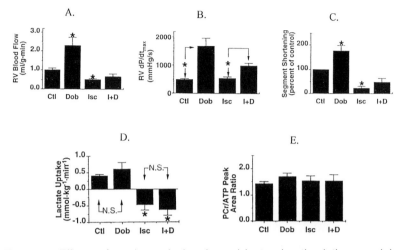

Figure 5. Effects of moderate ischemia and inotropic stimulation on global and regional RV function and energy metabolism of RV free wall. Measurements were made in 12 pigs under control conditions, during dobutamine infusion without RV ischemia (Dob), moderate RV free wall ischemia (Isc), and ischemia with inotropic stimulation (Isc + Dob). Regional blood flow in the RV free wall **(A)** decreased significantly during Isc, but was not significantly augmented during Isc + Dob. Global RV function, assessed by maximum RV dp/dt **(B)**, increased with dobutamine stimulation under both nonischemic and ischemic conditions. Regional function of the RV free wall, assessed by systolic segment shortening **(C)**, decreased during ischemia but showed no significant improvement during Isc + Dob. Thus, the improvement in global RV function during Isc + Dob can be attributed to stimulation of non-ischemic regions of the RV. The degree of ischemia was sufficiently severe to cause net lactate release from the RV free wall **(D)**, but the PCr/ATP ratio measured by ^{31}P NMR **(E)** was unchanged from baseline during Isc and Isc + Dob. The preservation of high energy phosphates indicates a metabolic adaptation of the RV myocardium to sustained, moderate ischemia. *$P<.05$ vs. control or for specific comparisons indicated.

Summary

    The RV both consumes and generates less chemical energy than the LV. Because of its lower intracavitary pressure and perfusion throughout the cardiac cycle, the RV is relatively resistant to ischemia at high cardiac workloads. As a consequence, physiological changes in energy metabolism in response to increased workload are less likely to be obscured by concomitant ischemic metabolic changes, making the RV an attractive model for the study of energetic regulation. However, the thinness of the RV free wall poses special challenges for *in vivo* NMR spectroscopy. NMR surface coils designed to be sensitive over a very limited depth are useful in overcoming this obstacle. In response to increased workload, RV PCr/ATP may either decrease or increase, implying increased or decreased free [ADP], respectively. The direction of the response depends upon the intervention employed to increase work and the prevailing milieu of carbon substrates. The results of studies of energetic regulation in the RV suggest multifactorial control of oxidative phosphorylation by ATP hydrolysis products and mitochondrial redox potential. The RV appears to undergo metabolic adaptation to prolonged, moderate ischemia by maintaining high energy phosphate concentrations despite reduced contractile function and accelerated anaerobic metabolism. Further studies of RV energy metabolism may prove useful in gaining a fuller understanding of the pathophysiology of common clinical conditions affecting the RV, including cor pulmonale and ischemic heart disease.

References

1. Goldstein JA, Tweddell JS, Barzilai B, et al. Importance of left ventricular function and systolic ventricular interaction to right ventricular performance during acute right heart ischemia. *J Am Coll Cardiol.* 1992;19:704–711.
2. Kusachi S, Nishiyama O, Yasuhara K, et al. Right and left ventricular oxygen consumption in open-chest dogs. *Am J Physiol.* 1982;243:H761–H766.
3. Schwartz GG, Greyson CR, Wisneski JA, et al. Relation among regional O_2 consumption, high-energy phosphates, and substrate uptake in porcine right ventricle. *Am J Physiol.* 1994;266:H521–H530.
4. Weiss HR, Neubauer JA, Lipp JA, Sinha AK. Quantitative determination of regional oxygen consumption in the dog heart. *Circ Res.* 1978;42:394–401.
5. Massie BM, Schwartz GG, Garcia J, et al. Myocardial metabolism during increased work states in porcine left ventricle in vivo. *Circ Res.* 1994;74: 64–73.
6. Gold FL, Bache RJ. Influence of systolic intracavitary pressure on right ventricular perfusion in the awake dog. *Cardiovasc Res.* 1982;16:467–472.
7. Singh S, White FC, Bloor CM. Myocardial morphometric characteristics in swine. *Circ Res.* 1981;49:434–441.
8. Karpova VV, Tverskaia MS, Virganskii AO, et al. The functional-morphological state of the myocardium in experimental massive embolism of the pulmonary artery. *Biul Eks Biol Med.* 1991;111:130–132.
9. Kainulainen H, Komulainen J, Leionen A, et al. Regional differences of substrate oxidation capacity in rat hearts: Effects of extra load and endurance training. *Basic Res Cardiol.* 1990;85:630–639.
10. Smith SH, Kramer MF, Reis I, et al. Regional changes in creatine kinase and myocyte size in hypertensive and nonhypertensive cardiac hypertrophy. *Circ Res.* 1990;67:1334–1344.
11. Lin L, Sylven C, Sotonyi P, et al. Lactate dehydrogenase and its isoenzyme activities in different parts of normal human heart. *Cardiovasc Res.* 1989;23: 601–606.
12. Brooks WW, Bing OHL, Blaustein AS, Allen PD. Comparison of contractile state and myosin isozymes of rat right and left ventricular myocardium. *J Mol Cell Cardiol.* 1987;19:433–440.

13. Bouvagnet P, Mairhofer H, Leger JOC, et al. Distribution pattern of α and β myosin in normal and diseased human ventricular myocardium. *Basic Res Cardiol.* 1989;84:91–102.
14. Perrault CL, Bing OHL, Brooks WW, Ransil BJ, Morgan JP. Differential effects of cardiac hypertrophy and failure on right versus left ventricular calcium activation. *Circ Res.* 1990;67:707–712.
15. Marcus ML. *The Coronary Circulation in Health and Disease.* New York: McGraw Hill; 1983, pp. 65–92.
16. Heineman FW, Balaban RS. Control of mitochondrial respiration in the heart in vivo. *Ann Rev Physiol.* 1990;52:523–542.
17. Jacobus WE. Respiratory control and integration of high energy phosphate metabolism by creatine kinase. *Ann Rev Physiol.* 1985;47:707–725.
18. Zhang J, Duncker DJ, Xu Y, et al. Transmural bioenergetic responses of normal myocardium to high workstates. *Am J Physiol.* 1995;268:H1891–H1905.
19. Hoffman JIE. Transmural myocardial perfusion. *Prog Cardiovasc Dis.* 1987;29:429–464.
20. Vlhakes GJ, Turley K, Hoffman JIE. The pathophysiology of failure in acute right ventricular hypertension: Hemodynamic and biochemical correlations. *Circulation.* 1981;63:87–95.
21. Gold FL, Bache RJ. Transmural right ventricular blood flow during acute pulmonary artery hypertension in the sedated dog. *Circ Res.* 1982;51:196–204.
22. Schwartz GG, Steinman S, Garcia J, et al. Energetics of acute pressure overload of the porcine right ventricle. *J Clin Invest.* 1992;89:909–918.
23. Kantor HL, Briggs RW, Balaban RS. In vivo ^{31}P nuclear magnetic resonance measurements in canine heart using a catheter-coil. *Circ Res.* 1984;55:261–266.
24. Schwartz GG, Steinman SK, Weiner MW, Matson GB. In vivo ^{31}P-NMR spectroscopy of right ventricle in pigs. *Am J Physiol.* 1992;262:H1950–H1954.
25. Marcus ML, Weiss RM. Evaluation of cardiac structure and function with ultrafast computed tomography. In: Marcus ML, Schelbert HR, Skorton DJ, Wolf GL, eds. *Cardiac Imaging.* Philadelphia, Saunders, 1991, pp. 669–681.
26. Nagel TL, Alderman DW, Schoenborn RR, et al. The slotted crossover surface coil: a detector for in vivo NMR of skin. *Magn Reson Med.* 1990;16:252–268.
27. Greyson C, Garcia J, Mayr M, Schwartz GG. Effects of inotropic stimulation on energy metabolism and systolic function of ischemic right ventricle. *Am J Physiol.* 1995;268:H1821–H1828.
28. Pantely GA, Malone SA, Rhen WS, et al. Regeneration of myocardial phosphocreatine in pigs despite continued moderate ischemia. *Circ Res.* 1990;67:1481–1493.
29. Heineman FW, Balaban RS. Phosphorus-31 nuclear magnetic resonance analysis of transient changes of canine myocardial metabolism in vivo. *J Clin Invest.* 1990;85:843–852.
30. Portman MA, Heineman FW, Balaban RS. Developmental changes in the relation between phosphate metabolites and oxygen consumption in the sheep heart in vivo. *J Clin Invest.* 1989;83:456–464.
31. Rattigan S, Appleby GJ, Clark MG. Insulin-like action of catecholamines and Ca^{2+} to stimulate glucose transport and GLUT4 translocation in perfused rat heart. *Biochim Biophys Acta.* 1991;1094:217–223.
32. Lassers BW, Kaijser L, Carlson LA. Myocardial lipid and carbohydrate

metabolism in healthy fasting men at rest: studies during continuous infusion of ³H-palmitate. *Eur J Clin Invest.* 1972;2:348–358.

33. Scholz TD, Laughlin MR, Balaban RS, et al. Effect of substrate on mitochondrial NADH, cytosolic redox state, and phosphorylated compounds in isolated hearts. *Am J Physiol.* 1995;268:H82–H91.

34. Hassinen I, Ito K, Nioka S, Chance B. Mechanism of fatty acid effect on myocardial oxygen consumption. A phosphorus NMR study. *Biochim Biophys Acta.* 1990;1019:73–80.

35. Starnes JW, Wilson DF, Erecinska M. Substrate dependence of metabolic state and coronary flow in perfused rat heart. *Am J Physiol.* 1985;249:H799–H806.

36. Schwartz GG, Greyson C, Wisneski J, Garcia J. Inhibition of fatty acid metabolism alters myocardial high-energy phosphates in vivo. *Am J Physiol.* 1994;267:H224–H231.

37. Balschi J, Hai J, Wolkowicz PE, Pohost GM. The effect of the inhibition of fatty acid oxidation on in vivo canine myocardial ¹H and ³¹P NMR spectra. *J Mol Cell Cardiol.* 1995;27:A9. Abstract.

38. Zehender M, Kasper W, Kauder E, et al. Right ventricular infarction as an independent predictor of prognosis after acute inferior myocardial infarction. *N Engl J Med.* 1993;328:981–988.

39. Schulz R, Guth BD, Pieper K, et al. Recruitment of an inotropic reserve in moderately ischemic myocardium at the expense of metabolic recovery. *Circ Res.* 1992;70:1282–1295.

40. Arai AE, Pantely GA, Anselone CG, et al. Active downregulation of myocardial energy requirements during prolonged moderate ischemia in swine. *Circ Res.* 1991;69:1458–1469.

## Chapter 28

Phosphorus Magnetic Resonance Spectroscopic Studies of Skeletal Muscle in Patients with Congestive Heart Failure
Contributions to the Understanding of the Pathophysiology of Exercise Intolerance

Barry M. Massie, MD

Exercise Intolerance in Congestive Heart Failure

Activity and exercise intolerance are the most frequent complaints of patients with congestive heart failure (CHF). For years, these symptoms were ascribed to the characteristic hemodynamic abnormalities of left ventricular dysfunction. It was thought that dyspnea was a product of elevated left atrial pressures and that exercise capacity was limited by impaired cardiac reserve, resulting in limitation of nutritive blood flow to exercising muscle. However, a series of studies demonstrating a poor relation between measurements of cardiac function and exercise capacity made it clear that additional factors were operative.[1,2] Although Zelis, Wilson and other investigators have demonstrated abnormalities of blood flow to exercising muscle and of peripheral vascu-

This work was supported by the Department of Veterans Affairs Research Service, Washington, D.C. and by Grant Number P01-HL25847 from the National Heart, Lung, and Blood Institute, Bethesda, Maryland.

From: Higgins CB, Ingwall JS, Pohost GM, (eds). *Current and Future Applications of Magnetic Resonance in Cardiovascular Disease.* Armonk, NY: Futura Publishing Company, Inc.; © 1998.

lar regulation in patients with heart failure,[3,4] these also have not been sufficient to explain the exercise limitation in many patients.[5] Therefore, there has been an increasing interest in determining whether abnormalities of skeletal muscle itself may play a role.

The focus on skeletal muscle in the syndrome of CHF coincided with the increasing utilization of [31]phosphorus-magnetic resonance spectroscopy (31P-MRS) for defining normal and pathological aspects of muscle metabolism.[6] This technique was found to be well suited for the assessment of oxidative and glycolytic metabolism during exercise in patients with heart failure, and rapidly became an important tool for investigating the pathophysiology of exercise intolerance in CHF.

^{31}P MRS Studies of Skeletal Muscle Metabolism in CHF

Wilson et al[6] were the first to study ^{31}P-MRS in patients with heart failure (6). They studied the forearm muscles of nine CHF patients and eight controls during a three-stage exercise protocol, using the relations between the ratio of inorganic phosphate (Pi) and creatine phosphate (PCr) and power output as a measure of muscle oxidative capacity. The CHF patients exhibited a more rapid rise in Pi/PCr in relation to the power output, indicating reduced adenosine triphosphate (ATP) synthesis and oxidative metabolism. In addition, there was a greater decline in pH in the patients.

Massie et al[8] used a bulb-squeezing protocol that allowed patients to determine their own work output. Although the 11 CHF patients performed much less work than the 7 controls, as evidenced by a 50% lower pressure-time integral during bulb squeezing, they exhibited a significantly greater decline in PCr (followed as the ratio of PCr/(PCr + Pi)), and a much greater decline in pH (Figures 1A and 1B). The pH decline was particularly marked and may have been the mechanism for the greater fatigue and reduced force development in the patients.

The same group then studied 22 patients and 11 age-matched controls during a gradual incremental finger flexion protocol that was carried to the end point of fatigue.[9] A number of new observations resulted. First, to account for the difference in strength, metabolism was examined at matched normalized workloads. PCr and pH were both significantly lower at 25%, 50%, and 75% of maximum (Figure 2). These findings suggest that the metabolic changes are probably not explained by differences in muscle mass. Second, the subgroup of patients with the more severe impairment of exercise capacity exhibited the greatest decline in pH at lower levels of exercise, again suggesting that rapid acidification may be one mechanism of early fatigue. Of particular in-

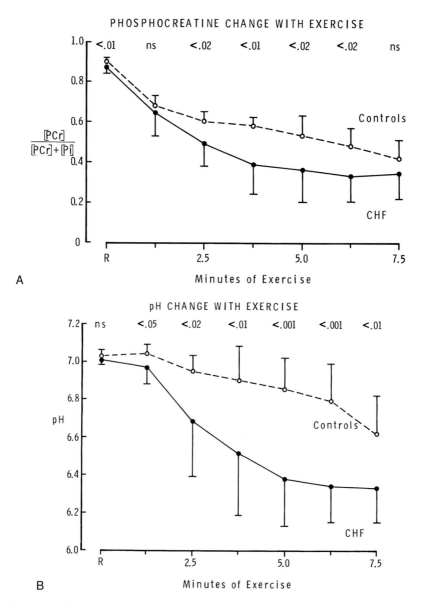

FIGURE 1. **(A)** illustrates the changes in the ratio of PCr/(PCr + ATP) during a bulb-squeezing program in 11 CHF patients and 7 age-matched sedentary controls. After the first minute, during which the PCr fell similarly in both groups, CHF patients displayed significantly greater decreases. In the final minute of exercise, when the patients were performing very little work because of more severe fatigue, the two curves converge. **(B)** illustrates the pH changes during exercise. Throughout exercise, pH was significantly lower in the patients. (Reproduced with permission from Reference 8.)

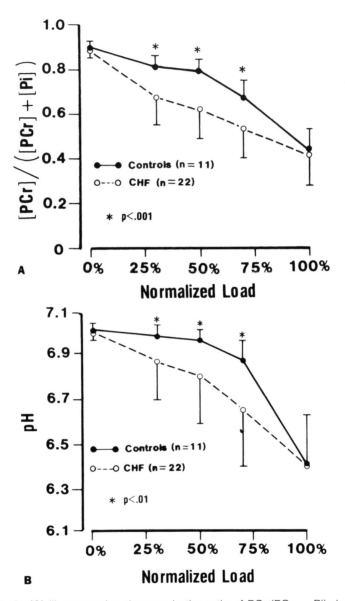

FIGURE 2. **(A)** illustrates the changes in the ratio of PCr/(PCr + Pi) during a gradually incremental finger flexion protocol. The metabolic measurements are plotted against relative workload, normalized for maximal tolerated load. Because the patients' maximal load was significantly lower than the controls, the absolute loads were lower at each point. Nonetheless, the PCr decline was more marked at submaximal levels. **(B)** illustrates the pH findings, using the same format. pH changes were also greater at submaximal levels of exercise. (Reproduced with permission from Reference 9.)

terest was the observation that patients with the most significantly reduced systemic exercise capacity also displayed the most marked decline in pH in finger flexor endurance. This observation suggests that
the metabolic changes in the forearm muscles reflect other muscle
groups and may be a determinant of systemic exercise capacity. Finally,
and most significantly, measurements of forearm blood flow during
the same exercise protocol showed no difference in forearm blood flow
between the patients and the controls at matched levels of exercise.
Thus, the metabolic changes could not be readily explained by differences in flow. Similar their conclusions were reached in a report by
Wiener et al[10]

This lack of difference in blood flow was unexpected, because impaired blood flow to exercising muscle was an obvious mechanism
for the metabolic abnormalities and previous studies showed reduced
blood flow during forearm exercises in patients with more severe heart
failure.[3] In addition, reduced exercise blood flow has been shown to
induce identical metabolic changes as those seen in CHF.[11] Therefore,
to definitively exclude reduced blood flow as a factor, Massie et al[12]
conducted a forearm exercise protocol with blood flow to the arm occluded by a cuff inflated above arterial pressure. Patients and controls
each exercised at a workload equivalent to 33% of their predetermined
maximum. During 3 minutes of exercise under ischemic conditions,
the ratio of PCr/(PCr + Pi) declined significantly more in patients than
controls to 0.38 ± 0.03 vs. 0.61 ± 0.09 ($P < .001$), as did pH to $6.52 \pm
0.31$ vs. 6.82 ± 0.11 ($P < .05$). Because oxidative metabolism ceases
during prolonged anaerobic exercise, it is possible to estimate the
amount of ATP use from the decline in PCr and the amount of lactate
produced, with the latter quantity estimated from the pH change and
the buffering capacity of muscle. Figure 3 illustrates estimates for the
metabolic changes during the final 2 minutes of ischemic exercise in
the CHF patients and controls. The greater rate of ATP consumption
for matched levels of exercise suggests reduced "efficiency" of work
output in relation to energy consumption. This finding is another piece
of evidence suggesting that heart failure causes intrinsic changes in
skeletal muscle.

Although this early work focused on the forearm muscles, it was
recognized that there may be important differences between the small
forearm muscles and large muscle groups of the lower extremities. In
particular, these larger muscles can consume a substantial proportion
of cardiac output during strenuous exertion. Mancini, et al[13] used a
"metabolic freeze" technique, in which exercise was conducted outside
of the magnet and then metabolism was evaluated by preventing recovery with rapid inflation of a cuff to supra-arterial pressure to prevent
oxidative metabolism. After both stair climbing and a plantar flexion

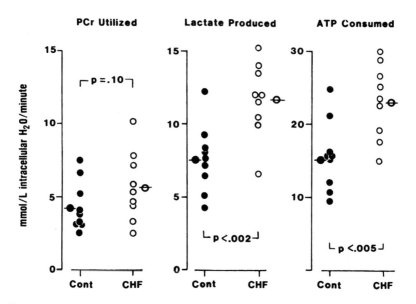

FIGURE 3. The three panels illustrate changes in the calculated rates of PCr use, lactate production, and ATP consumption during the final 2 minutes of forearm exercise conducted during ischemic conditions. Exercise was performed at equivalent normalized loads in the controls (Cont) and CHF patients. The differing rates of ATP consumption suggest less metabolic efficiency in the CHF group. (Reproduced with permission from Reference 12.)

protocol, CHF patients exhibited a much steeper Pi/PCr versus vs. VO_2 slope, just as was seen with forearm muscle exercise. Of note is that the recovery of Pi/PCr was prolonged in these patients, indicating impaired post-release blood flow or reduced oxidative capacity. In contrast, the previously cited studies of forearm muscle metabolism reported recovery rates generally, comparable between heart failure patients and controls, with rare exceptions among the most severely affected patients.

Subsequently, Arnolda et al[14] studied calf muscle metabolism in 7 CHF patients and 5 comparably aged controls, using a plantar flexion protocol conducted within the magnet. They observed significantly greater declines in PCr/(PCr + Pi) and pH in CHF patients, despite their lower work rate. As with the forearms, no differences in blood flow at matched work rates were observed. In contrast to the results of the previously cited Mancini's study, PCr recovery did not differ between patients in controls, a finding consistent with the lack of differences in blood flow. Recently, Chati et al[15] have studied calf muscle metabolism in a larger population of heart failure subjects. Although their overall findings were consistent with the previously cited studies, they identified a subgroup of patients who exhibited marked metabolic changes, including a decrease in ATP concentration. It was noted that these patients exhibited lower peak VO_2 values during systemic exercise testing, and also displayed impaired postexercise metabolic recovery. These findings demonstrate that there is considerable heterogeneity in skeletal muscle metabolic responses to exercise among CHF patients, with those demonstrating the most severe derangements also having the greatest impairment of exercise capacity. These results are consistent with the hypothesis that changes in skeletal muscle may play a role in determining exercise capacity, but alternatively could be explained by secondary muscle changes in response to reduced activity.

Mechanisms for Skeletal Muscle Abnormalities in CHF

The consistent finding of abnormal metabolic responses during ^{31}P-MRS studies of skeletal muscle in patients with CHF greatly accelerated the pace of investigation into the nature and mechanism of the changes in skeletal muscle in this condition. Table 1 lists some of the potential mechanisms that could explain the metabolic findings.

Blood Flow

As noted previously, impairment of blood flow to exercising muscle is perhaps the most obvious explanation for the metabolic abnormalities. However, although the evidence is somewhat conflicting, overall

---

TABLE 1

Potential Mechanisms for Abnormal
Muscle Metabolism in CHF

I. Reduced blood flow
   A. Due to reduced cardiac reserve
   B. Due to peripheral abnormalities
      a. Enhanced vasoconstriction
      b. Impaired vasodilation
      c. Microvascular abnormalities
II. Reduced muscle mass
III. Reduced oxidative capacity
   A. Altered fiber type distribution
   B. Reduced oxidative enzyme content
IV. Reduced metabolic efficiency

---

it is clear that abnormalities of blood flow cannot explain all of the observed metabolic alterations. This is certainly the case for systemic cardiac output, because a number of studies have shown modest relations between exercise cardiac output and exercise capacity.[1,2,5] More definitively, an elegant study by Jondeau et al,[16] using combined lower and upper limb exercise, demonstrated then that in patients with severe exercise impairment (peak VO_2 <15 mL/kg per minute) cardiopulmonary reserve is not exhausted during symptom-limited maximal lower limb exercise.

Blood flow to exercising muscle could also be impaired by abnormalities of the peripheral circulation.[3] There is also substantial evidence that this is not the sole mechanism for exercise impairment or the metabolic abnormalities observed by ^{31}P-MRS. Wilson et al[5] have shown that in a substantial subset of patients, exercise is limited by muscle fatigue despite normal increments in leg blood flow. Moreover, the previously cited studies by Massie, Wiener, and Arnolda noted metabolic abnormalities of exercising muscle despite lack of evidence of reduced limb blood flow.[9,10,14] Finally, abnormal muscle metabolism was observed even in protocols in which blood flow was occluded.[12] There is also little evidence that microcirculatory abnormalities which might impair oxygen uptake are important factors. Several muscle biopsies studies have not found a reduction in muscle capillarization.[17,18] The most definitive evidence against impaired oxygen delivery as a primary mechanism comes from a recent study by Mancini et al.[19] These investigators simultaneously performed near-infrared spectroscopy to measure deoxymyoglobin and ^{31}P-MRS during repetitive plantar flexion of the foot. As can be seen in Figure 4, CHF patients exhibited a more rapid rise in Pi/PCr, indicative of impaired oxidative metabolism, but no greater decrease in muscle oxygenation. The findings argue strongly against either in reduction in blood flow or impairment of oxygen uptake as the major mechanism for the metabolic abnormalities.

Muscle Atrophy

It is now recognized that muscle atrophy is common in patients with heart failure, even in the absence of cardiac cachexia or severe debilitation.[20,21] Massie and coworkers[9] minimized the contribution of muscle atrophy by evaluating patients and controls at matched relative workloads, and nonetheless found important metabolic differences with CHF. Mancini et al[20] found only a weak relation between the parity of metabolic changes and muscle volume measured by magnetic resonance imaging. A further strong argument against muscle atrophy

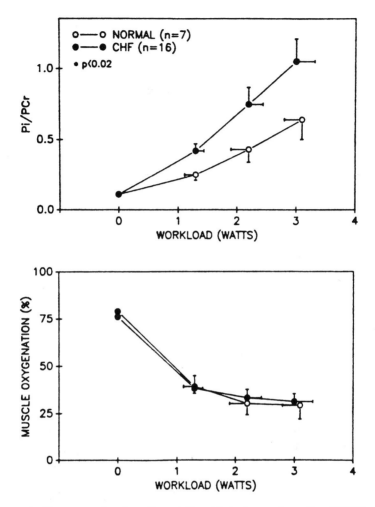

FIGURE 4. These graphs show the relationship between the ratio of Pi/PCr and workload in normal and heart failure subjects above and the relationship of muscle oxygenation assessed from 760- to 850-nm absorption below. Although the metabolic changes indicate reduced oxidative capacity in the CHF patients, there is no evidence of greater tissue deoxygenation. These findings suggest that the metabolic abnormality is intrinsic to the muscle rather than a result of reduce oxygen delivery. (Reproduced with permission from Reference 19.)

as a major factor underlying the metabolic abnormalities is provided as a study in which ^{31}P-spectra were obtained from the tibialis anterior muscle during peroneal nerve stimulation.[22] This protocol produced declines in PCr and pH quite similar to those observed during exercise protocols. However, since no external work was being performed, it is unlikely that the differences in muscle size could explain metabolic changes.

Reduced Muscle Oxidative Capacity

Because impairment of blood flow to exercising muscle is not the primary factor responsible for the metabolic changes, it must, at least in part, indicate reduced muscle oxidative capacity. This mechanism is supported by a growing number of biopsy studies. The most consistent finding has been a reduction in the percentage of type I slow twitch oxidative fibers and an increase in the proportion of fast twitch type II fibers.[17,18,23,24] In particular, there is an increase in the more glycolytic type IIb subtype and in intermediate staining type IIab fibers, which are thought to represent a transition from type IIa to type IIb fibers.[17,18,23] Because there is a stepwise decrease in oxidative capacity from type I to type IIa to type IIb fibers and since type II fibers exhibit more glycolytic metabolism, this change in muscle composition could explain the ^{31}P-MRS results. In addition, because type II fibers are more rapidly fatiguable, this phenomenon could also provide an explanation for the early onset of muscle fatigue. Other consistent findings from both human and animal studies have been a reduction in the content of a variety of oxidative enzymes in the skeletal muscles in CHF.[17,18,23,24]

Indeed, Arnolda et al,[25] used the rat infarct model of heart failure to demonstrate the relation between muscle metabolism and muscle biochemistry. Six to 8 weeks after myocardial infarction, ^{31}P-MRS spectra obtained from the distal hindlimb flexor muscles (gastrocnemius-plantaris-soleus group) during repetitive sciatic nerve stimulation demonstrated that the infarcted animals have a greater decline in PCr/(PCr + Pi) and in pH, as well as reduced force development. Changes were significantly correlated with the degree of heart failure, as assessed by measurements of infarct size. Most interestingly, there was a significant correlation between PCr concentration and the activity of citrate synthase, a mitochondrial oxidative enzyme (Figure 5). Although a similar relationship between ^{31}P-MRS findings in muscle biopsies from the human gastrocnemius muscle was not observed,[17] this may have represented a sampling error, because the gastrocnemius muscle is heterogenous and the spectra obtained by a surface coil may be contaminated by signal from the soleus muscle, which has substantially different fiber type composition.

Relationship of Oxidative Enzyme Activity to Muscle Metabolism in Rat CHF Model

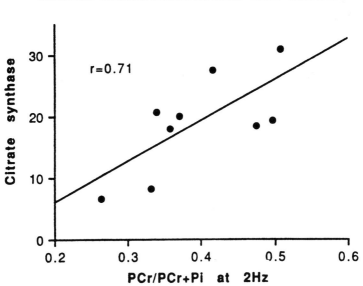

FIGURE 5. This plot illustrates the relation between citrate synthase activity and the ratio of PCr/(PCr + Pi) in rats with heart failure induced by left coronary artery ligation. Citrate synthase activity was measured in homogenates of the distal hindlimb flexor muscles, and ^{31}P-MRS spectra were obtained from the same muscle during repetitive sciatic nerve stimulation. The strong correlation suggests that the changes in energy-related phosphates may be determined by the oxidative capacity of the muscle. (Reproduced with permission from Reference 25.)

The importance of the reduced oxidative capacity of skeletal muscle is illustrated by the relation between succinate dehydrogenase activity in the quadriceps and systemic exercise capacity (Figure 6)[18] There was a strong correlation in CHF patients, but not in age-matched sedentary controls. This result suggests that the reduced ability of exercising muscle to use O_2 may limit exercise capacity in CHF patients, whereas exercise capacity is limited by cardiopulmonary focus in normal subjects.

Reduced Work Efficiency

As noted previously, some of the ^{31}P-MRS findings suggest a shift in the relationship between ATP consumption and force develop-

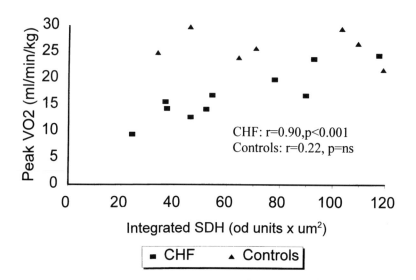

FIGURE 6. There is a strong relation between integrated succinate dehydrogenase (SDH) activity, which was reduced in all fiber types, and peak VO$_2$ in CHF patients ($r = 0.90$, $P < .001$). This finding suggests that the reduced oxidative capacity may be a limiting factor to these patients' exercise capacity. In contrast, there was no such relationship in the controls, indicating that their exercise tolerance is more likely limited by cardiopulmonary factors. (Reproduced with permission from Reference 18.)

ment.[12] This finding needs further confirmation, but it could be explained in part by early recruitment of the less efficient type IIb fibers at lower levels of exercise in heart failure patients. Another factor may be a degree of uncoupling between muscle activation and force development, which may be caused by alterations in the way that calcium is handled.[26,27]

^{31}P-MRS Studies of Exercise Training in Congestive Heart Failure

Although for many years it was considered prudent to limit the activity of patients suffering from CHF, the growing information about the changes in skeletal muscle has stimulated interest in exercise training in cardiac rehabilitation programs for these patients.[28,29] A number of studies have shown that an exercise training programs can be safely used and that they consistently improve exercise tolerance in patients with CHF. In addition, even in this population, many of the other goals of improved physical fitness can also be accomplished, including re-

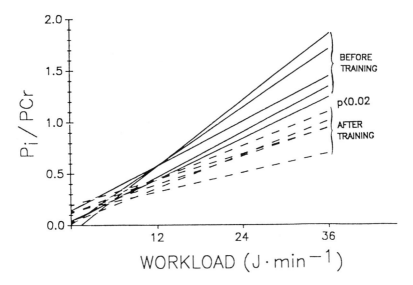

FIGURE 7. This graph shows the regression lines of the relationship of Pi/PCr vs. submaximal workload obtained from the forearm flexor muscles in five CHF patients before and after 1 month of low-level forearm training. Training resulted in a decreased slope in each patient, indicating improved oxidative metabolism. (Reproduced with permission from Reference 31.)

duced adrenergic nervous system activity, increased heart rate variability and improved ventilatory efficiency. Serial muscle biopsies performed during training demonstrate improved mitochondrial morphology and increased oxidative activity.[30] Several groups have studied ^{31}P-MRS spectroscopy before and after a period of training.[32–33] Figure 7 illustrates the improvement in oxidative metabolism observed in the forearm flexor muscles following a month period of low level forearm training.[31] The direction and the magnitude of these changes in heart failure patients are quite comparable to normal subjects undergoing training programs. Therefore, it is unclear whether the improved metabolism is the result of exercise training or if it is involved in the mechanism of improved exercise capacity.

Is There a Clinical Role for ^{31}P-MRS Congestive Heart Failure?

Thus far, this article has focused on the insights this technique has provided into the pathophysiology of exercise intolerance and skeletal muscle dysfunction in patients with heart failure. This reflects the fact that thus far, ^{31}P-MRS has been used solely as an investigational technique in this setting. However, a number of factors also make it unlikely that ^{31}P-MRS will have clinical application in this situation. First, this technique is somewhat cumbersome and technically demanding. There is also substantial variability in the spectroscopic results from day to day, with the results being effect by such factors as temperature, diet, and familiarity with the procedure. Second, heart failure is an extremely heterogenous syndrome. Muscle metabolism may be abnormal in mildly affected patients and be preserved in patients with relatively severe symptoms. Furthermore, it isn't clear whether clinical information which could impact on the management of individual patients can be provided by this technique, and if so, whether it offers any advantage to more traditional approaches to exercise testing. Lastly, many of the changes which are characteristic of patients with heart failure, namely more rapid PCr depletion and muscle acidification, are nonspecific. Similar findings have been reported in patients with peripheral vascular, pulmonary, and renal disease, and might be expected with anemia, muscle wasting, and many other conditions which often coexist with CHF.[34]

One group has used ^{31}P-MRS to evaluate patients after cardiac transplantation.[35] They observed that abnormalities observed prior to transplantation persisted and sometimes even appeared more severe, early (6 months) after transplantation. Among patients studied at later time points, several aspects of muscle metabolism remained abnormal, although the phosphocreatine resynthesis rate returned to normal, suggesting some late improvement in oxidative capacity. Thus, even in this setting where cardiac function is presumably normal or near normal, the recovery of muscle metabolism is quite variable. It is likely that this reflects an effect of immunosuppressive medications, such as corticosteroids and cyclosporin, and the variable levels of activity in posttransplantation patients.

Altered Muscle Metabolism in Congestive Heart Failure: Mechanism or Manifestation?

The results of the studies summarized above lead to the critical question of whether the abnormalities in skeletal muscle in CHF represent an important mechanism for exercise intolerance or whether they merely reflect the limited level of activity in these patients. Although, the data indicate that the changes are not solely due to reduced in blood flow to exercising muscle, the impaired oxidative capacity and increased glycolytic metabolism characteristic of heart failure patients are also expected responses to detraining and can be reversed by training protocols. As discussed previously, there is certainly circumstantial evidence that the muscle changes may play a role in the limitation of exercise in CHF. Unfortunately, ^{31}P-MRS alone cannot distinguish between these two possibilities. However, there is little doubt that this technique has played an important role in advancing our knowledge of the mechanisms of exercise intolerance in patients with CHF and has stimulated investigators to use other innovative approaches, often as adjuncts to ^{31}P-MRS, in addressing this problem.

In the end, it is likely that the missing answers will become apparent when the basic mechanisms governing the muscle changes at the molecular level are unraveled. We have used an animal model to examine the changes in skeletal gene expression in relationship to the severity of heart failure and monitored levels of activity.[36] In rats with hemodynamic evidence of heart failure 8 weeks after left coronary ligation, we found a changes in contractile protein and oxidative enzyme expression in the soleus and plantaris muscles compared with sham-operated controls. Succinate dehydrogenase activity and mRNA for cytochrome oxidase were reduced in both muscles. Importantly, the magnitude of these changes in gene expression correlated significantly with the severity of the heart failure, but was unrelated to quantitative measures of locomotor activity. These findings can best be explained by a primary abnormalities of skeletal muscle and highlight the significance of the original observations of the altered muscle metabolism in patients with CHF.

References

1. Franciosa JA, Park M, Levine TB. Lack of correlation between exercise capacity and indexes of resting left ventricular performance in heart failure. *Am J Cardiol.* 1981;47:33–39.
2. Szlachcic J, Massie BM, Kramer B, et al. Correlates and prognostic implication of exercise capacity in chronic congestive heart failure. *Am J Cardiol.* 1985;55:1037–1042.
3. Zelis R, Nellis SH, Longhurst J, et al. Abnormalities in the regional circulations accompanying congestive heart failure. *Prog Cardiovasc Dis.* 1975;72: 494–510.
4. Wilson JR, Martin JL, Schwartz D, Ferraro N. Exercise intolerance in patients with chronic heart failure: role of impaired nutritive flow to skeletal muscle. *Circulation.* 1984;69:1079–87.
5. Wilson JR, Mancini D, Dunkman B. Exertional fatigue due to intrinsic skeletal muscle dysfunction in patients with heart failure. *Circulation.* 1993;87: 470–475.
6. Taylor D, Bore PJ, Styles P, et al. Bioenergetics of intact human muscle a 31P nuclear magnet resonance study. *Mol Biol Med.* 1983;1:77–94.
7. Wilson JR, Fink L, Maris J, et al. Evaluation of energy metabolism in skeletal muscle of patients with heart failure with gated phosphorus-31 nuclear magnetic resonance. *Circulation.* 1985;71:57–62.

8. Massie BM, Conway M, Yonge R, et al. ^{31}P nuclear magnetic resonance evidence of abnormal skeletal muscle metabolism in patients with congestive heart failure. *Am J Cardiol.* 1987;60:309–315.
9. Massie BM, Conway M, Yonge R, et al. Skeletal muscle metabolism in patients with congestive heart failure. Relation to clinical severity and blood flow. *Circulation.* 1987;76:1009–1019.
10. Wiener DH, Fink LI, Maris J, et al. Abnormal skeletal muscle bioenergetics during exercise in patients with heart failure: role of reduced muscle blood flow. *Circulation.* 1986;73:1127–1136.
11. Wiener DH, Maris J, Chance B, Wilson JR. Detection of skeletal muscle hypoperfusion during exercise using phosphorus-31 nuclear magnetic resonance spectroscopy. *J Am Coll Cardiol.* 1986;7:793–799.
12. Massie BM, Conway M, Rajagopalan B, et al. Skeletal muscle metabolism during exercise under ischemic conditions: Evidence for abnormalities unrelated to blood flow. *Circulation.* 1988;78:320–6.
13. Mancini DM, Ferraro N, Tuchler M, et al. Detection of abnormal calf muscle metabolism in patients with heart failure using phosphorus-31 nuclear magnetic resonance. *Am J Cardiol.* 1988;62:1234–1240.
14. Arnolda L, Conway M, Dolecki M, et al. Skeletal muscle metabolism in heart failure: A ^{31}P nuclear magnetic resonance spectroscopy study of leg muscle. *Clin Science.* 1990;79:583–589.
15. Chati Z, Zannad F, Robin-Lherbier B, et al. Contribution of specific skeletal muscle metabolic abnormalities to limitation of exercise capacity in patients with chronic heart failure: A phosphorus 31 nuclear magnetic resonance study. *Am Heart J.* 1994;128:781–792.
16. Jondeau G, Katz SD, Zohman L, et al. Active skeletal muscle mass and cardiopulmonary reserve. Failure to attain peak aerobic capacity during maximal bicycle exercise in patients with severe congestive heart failure. *Circulation.* 1992;86:1351–1356.
17. Mancini DM, Coyle E, Coggan A, et al. Contribution of intrinsic skeletal muscle changes to 31P skeletal muscle metabolic abnormalities in patients with chronic heart failure. *Circulation.* 1989;80:1338–1346.
18. Massie BM, Simonini A, Sahgal P, et al. Relation of systemic and local muscle exercise capacity to skeletal muscle characteristics in men with congestive heart failure. *J Am Coll Cardiol.* 1996;27:140–145.
19. Mancini DM, Wilson JR, Bolinger L, et al. In vivo magnetic resonance spectroscopy measurement of deoxymyoglobin during exercise in patients with heart failure. Demonstration of abnormal muscle metabolism despite adequate oxygenation. *Circulation.* 1994;90:500–508.
20. Mancini DM, Walter G, Reichek N, et al. Contribution of skeletal muscle atrophy to exercise intolerance and altered muscle metabolism in heart failure. *Circulation.* 1992;85:1364–1373.
21. Minotti JR, Pillay P, Oka R, et al. Skeletal muscle size: relationship to muscle function in heart failure. *J Appl Physiol.* 1993;373–381.
22. Kao W, Helpern JA, Goldstein S, et al. Abnormalities of skeletal muscle metabolism during nerve stimulation determined by 31P nuclear magnetic resonance spectroscopy in severe congestive heart failure. *Am J Cardiol.* 1995;76:606–609.
23. Sullivan MJ, Green HJ, Cobb FR. Skeletal muscle biochemistry and histology in ambulatory patients with long-term heart failure. *Circulation.* 1990; 81:518–27.
24. Drexler H, Riede U, Munzel T, et al. Alterations of skeletal muscle in chronic heart failure. *Circulation.* 1992;85:1751–1759.

25. Arnolda L, Brosnan J, Rajagopalan B, Radda GK. Skeletal muscle metabolism in heart failure in rats. *Am J Physiol.* 1991;261:H434–H442.
26. Perreault CL, Gonzalez-Serratos H, Litwin SE, et al. Alterations in contractility and intracellular Ca^{2+} transients in isolated bundles of skeletal muscle fibers from rats with chronic heart failure. *Circ Res.* 1993;73:405–412.
27. Simonini A, Long CS, Yue P, et al. Expression of skeletal muscle sarcoplasmic reticulum Ca^{2+}-ATPase is reduced in experimental heart failure. *Circulation.* 1995;92(Suppl I):I258–9. Abstract.
28. Coats AJS. Exercise rehabilitation in chronic heart failure. *J Am Coll Cardiol.* 1193;32(Suppl A):172A–177A.
29. McKelyie RS, Teo KK, McCartney N, et al. Effects of exercise training in patients with congestive heart failure: A critical review. *J Am Coll Cardiol.* 1995;25:789–796.
30. Hambrecht R, Niebauer J, Fiehn E, et al. Physical training in patients with stable chronic heart failure: Effects on cardiorespiratory fitness and ultrastructural abnormalities of leg muscles. *J Am Coll Cardiol.* 1995;25:1239–1249.
31. Minotti JR, Johnson EC, Hudson TL, et al. Skeletal muscle response to exercise training in congestive heart failure. *J Clin Invest.* 1990;86:751–758.
32. Adamopoulos S, Coats AJS, Brunotte F, et al. Physical training improves skeletal muscle metabolism in patients with chronic heart failure. *J Am Coll Cardiol.* 1993;21:1101–1106.
33. Stratton J, Dunn JF, Adamopoulos S, et al. Training partially reverses skeletal muscle metabolic abnormalities during exercise in heart failure. *J Appl Physiol.* 1994;76:1575–1582.
34. Kent-Braun JA, Miller RG, Weiner MW. Magnetic resonance spectroscopy studies of human muscle. *Radiology Clin North Am.* 1994;32:313–335.
35. Stratton J, Kemp GJ, Daly RC, et al. Effects of cardiac transplantation on bioenergetic abnormalities of skeletal muscle in congestive heart failure. *Circulation.* 1994;89:1624–1631.
36. Simonini A, Long CS, Yue P, et al. Heart failure in rats causes changes in skeletal muscle morphology and gene expression which are not explained by reduced activity. Circ Res. 1996;79:128–136.

## Chapter 29

Critical Oxygen and Myoglobin Function in Myocardium

Youngran Chung, MD, PhD
and Thomas Jue, PhD

Detection of Intracellular Myoglobin by 1H Nuclear Magnetic Resonance

The ^{1}H nuclear magnetic resonance (NMR) signals of cytosolic myoglobin (Mb) offer an opportunity to observe intracellular oxygenation in the myocardium.[1-3] Oxygen is fundamental in maintaining cellular viability and is central to the bioenergetics of oxidative phosphorylation. Yet the presumed familiarity with its importance often overlooks the numerous uncertainties about its cellular interactions *in vivo*. Measuring the intracellular oxygen (O_2) level has been a major stumbling block. What is the critical oxygen level that limits respiration *in vivo*? How does the cell sense limiting oxygen concentration and signal the appropriate cellular response? Does myoglobin facilitate oxygen transport in the myocyte, especially during postischemic reperfusion? Only a reliable measurement of intracellular oxygen under various physiological conditions will remove some of the uncertainties and the questions.

Because ^{1}H NMR can detect myoglobin signals in the intact muscle tissue, certain spectral changes can now reflect the intracellular oxygen tension (pO_2). Ligated with oxygen, the heme Fe(II) electrons are paired ($S=0$), and MbO_2 is diamagnetic. Unligated with oxygen, the heme Fe(II) electrons are unpaired ($S=2$), and deoxy Mb is paramagnetic.

Grant Support: NIH GM 44916, American Heart Association Grant, CA Affiliate 92-221A, National Research Service Award, NZH HL09274 (YC).

From: Higgins CB, Ingwall JS, Pohost GM, (eds). *Current and Future Applications of Magnetic Resonance in Cardiovascular Disease.* Armonk, NY: Futura Publishing Company, Inc.; © 1998.

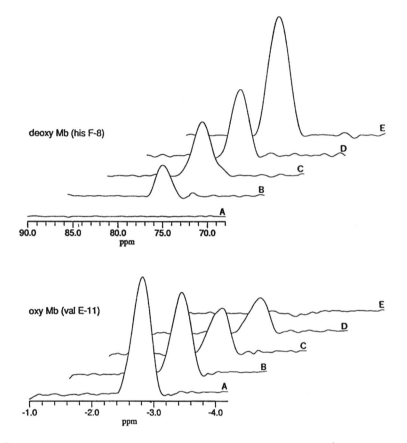

FIGURE 1. Mb histidyl NH and Val E11 signals from myocardium. ^1H NMR spectra of MbO_2 and deoxy Mb in myocardium under various ischemic conditions: Hearts were perfused at different flow rate, 11 mL/min **(A)**, 3 mL/min **(B)**, 2 mL/min **(C)**, 1 mL/min **(D)**, and 0 mL/min **(E)**. Top trace shows the response of the proximal histidyl NH signal; bottom trace, the Val E11 signal. The Val E11 signal intensity decreases with decreasing flow rate or oxygenation, the proximal histidyl NH signal varies inversely (Reproduced with permission from Reference 3.)

The shift in the Fe electronic state gives rise to contrasting electron-nuclear interactions with the F8 proximal histidine, such that in the deoxygenated state the distinct NH reporter signal appears and reflects the extent of cellular deoxygenation in the myocardium.[3,4]

Figure 1 shows a bank of spectra from an approximately 1-g perfused rat heart under graded ischemic conditions. The top panel shows the spectral region between 100–60 ppm. Under well-oxygenated conditions no signal appears. As the perfusion flow rate decreases, the proximal histidyl NH signal at 80 ppm increases, reaching maximum intensity at 0 mL/min perfusate flow (Figure 1E). The signal disappears on 11 mL/min reflow with oxygen saturated buffer. A similar spectral pattern is observed during graded hypoxia.[5] In these experiments, the signal intensity under 0 mL/min perfusate flow is normalized to 100% signal intensity, which in turn is the basis to determine the MbO_2 fraction as well as cellular oxygenation at the intermediate experimental points, given the $[pO_2]_{50}$ value of 1.5 mm Hg.[3,4]

However, using only the proximal histidyl NH signal to measure intracellular oxygen has two drawbacks. The 100% normalization point is required to quantitate the oxyMb fraction. In many *in vivo* and potential clinical applications, assessing the signal intensity during total ischemia or 100% desaturation point is impractical and is unachievable. Moreover, the deoxy Mb signal intensity has its maximum signal to noise only when the myocytes are severely hypoxic or ischemic. For the clinically relevant cases where the detection of the mild hypoxic/ischemic myocardium is critical, the deoxy Mb signal has its lowest signal to noise.

Detecting the Val E11 γ-CH_3, an oxyMb reporter signal, has alleviated many constraints associated with using the Mb technique to detect the full range of the physiologically relevant tissue oxygenation. Figure 1, bottom panel, shows that the Val E11 signal, reflecting the oxygenated state, is also detectable in perfused rat myocardium.[3] Under well-oxygenated conditions, the Val E11 signal is detected at -2.8 ppm, whereas the proximal histidyl NH signal at 80 ppm is not (Figure 1). Conversely, at 0 mL/min, the proximal histidyl NH signal intensity reaches the maximum, and the Val E11 signal becomes undetectable. A dynamic equilibrium exists between the Val E11 and His F8 signals, such that one resonance's intensity is balanced by the other under all oxygenation conditions. The sum of the signal intensities of the two Mb peaks is constant. On reoxygenation, the Val E11 signal reappears at the same chemical shift position. Introducing carbon monoxide into the perfusate shifts the Val E11 signal to -2.4 ppm, as assigned in NMR protein studies.[6]

Critical pO_2 and Energy Metabolism in the Myocardium

Critical pO_2 in Hypoxic Myocardium

The myocardial Mb signals provide a unique opportunity to measure the *in vivo* critical pO_2, the oxygen level when cellular respiration

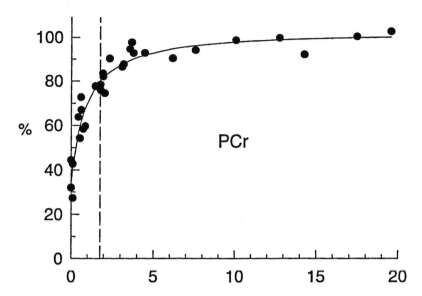

FIGURE 2. Graph of PCr versus pO_2. The interaction between PCr and intracellular oxygen level. PCr was measured from the ^{31}P spectra, the oxygen level from the 1H NMR signal of Mb Val E11. The critical pO_2 is ~1.8 mm Hg. Y axis refers to percent PCr normalized to control value; x axis refers to pO_2 in mm of Hg (Reproduced with permission from Reference 5).

becomes limiting. Figure 2 shows a correlation between phosphocreatine (PCr) and intracellular oxygen level, derived from NMR observations. PCr is readily detectable in the phosphorus (^{31}P) NMR spectra. Above 1.8 mm Hg of oxygen the PCr level remains stable. However, below the 1.8 mm Hg threshold, the PCr level drops precipitously. Graphs displaying the interactions between the intracellular oxygen versus ATP level, oxygen consumption (MVO_2), rate pressure product (RPP), all exhibit a critical pO_2. However, the exact points appear at different cellular pO_2.[5,7] Limiting oxygenation produces a series of sequential responses in hypoxic or ischemic myocardium, starting first with changes in RPP and lactate and then following with decreases in MVO_2 and PCr (Table 1). Moreover ischemic myocardium shows a critical pO_2 in its RPP, lactate, MVO_2 and PCr responses at a higher oxygen concentration than hypoxic myocardium.[7]

The metabolic and functional responses elicited under hypoxia and ischemia may contribute to the contrasting critical pO_2 points. Ischemic myocardium often suffers more damage than hypoxic myocardium due to a delayed metabolite clearance, which contributes to a pronounced intracellular H^+ accumulation. In the ischemic myocardium pH de-

TABLE 1

Physiological Index versus MbO$_2$ Saturation

Metabolic inc	n	Slope ± S.E.	y intercept ± S.E.	r	MbO$_2$ 50%	pO$_2$ 50%
			Control			
RPP	4	1.24 ± 0.10	−21.44 ± 8.13	0.933	57.6	2.04
PCr	5	0.63 ± 0.03	33.19 ± 2.23	0.970	26.7	0.55
Pi	5	−0.20 ± 0.02	31.06 ± 1.44	0.892	77.7	5.21
pH	5	0.002 ± 0.0003	7.03 ± 0.02	0.814		
Lactate	6	−0.08 ± 0.01	10.06 ± 0.47	0.981	62.9	2.54
mVO$_2$	6	0.96 ± 0.06	1.99 ± 4.81	0.967	50.0	1.50
			Postischemic			
RPP	24					
PCr	23	0.71 ± 0.05	26.72 ± 3.26	0.951	32.8	0.73
Pi	24	−0.18 ± 0.03	28.16 ± 1.65	0.833	78.2	5.39
pH	20	0.002 ± 0.0004	7.05 ± 0.02	0.809		
Lactate	4	−0.08 ± 0.01	9.37 ± 0.67	0.967	58.6	2.12
mVO$_2$	15	1.05 ± 0.06	−0.63 ± 4.39	0.977	48.2	1.40

* PCr, RPP, and MVO$_2$ values are normalized to control values as 100%. For Pi, the values are normalized to control PCr. Lactate is reported as μmol/min/g dry wt. The pH value is calculated from the chemical shift of Pi. The Mb saturation and pO$_2$ points are reported at 50% of maximal value.

clines from 7.27 to 7.03, as MbO$_2$ saturation approaches 0.[5,7] In contrast, the hypoxic myocardium maintains a relatively constant pH between 7.17 and 7.21 throughout a wide range of oxygenation conditions.

When plotted against MbO$_2$ saturation, all the metabolic indices measurable by ^{31}P NMR, MVO$_2$, and RPP display a linear relation.[5,7] The linear relation between MVO$_2$ and Mb saturation implies a steep O$_2$ gradient between the cytosolic and mitochondrial compartments even at low temperature, 25°C. Normalized MVO$_2$ (%) maintains one-to-one relation with MbO$_2$ saturation with the y intercept = 0 (Figure 3), even though the [pO$_2$]$_{50}$ for Mb is 1–2 mm Hg, whereas [pO$_2$]$_{50}$ for cytochrome oxidase is approximately ~0.1 mm Hg.[8] An order of magnitude difference in [pO$_2$]$_{50}$ values then requires that the cytosol maintains a substantially higher O$_2$ concentration than the mitochondrial compartment under a wide oxygenation range.[9,10]

The widespread linear relation between the physiological/metabolic indices versus percent MbO$_2$ saturation reveals a potential coherent metabolic and physiological response to cellular oxygenation, which may involve a common effector, such as nicotinamide adenine dinucleotide (NADH).[7,8]

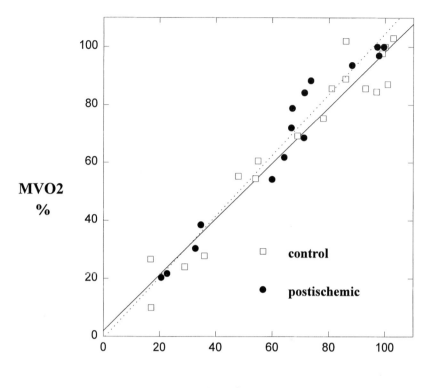

MVO2 %

MbO2, %

FIGURE 3. Oxygen consumption vs. MbO$_2$ saturation in both the control (□) and postischemic hearts (●). Oxygen consumption also shows a linear relationship with Mb oxygen saturation, which shows no significant deviation between the control (———) and postischemic (⋯⋯⋯) hearts (Reproduced with permission from Reference 7).

Critical pO$_2$ in the Postischemic Myocardium

Intracellular Oxygen Level in the Postischemic Myocardium

With a sudden onset of global ischemia, myocardial MbO$_2$ desaturates completely within minutes.[7] The Mb desaturation and the left ventricular developed pressure (LVDP) reduction curves coincide and drop to 0 within 15 minutes. Heart function in the initial phase of ischemic decline, therefore, seems to be largely determined by intracellular O$_2$ availability. The extrapolated curves indicate an apparent t$_{50\%}$ (time to reach 50% of the control level) of 0.9 minutes. The analysis yields a time frame for metabolic decline after ischemia that is consistent with the reported $t_{50\%}$ approximately 2.5 minutes for PCr depletion.[11]

During postischemic reperfusion intracellular oxygen is rapidly replenished.[7] The final steady state intracellular oxygen level is reached within 5 to 10 minutes after reperfusion. The steady-state values of intracellular oxygen in the postischemic myocardium, however, are consistently lower than the ones observed in the control ischemic myocardium (Figure 4A). Only at high flow rate reperfusion, 12 mL/min, does the postischemic value begin to approach the control one. In the control heart, a 12 mL/min perfusion with fully oxygenated buffer delivers 685 mm Hg O_2 to saturate cellular myoglobin at 25°C. Despite the common notion that the oxygen supply in blood-free buffer perfusion is inadequate,[12] no significant increase in the oxyMb Val E11 signal is noted above the perfusion flow rate of 6 mL/min at 25°C, indicating fully saturated MbO_2 (Figure 4A). At approximately 2.5 mL/min perfusion flow rate, the Mb saturation reduces to 80% of control and thereafter decreases rapidly. In contrast, the profile for the postischemic myocardium shows consistently lower steady-state value of Mb saturation at each corresponding flow rate. The critical flow rate, defined as the flow rate corresponding to 80% of maximum MbO_2 saturation, has shifted from 2.5 mL/min to 6 mL/min.[7]

Depressed intracellular oxygenation in the postischemic myocardium may arise from either altered cellular bioenergetics or vascular impedance. MVO_2 versus Mb saturation relation in the postischemic myocardium favors a vascular, rather than a cellular, site for O_2 resistance in the postischemic myocardium. MVO_2 profiles in the control and postischemic myocardium (Figure 3), match closely and show no significant differences in their responses to varying oxygen levels. A similar pattern appears when other metabolite indices are correlated with MbO_2 saturation. Postischemic oxygen consumption per given intracellular O_2 and its cellular oxygen gradient have not changed significantly. The results suggest that the depressed postischemic O_2 level originates from an alteration in vascular O_2 conductance.[13]

Researchers have already demonstrated that prolonged myocardial ischemia can produce irreversible cellular damage and persistent structural and functional derangement in the coronary vasculature even after full reperfusion.[14] However, they have not reached consensus on the effect of transient, reversible ischemia. Some studies report normal resting coronary reflow in the stunned myocardium, while others have observed a decreased reflow rate.[15] The ^{1}H NMR results are consistent with a vascular resistance in supplying reperfused oxygen, which is pronounced at low reflow.[7]

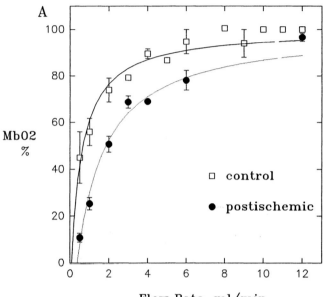

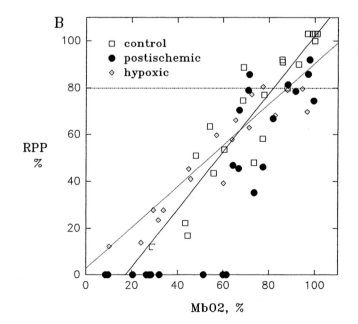

Critical pO_2 of Functional and Metabolic Recovery in the Postischemic Myocardium

Despite rapid entry of O_2 after reperfusion, the postischemic RPP remains depressed. Such prolonged postischemic RPP depression is characteristic of the stunned myocardium.[16] In addition to the classic description of stunned myocardium, a postischemic condition with adequate O_2 supply, postischemic reperfusion at reduced flow rates appears to completely block myocardial recovery.[7] Myocardial function does not recover below reperfusion flow rate, 3 mL/min, which coincides with 2.5 mm Hg pO_2 or 63% MbO_2 saturation (Figure 4B). Above the threshold point, RPP recovers abruptly. At 3 mL/min reperfusion, RPP reaches only 43% of control. From 4 mL/min to 12 mL/min reflow, the RPP remains at 80% of control.

Figure 4B also shows the RPP response to the varying O_2 concentrations at a constant reflow rate, 12 mL/min, which creates a graded hypoxic reperfusion rather than an ischemic one. Reperfusion with graded oxygenated buffer and at 12 mL/min flow rate permits the myocardium to maintain a linear relation between RPP and MbO_2 saturation. The O_2 threshold phenomenon is no longer present. Limitation in the intracellular oxygen level does not appear to be the sole basis for the threshold phenomenon noted under graded flow reperfusion with fully oxygenated buffer. The failure of functional recovery under <3 mL/min reperfusion also does not appear to coincide with H^+ clear-

◄────────────────────────────

FIGURE 4. **A:** Mb oxygen saturation versus flow rate in both the control (□) and postischemic hearts (●). In the control heart, the graph of MbO_2 versus flow rate shows that the 80% Mb saturation point is slightly below 2.4 mL/min and conforms closely to a hyperbolic curve. In the postischemic heart, the 80% point has shifted substantially to 6.3 mL/min, but still follows a hyperbolic curve. At all flow rates below 6 mL/min, however, the postischemic myocardium displays a significantly lower Mb oxygen saturation level than control. **B:** RPP versus Mb oxygen saturation in control heart (□), in the postischemic heart reperfused with O_2 saturated buffer at different flow rates (●), and in the postischemic heart reperfused with different concentration of O_2 buffer at a constant 12 mL/min flow rate (◇). RPP is a linear function of Mb oxygen saturation level in the control heart and drops to 0 when MbO_2 is at 17% saturation. In the postischemic myocardium RPP does not recover until MbO_2 saturation reaches a threshold of 63%. At that point, the RPP begins abruptly. At 3 mL/min reperfusion, RPP reaches 43% of control. With reperfusion rates from 4–12 mL/min, RPP recovers only to 80% of control level, even though increasing flow rates elevates the intracellular oxygen level (see Figure 4A). Reperfusion with different concentrations of O_2 buffer at 12 mL/min flow rate produces a linear relationship that does not show a threshold effect (Reproduced with permission from Reference 7.)

ance or inorganic phosphate (Pi) accumulation. Although researchers have implicated Pi and proton as significant inhibitors of myofibril contraction,[17,18] neither Pi nor pH relation with intracellular oxygen in the postischemic myocardium deviates significantly from the control myocardium.[7] The potential accumulation of H^+ and/or Pi, therefore, fails to provide a satisfactory explanation for the postischemic functional depression at high flow reperfusion as well as total lack of recovery during low flow reperfusion.

Energy Production versus Utilization in Postischemic Myocardium

A comparable relation between MVO_2/PCr and percent MbO_2 saturation in both the control and the postischemic myocardium implies that the respiration and the oxidative energy production in the postischemic myocardium is not disrupted.[7] In addition, the control and the postischemic hearts show a similar nonoxidative energy capacity. As O_2 and MVO_2 approach 0 the cell can still provide a residual nonoxidative source of energy, as reflected in the >5 time increase (1.78 to 10 μmol/min/g dry weight) in lactate formation, to maintain the PCr level at 33% of control, despite the demands from ion pumps and the losses in the adenine nucleotide pool.[7]

In addition to glycolytic supplementation, myocardium appears to conserve energy by reducing the contractile work. Figure 4B shows that RPP reduces to 0, reaching a basal quiescent state, when Mb saturation is still at 17%. The corresponding MVO_2 in the noncontracting quiescent state is 19% of the control MVO_2, 2.6 μmol O_2/min/g dry weight.[7,19] The lactate formation rate when MbO_2 saturation reaches 17% is 9 μmol/min/g dry weight. With an assumed P/O ratio 3:1, the total ATP synthesis rate, oxidative and non-oxidative, is then 24.6 μmol/min/g dry weight, a basal energy requirement in the noncontracting heart. In the hypoxic myocardium, which maintains contractile activity until the MbO_2 reaches 0 a quiescent state, defined as a noncontracting yet O_2 consuming state, is virtually absent. A pronounced intracellular acidification in the ischemic myocardium may produce a premature cessation of myocardial contraction in response to O_2 limitation.

Because the cellular energy production in the postischemic myocardium remains intact, the depressed RPP even at high flow reperfusion arises most likely from an altered energy utilization. Reduced Ca^{++} sensitivity of contractile proteins or free radical damage may be the causal links to the impaired energy utilization in the stunned myocardium, even though the specific relationship to cellular pO_2 is presently unclear.[16]

Physiological Role of Myoglobin Probed by *in vivo* Nuclear Magnetic Resonance

Introduction

According to the conventional biochemical view, the primary physiological role of myoglobin is oxygen storage. Researchers also have postulated that it can facilitate oxygen diffusion through the sarcoplasm.[20] Recent myocyte studies, however, have challenged that view. Under oxygenation conditions that far exceed mitochondrial demand, as reflected by an unperturbed cytochrome aa_3 state, either nitrite or carbon monoxide inhibition of the oxygen binding function of Mb produces a decline in MVO_2 and phosphocreatine.[21–23] Even though Mb will no longer facilitate O_2 diffusion under these nonlimiting O_2 conditions, it appears to have a role in directly regulating respiration.[22,23]

So far, mainly myocyte nitrite inhibition experiments have supported the hypothesis. In contrast, perfused myocardium results are equivocal.[24–26] The ambiguous results arise potentially from the uncertain extent of nitrite inhibition of Mb in the myocardium, because previous techniques cannot confidently detect Mb oxidation kinetics *in vivo*. Even though the nitrite oxidation reaction from Fe(II) MbO_2 to Fe (III) metMb is a well-established one *in vitro*, the *in vivo* kinetics is uncertain, given that the contribution from nitrite transport, nitrite reductase as well as metMb reductase activity *in vivo* is poorly characterized.[27,28] As a result the postulated new role of Mb in regulating respiration needs clarification by studying the function of Mb *in vivo*.

Nitrite Inactivation of Myocardial Mb

Oxidation of Mb in the Perfused Myocardium

Figure 5 shows ^1H and ^{31}P NMR spectra of control and nitrite perfused heart. During the control period, O_2 saturated perfusate flowing at 16 mL/min keep the myocardium well oxygenated. At 37°C, MbO_2 signal is kept high until the perfusion flow rate is reduced to 12 mL/min. Reference ^1H NMR spectrum shows fully saturated MbO_2 signal (Figure 5a′). Even with 10 mM nitrite, Mb oxidation does not proceed as indicated by the constant signal intensity of the γ-CH$_3$ Val

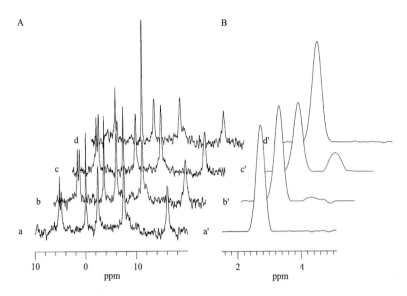

FIGURE 5. ^1H and ^{31}P NMR spectra of perfused myocardium infused with varying concentrations of nitrite. **A:** The ^{31}P spectra are shown from a-d. **(a)** control; **(b)** 10 mM nitrite; **(c)** 30 mM nitrite **(d)** reperfusion. **B:** The corresponding ^1H spectra are shown from a'-d'. **(a')** control ^1H spectrum from myocardium perfused with nitrite-free, oxygen saturated buffer flowing at 16 mL/min. The γ-CH$_3$ Val E11 signal of MbO$_2$ appears at -2.8 ppm and reflects full oxygen saturation. **(b')** With 10 mM nitrite infusion, the ^1H spectrum shows a modest decrease in the γ-CH$_3$ Val E11 signal of MbO$_2$. A signal corresponding to metMb emerges at -3.9 ppm. **(c')** With 30 mM nitrite infusion, the -3.9 ppm signal of metMb becomes prominent. The signal intensity increase in the metMb signal matches the decrease in the MbO$_2$ signal. **(d')** Upon reperfusion with nitrite free, oxygen saturated buffer, the metMb signal disappears and the γ-CH$_3$ Val E11 signal of MbO$_2$ regains its full intensity (Reproduced with permission from Reference 26.)

E11 peak (Figure 5b'). However with 30 mM nitrite, Mb oxidation is noticeable. The oxy Mb Val E11 signal decreases to 65% of control level, while a peak at -3.9 ppm, assigned to a three-proton amino acid residue in metMb, increases to 24% with respect to the fully saturated γ-CH$_3$ Val E11 signal of MbO$_2$ (Figure 5c').[29] The half-height linewidth ratio of the metMb/MbO$_2$ reporter signals is 1.6/1, consistent with the contrasting relaxation of the paramagnetic metMb relative to the diamagnetic MbO$_2$. Upon reperfusion with oxygen saturated, but nitrite free buffer, the Mb oxidation is reversed, and the γ-CH$_3$ Val E11 signal intensity recovers fully, while the metMb signal disappears (Figure 5d').

In vitro experiments indicate that a 2/1 stoichiometry of NO$^-_2$/MbO$_2$

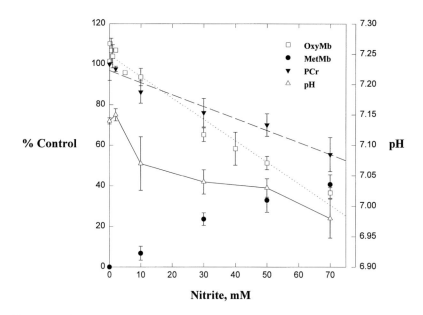

Nitrite, mM

FIGURE 6. Graphs of the metabolic responses in the myocardium upon infusion with nitrite. The MbO_2, metMb, PCr, and pH response. MbO_2 and metMb levels are reflected by the γ-CH_3 Val E11 and the metMb reporter signal at -2.8 and -3.9 ppm, respectively (Reproduced with permission from Reference 26.)

is sufficient to completely oxidize Mb to metMb.[27] With 0.4 mM infused nitrite, myocardial MbO_2 should convert completely then to metMb. Surprisingly, Figure 5B shows that nitrite does not significantly alter either the MbO_2 signal or produce any evidence of a metMb peak until the nitrite concentration exceeds 10 mM. The result is in contrast to previous studies, which report Mb oxidation with nitrite concentration at less than 10 mM.[24,25]

The fraction of Mb converted to metMb depends linearly on the infused nitrite concentrations, Figure 6. Nitrite oxidation, however, does not seem to convert stoichiometrically MbO_2 to metMb, as indicated by the differences in the slopes of their changes, $Y = -1.10X + 105$ for MbO_2 and $Y = 0.59X + 1.9$ for metMb (Figure 6). Nitrite oxidation of Mb may include side reactions, such as nitrimyoglobin formation.[30]

The high nitrite concentration required for oxidizing cellular MbO_2 may imply the presence of an extremely robust metMb reductase activity or limitation in nitrite transport. Complete oxidation would require over 160 mM infused nitrite, as extrapolated from the metMb graph in Figure 6. Although limitation in nitrite transport could explain in part the contrasting perfused myocardium and myocyte results, it is likely that sufficient nitrite, even at low concentration, has entered the cell to produce a distinct RPP response with a biphasic junction point at 0.4 mM nitrite. Infusing the myocardium with 0.05 mM nitrite already elicits a significant drop in RPP.[26] These observations tend to argue against a transport limitation, even though the direct experimental evidence is still required.

If nitrite transport is not limiting, then 30 mM infused nitrite oxidizes MbO_2 to metMb in the myocardium to yield a product ratio of metMb/MbO_2 of 0.37. MetMb/MbO_2 equilibrium *in vivo*, therefore, is shifted in favor of MbO_2, from the near-complete conversion to metMb expected from the *in vitro* oxidation kinetics.[26–28] The presence of a robust metMb reductase activity is also supported by reperfusion data. Immediately after reperfusion with nitrite-free medium, after a period of 70 mM nitrite infusion, the metMb signal disappears within 5 minutes.

Mb Role in Mediating Oxidative Phosphorylation

Even though some myocyte studies have indicated that nitrite oxidation of Mb can inhibit respiration under nonlimiting oxygen condition, perfused heart data suggest that the interaction is somewhat different.[24–26] In the perfused myocardium, neither the ^{31}P metabolite signal intensities nor the pH exhibits any significant changes with 0–5 mM nitrite infusion. MVO_2 remains constant, but RPP starts to decline at nitrite concentration as low as 0.05 mM.[26] At 5 mM infused nitrite, RPP decreases by 26%. With increasing nitrite infusion, 10 mM − 70 mM, RPP continues to decline, reaching 64% of control at 30 mM nitrite. MVO_2 is still unperturbed while the ^{1}H NMR spectra indicate the increasing presence of metMb. At 30 mM nitrite, both the PCr concentration and pH show significant changes from the control values (Figure 5c). At 70 mM nitrite, RPP has dropped to 40% of resting level, and MVO_2 shows a slight rise. Upon reperfusion with nitrite free, oxygen saturated buffer, the PCr signal intensity reaches 123% of control, while the ATP level is depressed, 81% of control (Figure 5d). The RPP returns only to 75% of the control value.[26]

The perfused myocardium results are in contrast to the observations of isolated myocyte studies. These myocyte studies have reported a 30% MVO_2 and PCr decrease on 2 mM nitrite infusion.[22,23] The perfused myocardium exhibits no corresponding alterations under similar experimental conditions. Presently it is uncertain what gives rise to the contrasting observations in myocytes and perfused hearts.

Changes in both Mb signals and PCr at high concentration nitrite are linearly dependent on nitrite concentration. As a result, PCr decreases linearly with MbO_2 desaturation, $Y = 0.62X + 35.1$, where $Y = \%PCr$ and $X = \%MbO_2$.[26] The linear extrapolation to 0% MbO_2 saturation indicates that non-Mb dependent reactions can still supply sufficient energy to maintain the residual PCr at 35% of control. The same results are observed in myocardium perfused with decreasing oxygenated buffer ($Y = 0.63X + 33$).[5,7] The similarity in PCr responses between Mb inhibited, normoxic heart, and hypoxic myocardium suggests that Mb inhibition does affect oxidative phosphorylation, as if corresponding amount of oxygen were limiting. On the other hand, MVO_2 is constant throughout the wide ranges of MbO_2 saturation. At 70 mM nitrite, MVO_2 even rises slightly. The constant MVO_2 is certainly consistent with a nonlimiting oxygen condition and is in agreement with the observation that Mb may not significantly contribute to the facilitated O_2 diffusion under normoxic condition.[25]

To compensate for the PCr drop, an enhanced glycolytic ATP production should occur. Indeed lactate formation rate increases dramatically upon Mb oxidation.[26] Intracellular pH also drops significantly from 7.14 to 6.98 at 70 mM nitrite (Figure 6). Even though MVO_2 is constant, PCr level still declines, despite stimulated glycolytic ATP production. Such observations suggest that Mb oxidation may uncouple the respiration from oxidative ATP synthesis. The contribution from a nonspecific nitrite effect and the biochemical mechanism underlying the energy uncoupling are uncertain at this time.

As in hypoxic/ischemic myocardium, nitrite inhibited myocardium exhibits the asynchronous metabolic responses to limiting O_2.[26] RPP is reduced even at very low nitrite concentration, lactate production then increases, followed by decrease in PCr. The sequential metabolic/physi-ological response to nitrite parallels the one observed in hypoxic/ischemic myocardium, which shows RPP decline and lactate increase before MVO_2 and PCr decrease.[5,7]

Transient Effect of Nitrite

Aside from modulating respiration, nitrite or nitrite oxidation of Mb affects the myocardium as if it were stunned. In the stunned myocardium, reperfusion after a transient global ischemia produces a prolonged RPP depression. After the reperfusion, PCr characteristically overshoots and MVO_2 returns to its control level, but ATP level remains depressed.[31] The myocardial recovery after nitrite exposure shows a similar manifestation. Infusion of high concentration of nitrite causes a drop in RPP, PCr, and intracellular pH. Reperfusion with nitrite-free buffer elicits a PCr overshoot initially to 123%, which returns gradually to control level; ATP remains depressed at 81% of control. RPP never recovers fully, but reaches only 75% of the control level. The functional depression may point to the involvement of metMb, whose Fe(III) can participate in free radical generation.[32] However, at present the relation between free radicals, metMb, and the myocardial response to a nitrite challenge is currently uncertain.

Summary

^{1}H NMR can detect myoglobin signals in the myocardium. These signals reflect the oxygen tension in the muscle tissue, including perfused myocardium and *in situ* skeletal muscle. The technique offers an opportunity to investigate a wide range of physiological and relies on the quantitative measurement of the Val E11 γ-CH3 signal from oxyMb and His F8 NH signal from deoxyMb. The intracellular pO_2 then is obtained, based on the $[pO_2]_{50}$.

In the myocardium, the critical pO_2s, the partial pressure of oxygen when the metabolite or physiological indices fall to 80% of their control values, are not identical. They show an asynchronous response. Moreover the critical pO_2 for the ischemic heart occurs at a higher oxygen tension than the corresponding hypoxic heart. On the other hand, postischemic reperfusion after a transient ischemic episode does not shift any of the metabolic/physiological critical pO_2 values. However, the cellular oxygen is depressed relative to the control myocardium, despite a rapid oxygen reentry. The experimental results implicate an alteration in the vascular O_2 conductance.

Nitrite inactivation of Mb indicates that Mb maybe involved in modulating oxidative phosphorylation. High-energy reserves decline in the nitrite inhibited myocardium with no comparable changes in the oxygen consumption. Although the contribution from the nonspecific nitrite effect is currently unclear, either the loss of MbO_2 or the presence of metMb triggers an uncoupling of mitochondrial oxidative phosphorylation. Moreover, the metMb reductase activity in the myocardium appears to be extremely robust.

References

1. Jue T, Anderson S. [1]H observation of tissue myoglobin: an indicator of intracellular oxygenation in vivo. *Magn Res Med.* 1990;13:524–528.
2. Wang Z, Noyszewski EA, Leigh JS. In vivo MRS measurement of deoxymyoglobin in human forearms. *Magn Res Med.* 1990;14:562–567.
3. Kreutzer U, Wang DS, Jue T. Observing the 1H NMR Signal of the myoglobin val E11 in myocardium: An index of cellular oxygenation. *Proc Natl Acad Sci USA.* 1992;89:4731–4733.

4. Kreutzer U, Jue T. 1H nuclear magnetic resonance deoxymyoglobin signal as indicator of intracellular oxygenation in Myocardium. *Am J Physiol.* 1991; 30:H2091–H2097.
5. Kreutzer U, Jue T. Critical intracellular oxygen in the myocardium as determined with the 1H NMR signal of myoglobin. *Am J Physiol.* 1995;268: H1675–H1681.
6. Shulman RG, Wuthrich K, Yamane T, et al. Nuclear magnetic resonance determination of ligand-induced conformational changes in myoglobin. *J Mol Biol.* 1970;53:143–157.
7. Chung Y, Jue T. Cellular response to reperfused oxygen in the postischemic myocardium. *Am J Physiol.* 1996;271:H687–H695.
8. Heineman FW, Balaban RS. Control of mitochondrial respiration in the heart in vivo. *Annu Rev Physiol.* 1990;52:523–542.
9. Tamura M, Hazeki O, Nioka S, et al. In vivo study of tissue oxygen metabolism using optical and nuclear magnetic resonance spectroscopies. *Annu Rev Physiol.* 1989;51:813–834.
10. Tamura M, Oshino N, Chance B, et al. Optical measurements of intracellular concentration of rat heart in vitro. *Arch Biochem Biophys.* 1978;191:8–22.
11. Clarke KA, O'Connor J, Willis, RJ. Temporal relation between energy metabolism and myocardial function during ischemia and reperfusion. *Am J Physiol.* 1987;253:H412–H421.
12. Chemnitius JM, Burger W, Bing RJ. Crystalloid and perfluorochemical perfusates in an isolated working rabbit heart preparation. *Am J Physiol.* 1985; 249:H285–H292.
13. Honig CR, Gayeski TEJ. Resistance to O_2 diffusion in anemic red muscle: roles of flux density and cell pO_2. *Am J Physiol.* 1993;265:H868–H875.
14. Cobb FR, Bache RJ, Rivas F, et al. Local effects of acute cellular injury on regional myocardial blood flow. *J Clin Invest.* 1976;57:1359–1368.
15. Triana JF, Bolli R. Decreased flow reserve in "stunned" myocardium after a 10 min coronary occlusion. *Am J Physiol.* 1991;261:H793–H804.
16. Kusuoka H, Marban E. Cellular mechanism of myocardial stunning. *Annu Rev Physiol.* 1992;54:243–256.
17. Jacobus WE, Pores IH, Lucas SK, et al. Intracellular acidosis and contractility in the normal and the ischemic heart as examined by ^{31}P NMR. *J Mol Cell Cardiol.* 1982;14:Suppl3:13–20.
18. Nosek TM, Fender KY, Godt RE. It is the diprotonated form of inorganic phosphate that causes force depression in skinned skeletal muscle fiber. *Science.* 1987;236:190–193.
19. Zimmer SD, Ugurbil K, Michurski SP, et al. Alterations in oxidative function and respiratory regulation in the post-ischemic myocardium. *J Biol Chem.* 1989;264:12402–12411.
20. Wittenberg BA, Wittenberg JB. Transport of oxygen in muscle. *Annu Rev Physiol.* 1989;51:857–878.
21. Wittenberg BA, Wittenberg JB. Myoglobin-mediated oxygen delivery to mitochondria of isolated cardiac myocytes. *Proc Natl Acad Sci USA.* 1987; 84:7503–7507.
22. Doeller J, Wittenberg BA. Myoglobin function and energy metabolism of isolated cardiac myocytes:effect of sodium nitrite. *Am J Physiol.* 1991;261: H53–H62.
23. Gupta R, Wittenberg BA. 31P NMR studies of isolated adult heart cells: effect of myoglobin inactivation. *Am J Physiol.* 1991;261:H1155–H1163.
24. Cole RP, Wittenberg BA, Caldwell PRB. Myoglobin function in the isolated fluorocarbon-perfused dog heart. *Am J Physiol.* 1978;234:H567–H572.

25. Taylor DJ, Mathews PM, Radda GK. Myoglobin-dependent oxidative metabolism in the hypoxic rat heat. *Resp Physiol.* 1986;63:275–283.
26. Chung Y, Xu D, Jue T. Myoglobulin mediates energy coupling in myocardial respiration. Am J Physiol. 1996;271:H1166–H1173.
27. Steinhaus RK, Baskin SI, Clark JH, et al. Formation of methemoglobin and metmyoglobin using 8-aminoquinoline derivatives or sodium nitrite and subsequent reaction with cyanide. *J Appl Toxicol.* 1990;10:345–351.
28. Taylor DJ, Hochstein P. Reduction of metmyoglobin in myocytes. *J Mol Cell Cardiol.* 1982;14:133–140.
29. La Mar GN, Budd DL, Smith KM, et al. Nuclear magnetic resonance of high-spin ferric hemoproteins. Assignment of proton resonances in met-aquo myoglobins using deuterium-labeled hemes. *J Am Chem Soc.* 1980; 102:1822–1827.
30. Bondoc LL, Timkovich R. Structural characterization of nitrimyoglobin. *J Biol Chem.* 1989;264:6134–6145.
31. Ambrosio G, Jacobus WE, Mitchell MC, et al. Effects of ATP precursors on ATP and free ADP content and functional recovery of postischemic hearts. *Am J Physiol.* 1989;256:H560–H566.
32. Hogg N, Rice-Evans C, Darley-Usmar V, et al. The role of lipid hydroperoxides in the myoglobin-dependent oxidation of LDL. *Arch Bioch Biophys.* 1994;314:39–44.

## Chapter 30

Dynamic Analysis of Tricarboxylic Acid Cycle Flux and Substrate Selection Under *In Vivo* Conditions

Pierre-Marie Robitaille, PhD

More than 50 years have passed since Hans Krebs first described the series of reactions which came to be known as the tricarboxylic acid (TCA) cycle. In studying the discovery of the TCA cycle,[1,2] both the tenacity of the investigators and the inherent simplicity of their methods become apparent. Every step of the cycle (Figure 1) was painfully brought to light through the biochemical analysis of extracts. This is in sharp contrast to modern *in vivo* nuclear magnetic resonance spectroscopy; a seemingly complex methodology that enables scientists to probe simultaneously and noninvasively, in a living and working heart, many of the reactions associated with the TCA cycle. It is also interesting to ponder how Krebs would react to our continued studies of this series of reactions. In many respects, a pathway that long ago seemed well understood, remains filled with mystery. Consequently, scientists continue to strive for a deeper understanding of the details of its regulation, its adaptation to the demands of increased work, and the complexities of its substrate selection. From these studies, it is apparent that we are embarking on a new age in the analysis of the TCA cycle, wherein the workings of the cycle in the test tube will be intertwined with the complexities of whole organ physiology and function in the context of a living being.

Krebs once stated: "Those ignorant of the historical development

This work was supported in part by NIH grant #HL-45120.

From: Higgins CB, Ingwall JS, Pohost GM, (eds). *Current and Future Applications of Magnetic Resonance in Cardiovascular Disease.* Armonk, NY: Futura Publishing Company, Inc.; © 1998.

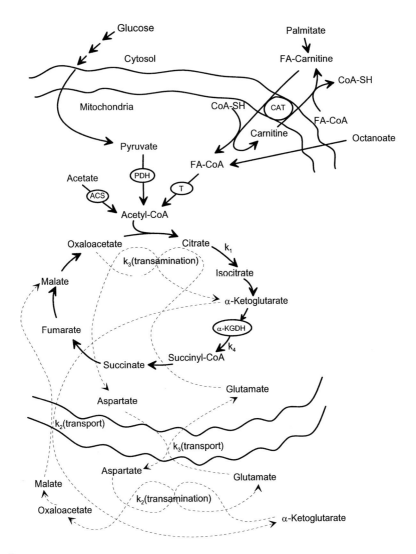

FIGURE 1. Schematic representation of the tricarboxylic acid cycle, the malate-aspartate shuttle, β-oxidation, glycolysis, anaplerotic and associated pathways. Labeled enzyme systems correspond to carnitine acyl transferase (CAT), thiolase (T), pyruvate dehydrogenase (PDH), acetyl Co-A synthetase (ACS), and α-ketoglutarate dehydrogenase (α-KGDH). Rate constant for transamination and transport steps of the malate-aspartate shuttle and TCA cycle flux correspond to previously applied conventions.[19]

of science are not likely ever to understand fully the nature of science and scientific research."[2] In this respect, the rich history of carbon nuclear magnetic resonance (^{13}C-NMR) spectroscopy cannot be dismissed. Many of the advancements currently made in the heart hold their origins in efforts that often appear distant. Whereas it is difficult to recount the many studies that have shaped modern ^{13}C-NMR, it is useful to review some of the key efforts in this area. It is clear that the earliest examples of the power of ^{13}C-NMR for the study of intermediary metabolism can be found in studies of the microorganism *S. cerevisiae*,[3,4] the isolated liver,[5–7] and the isolated perfused heart.[8–11] Shulman and Radda were instrumental in many of these studies. Their laboratories also shared the common understanding that ^{13}C-NMR could be used to probe intermediary metabolism and investigate metabolic flux at a previously unattainable level. They also were the first to note the importance of labeling patterns within glutamic acid as well as other metabolites.

The analysis of the TCA cycle with ^{13}C-NMR methods was further advanced when Chance[12] provided an elaborate mathematical analysis of isotope labeling in the citric acid cycle. This work emphasized the power of isotopomer analysis and the dynamic nature of the changes in signal intensity. While these two phenomena had been well recognized by other investigators, Chance's work can be viewed as an important branch point that launched two distinct approaches to the analysis of the TCA cycle: isotopomer analysis and dynamic methodology. It is now clear that through the use of the stable ^{13}C isotope, metabolic labeling studies[8,9,12–16] can be performed to monitor substrate flow through the major pathways of intermediary metabolism including glycogen synthase, glycolytic and anaplerotic pathways, and most importantly, the tricarboxylic acid cycle.

^{13}C-NMR Spectroscopy

Isotopomer Methods

One of the unique features of metabolic studies with NMR is the presence of metabolic isotopomers. Isotopomers are molecules that differ only in their ^{13}C enrichment at one or more atomic sites. Isotopomer analysis has been extensively applied to the study of substrate selection in the isolated perfused heart and much of the progress in this area can be attributed to the efforts of Malloy and Sherry[15,16] whose contributions in this area have had a profound impact on the field of ^{13}C-NMR.

Unfortunately, whole organ isotopomer based ^{13}C-NMR studies are restricted by the fact that glutamate tends to be the only isotopomer that can easily be resolved by magnetic resonance in the perfusion setting. As a result, isotopomer-based studies may lack the complement of information required to extract true flux measurements. In addition, isotopomer methods are somewhat difficult to apply under *in vivo* conditions, due to the broadened linewidths experienced in this setting. This unfortunate limitation may not be easily resolved even with homonuclear decoupling. Nonetheless, isotopomer methods continue to provide valuable confirmatory information in the analysis of extracts typically obtained following *in vivo* experiments.[15,16]

Isotopomers have also been analyzed with mass spectroscopy.[17] In studies of gluconeogenesis in the rat liver, many more intermediates could be isolated, and their isotopomer patterns analyzed to yield true flux measurements.[17] Consequently, while studies with mass spectroscopy require tissue digestion, they are able to provide much more specific information about intermediary metabolism.[17]

Dynamic Methods

In addition to difficulties in achieving narrow linewidths, the analysis of the TCA cycle in the *in vivo* myocardium is experimentally complex.[18,19] In animal studies, the subject typically is anaesthetized and undergoes extensive surgical preparation prior to each study. An angiocatheter is usually inserted into the proximal left anterior descending coronary artery (LAD) while the heart is still beating normally. This catheter is used to infused ^{13}C enriched substrates. Each radiofrequency (RF) surface coil,[20] prepared in the investigator's laboratory, is mounted on the heart and a decoupler coil is positioned inside the thoracic cavity. Cardiac gating procedures are also invoked to fully coordinate cardiac and respiratory motion.[21] Adiabatic spin excitation is typically used.[22–25] In addition, under *in vivo* conditions, the experimentalist cannot control the nature of the oxidized substrate. Hence, physiological determinants of substrate utilization are likely to be much more important under these conditions. This is in contrast to the Langendorff perfused heart.[26]

Because isotopomer methods cannot be simply applied under *in vivo* conditions, studies must be centered on the so-called dynamic methods[12,19,27–31]; namely pre-[12,27–31] and post-steady state[19] analysis. Nonsteady state dynamic methods have extended several aspects of Chance's work[12] to the dynamic analysis of substrate selection and TCA cycle fluxes in the isolated myocardium.[29–31] Using these methods,[29–31] it has been demonstrated, under widely varying workloads, that the myocardium displayed unchanging fractional enrichments and glutamate pool sizes. In addition, since pre-steady state ^{13}C-NMR approaches were independent of carbon-carbon coupling constants, they could be extended to the *in vivo* situation.[12,19,27–31] Pre-steady state and post-steady state methods also had the advantage of yielding information on Krebs cycle activity that was independent of intermediate pool size and fractional enrichment.[19,29–31]

In conducting the post-steady state experiments,[19] ^{13}C enriched substrate is initially infused into the coronary circulation under basal work conditions. To help ensure that post-steady state kinetics will not be complicated by transport processes, the infused substrate is typically acetate, and glucose is usually avoided. Once steady state in ^{13}C labeling is achieved and the glutamate intensity in the ^{13}C-NMR spectrum is no longer changing, the infused substrate is switched to the unlabeled form, thereby initiating the post-steady state experiment. The rate of label washout from the C4 carbon of glutamic acid is then monitored to assay the flux through α-ketoglutarate dehydrogenase and the malate-aspartate shuttle as previously described.[19] Initial labeling of the glutamate pool at low rate pressure products can then be repeated in the same animal. Thus, following steady-state labeling under basal conditions, the rate pressure product is elevated using a dobutamine infusion and the entire post-steady state experiment is reinitiated by infusion of unlabeled substrate.

As previously described,[19] the power of post-steady state analysis lies in the fact that this treatment provides an exact closed form mathematical expression describing the rate of label washout from the C4 carbon of glutamic acid through the malate-aspartate shuttle and then through α-ketoglutarate dehydrogenase. As such, this closed form expression can be used to determine not only TCA cycle flux activity, but also the rate of α-ketoglutarate/glutamate exchange across the mitochondrial membrane. Therefore, post-steady state methods also have the advantage of being able to more directly monitor the flux through α-ketoglutarate dehydrogenase a key regulatory step in the TCA cycle. Simple mathematical solutions are not yet available for isotopomer and pre-steady state methods.[19]

Interestingly, since the *in vivo* myocardium maintains full latitude in substrate selection, pre-steady state methods cannot be used to monitor TCA cycle flux under *in vivo* conditions. This is because the heart may select a substrate for oxidation at low workloads that is specifically excluded at high work, thus preventing analysis over the full range of workloads. This problem is not an issue with post-steady state analysis[19] because the labeling in this setting is always performed at low work. Therefore, post-steady state methods also have the advantage of being largely independent of substrate selection. The ability of the heart to change substrates as a function of rate pressure products is a distinct feature of this organ that is not shared by the brain. It is well established that the brain will primarily oxidize glucose and it is precisely for this reason that pre-steady state approaches remain valid in this organ.[27]

The Malate-Aspartate Shuttle

The importance of the transaminases and transport processes (Figure 1) in ^{13}C-NMR has recently received increased attention in the NMR literature. This is because ^{13}C-NMR measurements of TCA cycle flux obtained by measuring glutamic acid would be invalid if the glutamate/ketoglutarate exchange is slow relative to TCA cycle flux.[19] The coupling of the malate-aspartate shuttle to the TCA cycle is important in this exchange[19] and has been reviewed.[32] Importantly, in bringing reduction equivalents into the mitochondrial matrix, the shuttle relies on the electrogenic glutamate-aspartate carrier, which operates unidirectionally.[33-35] There is serious reason to believe that glutamate transport is operating slowly in the mitochondria[33-37] and this further highlights the need for caution in this area. Weiss et al[28] have recognized the importance of the transaminases in their work and have determined that in the isolated pyruvate/acetate perfused heart these equilibria appear to be rapid. Unfortunately, these insightful measurements appear to have been made under low workload conditions and do not completely resolve these questions.

Because the malate-aspartate shuttle is responsible for bringing reduction equivalents generated in the cytosol into the mitochondria, the nature of the oxidized substrate examined can greatly influence the rate of α-ketoglutarate/glutamate exchange. It is expected, for instance, that this rate of exchange may be more rapid under glucose, lactate, and pyruvate oxidation because all of these substrates generate reduction equivalents in the cystosol. Indeed, it was previously observed that "... the rate of label washout depends not only on the flux through α-ketoglutarate dehydrogenase, but most importantly on the activity of the malate-aspartate shuttle as determined by the forward and reverse fluxes through the transaminases and by the rate of transport of glutamate and α-ketoglutarate across the mitochondrial membrane."[19] This statement also applies to the pre-steady state methods.

It has recently been observed that the malate-aspartate shuttle equilibria are operating in the slow domain,[38] however, these measurements were performed under acetate and β-hydroxybutyrate perfusion. These conditions are not expected to result in high malate-aspartate shuttle activity, because no reduction equivalents would be generated in the cytosol. Interestingly, it has recently been demonstrated that the pre-steady state rate of label incorporation into the C4 carbon of glutamic acid can be accelerated in the butyrate perfused heart once the heart is challenged with lactic acid.[39]

There can be significant differences between the malate/aspartate shuttle activity in the brain and that noted in the heart. This stems from the fact that the brain is using glucose as its primary substrate. Moreover, because the brain will never experience the drastic increases in workload that are possible in the heart, the condition that the α-ketoglutarate/glutamate exchange rate be rapid relative to the TCA cycle flux should be much easier to fulfill. It should be noted that Mason et al[27] have estimated this rate of exchange to be approximately 89 to 126 times faster than the TCA cycle flux in the brain.

Some progress has been made with regard to the rate of α-ketoglutarate/glutamate exchange, but it is doubtful that this question can be adequately addressed in the perfused heart as the rate of exchange is inherently linked to the nature of the oxidized substrate. Because the myocardium has such a dynamic ability to alter its substrate under *in vivo* conditions, the rate of α-ketoglutarate/glutamate exchange can only be properly addressed under *in vivo* conditions. Moreover, this must be accomplished over a range of physiological workloads that takes into account possible changes in substrate selection.

In Vivo ^{13}C-NMR Analysis of Substrate Selection

As previously mentioned, pre-steady state methods cannot easily be used to assay TCA cycle flux in the *in vivo* myocardium as the heart has the ability to change the nature of its oxidized substrate under *in vivo* conditions. Consequently, a substrate that is oxidized at low workloads may not be oxidized at higher workloads. Such a substrate could not be used to study TCA cycle flux over a wide range of oxygen consumption. It is precisely for this reason that pre-steady state methods can be used to examine substrate selection. Post-steady state[19] methods, however, can be used to assay TCA cycle flux *in vivo*. It should be realized that there is an important difference between substrate selection and TCA cycle flux measurements.

In ^{13}C-NMR based substrate selection studies, the ability of each substrate to compete for oxidation in the TCA cycle is analyzed both at low and elevated workloads using pre-steady state methods. The degree to which a particular substrate can compete is assessed *in vivo* by noting the intensity change in the glutamate resonance as a function of rate pressure product. Importantly, fractional enrichment measurements, based on isotopomer analysis and performed in extracts, are then applied to confirm these results.

In conducting substrate selection studies based on pre-steady state experiments, a set of control data is typically acquired for approximately 40 minutes with the infusion of unenriched substrate (RPP≤10,000 mm Hg/min). The infused substrate is then changed to its enriched form and acquisition resumed for 40 minutes. At this stage, the RPP is elevated using a dopamine drip and the substrate changed to its unlabeled form. After 40 minutes of equilibration the infused substrate will then be correspondingly changed to a proportionately correct amount of its enriched form and acquisition resumed for 40 minutes. The extent of glutamate or aspartate pool labeling is then compared with results obtained under basal workload conditions.

Using pre-steady state substrate selection studies it has been demonstrated that the *in vivo* canine myocardium excludes acetate oxidation as rate pressure products are increased.[18] In this respect, it is interesting to note that a canine heart that can have a 90% fractional enrichment of glutamate at a rate pressure product of 10,000, will have absolutely no enrichment above 25,000.[18] Thus, over less than a threefold change in work, the fractional enrichment drops to 0, not to 30%. This occurred in spite of the fact that the rate of acetate infusion has been tripled, which theoretically should have resulted in little or change in fractional enrichment.[18] These results cannot be explained by a drop in glutamate pool size because this pool was found to remain relatively constant under *in vivo* conditions as a function of work.[40] In the canine heart for instance, it has been observed that over an eight fold change in RPP (5,000–40,000) there is about a 25% change in the mean glutamate pool (from 2.0 to 1.5). Studies in the perfused heart also revealed that glutamate pools do not change with workload.[29–31]

The fact that the myocardium excludes acetate from oxidation by the TCA cycle in the canine has also been confirmed in the swine as previously reported in part.[41] In one swine for instance,[41] the glutamate pool was extensively labeled by the infusion of 8 mM acetate at a workload of slightly more than 9,000. The experiment was then repeated in the same animal at a rate pressure product of slightly more than 14,000 using an infusion of 20 mM acetate. This corresponds to an increase in RPP of about 50% accompanied by a 2.5-fold increase in acetate infusion. Yet little or no labeling of the glutamate pool was observed at the higher workload and the glutamate pool sizes determined by chemical assay in these animals was fairly constant. This is truly a remarkable finding.

The observation that the canine and porcine myocardia limit acetate oxidation by the TCA cycle at elevated workloads supports the hypothesis that the selection of substrate for condensation with CoA-SH and subsequent oxidation in the TCA cycle is regulated kinetically through the K_M values of the appropriate condensation enzymes and through the absolute levels of free CoA-SH in the mitochondria.[18] In addition, because it has been demonstrated[18] that the rate of enriched carbon incorporation into the glutamate pool is not a direct reflection of Krebs cycle activity as previously proposed,[29–31] these findings illustrates that pre-steady state methods cannot be used to assay TCA cycle flux under *in vivo* conditions. This is because the experimentalist has no control over substrate selection under these conditions. The finding that some animals do not take up acetate even at the lowest workloads indicates that some caution may need to be exercised with ^{11}C acetate based positron emission tomographic (PET) studies.

Extensive studies of substrate selection have also been performed with lactate and pyruvate. As expected, these metabolites were typically able to label the glutamate pool at basal workloads.[42] However, the extent of this labeling was highly variable and could usually be increased with the addition of dichloroacetic acid, a well-know indirect activator of pyruvate dehydrogenase, through its action on pyruvate dehydrogenase kinase. It interesting to note that some animals were unable to oxidize pyruvate even at the lowest workload.[42] Without making any changes in the pyruvate infusion, dichloroacetic acid (DCA) was infused in these same animals. DCA indirectly activated pyruvate dehydrogenase (PDH) and as a result, pronounced labeling of glutamate was observed. This is a clear indication of kinetic inhibition of pyruvate oxidation controlled at PDH. It is also noteworthy that not all animals responded to DCA infusion. Some animals simply would not oxidize pyruvate at basal workloads under any circumstance.[42] In these studies it was also demonstrated that pyruvate oxidation was reduced at elevated workloads in a manner similar to that observed with acetate.[42] Importantly, this selection against pyruvate at very high workloads cannot be reversed even with the infusion of dichloroacetic acid. Similar findings were obtained when examining the oxidation of lactic acid.

These NMR experiments help bring to light our incomplete understanding of the regulation of substrate selection in the normal in-vivo myocardium. It is clear that free acetate and pyruvate levels are very low in normal blood. In the fasted state, normal free acetate concentrations in human blood are approximately 13 mg/L,[43] which corresponds to a molar concentration of 0.22 mM. These values should represent an upper limit in acetate concentrations relative to a nonfasted state. Similarly, free blood pyruvate concentrations are only 5.6 mg/L in the fasted state,[43] which corresponds to molar concentrations of less 0.06 mM. Therefore, in these *in vivo* experiments, acetate and pyruvate were presented in excess and at final concentrations that greatly exceed anything the heart can ever expect to encounter. Experiments have been performed (unpublished observations) using infusions of 0.1M acetate at a rate of 10 mL/min directly into the LAD. This results in a final concentration of about 15 mM in the blood distal to the infusion point. Even under these extreme circumstances, the heart was observed to select against acetate oxidation at high work. Because the myocardium will never see such high concentrations, this selection against acetate is dramatic and complete. It is also interesting to note that in all experiments where changes in rate pressure product occurred, the acetate infusion was proportionately increased. Because there is a well-established relation between increases in oxygen consumption, workload, and increases in blood flow, this approach should fully account for expected changes with increasing work. Clearly, while ^{13}C-NMR studies of substrate selection under *in vivo* conditions are just beginning, noninvasive NMR methods should provide significant new scientific insights in this exciting area.

Models of Myocardial Metabolism

Bing[44] initiated the study of *in vivo* myocardial biochemistry with his analysis of myocardial substrate selection in the *in vivo* heart. These seminal experiments were conducted by monitoring aortic/sinus differences in substrate concentrations. Ingenuously, the exact fate of a given metabolite was inferred from a rather elaborate chemical analysis rather than directly visualized. Whereas there has been considerable progress in our understanding of myocardial substrate selection since this classic study was published, many of its aspects remain largely unexplored under in-vivo conditions.[45] This is particularly true as it relates to substrate selection in response to changes in cardiac workload. In sharp contrast, substrate selection has been extensively studied under perfusion conditions and direct visualization of the metabolic fate of a given substrate has become possible through the application of high resolution NMR isotopomer and pre-steady state studies. However, the analysis and understanding of myocardial substrate selection remains clouded by the use of physiologically nonideal models. In their constant search for "the simplest relevant model," scientists have often invoked the use of preparations that partially compromise the physiological and neurohumoral conditions which surround the normal *in vivo* myocardium.

In this regard, while they have contributed extensively to the analysis of substrate selection in the myocardium, perfused heart experiments can bring only limited insight into this area. In many respects, these experiments must deal with a large number of complications. For instance, the oxygen carrying capacity of crystalline buffers, which are frequently used in these experiments, does not approach that of normal blood. This limitation becomes particularly important at high workloads. In addition, the perfused heart setting cannot easily duplicate the enormous variety of substrates (glucose, fatty acids of various lengths and with varying degrees of saturation, lactate, amino acids, and numerous other byproducts of catabolism) available to the normally functioning *in vivo* myocardium. A further complication is that the delivery of fatty acids from the coronary circulation to the mitochondria is a highly complex process, potentially involving a variety of carrier molecules.[46–50] This intricate transport process is likely to become disrupted once the *in vivo* myocardium is excised.

In many studies of substrate selection, two or three substrates are usually offered and their relative rates of oxidation are compared. Yet, in the perfused setting, the heart may actually prefer to oxidize a metabolite absent from the perfusate. Moreover, these experiments are also complicated by changes in workload brought about by increasing pressure heads or cardiac pacing. Both of these methods have the potential to bypass important intracellular cascades that would normally be activated in the *in vivo* setting. Because perfused heart experiments cannot easily mimic hormonal and substrate concentrations available to the myocardium *in vivo*, a model must be found where the heart is permitted to maintain full latitude in substrate selection under normal physiological conditions.

In this sense, *in vivo* animal models are perhaps more attractive for studying substrate selection as the *in vivo* myocardium is surrounded by a full complement of oxidizable substrates and maintains complete latitude in selecting between these metabolites. The *in vivo* setting can be used to monitor how well one substrate can compete for oxidation relative to endogenous substrates under nearly normal physiological conditions. Nonetheless, while it can be argued that *in vivo* models are more physiologically appropriate for studies of substrate competition, substrate use is a highly complex issue that must depend on the dietary state of the animal (fasted versus nonfasted), the workload change, and whether this change is physiologically relevant or not. In addition, *in vivo* animal models must also deal with surgical and anaesthetic issues. For instance, important biochemical differences have previously been noted in the *in vivo* canine myocardium under sodium pentobarbital versus α-chloralose anesthesia.[51] Hence, while it can be argued that *in vivo* animal models are more physiologically relevant in studying these issues, we remain one step away from the true subject of interest: the normal human heart.

Acknowledgments

I would like to take this opportunity to thank the many members of the Division of MR Research at The Ohio State University who have made this work possible and recognize the contribution of Mr. Ryan Augé in the preparation of Figure 1. This work is dedicated to the memory of my mother, Jacqueline Roy.

References

1. Krebs HA, Johnson WA. The role of citric acid in intermediate metabolism in animal tissues. *Enzymologia.* 1937;4:148–156.
2. Krebs HA. The history of the tricarboxylic acid cycle. *Perspect Biol Med.* 1970;154–170.
3. Dickerson JR, Dawes IW, Boyd ASF, Baxter RL. ^{13}C NMR studies of acetate metabolism during sporulation of Saccharomyces cerevisiae. *Proc Natl Acad Sci USA.* 1983;80:5847–51.
4. Den Hollander JA, Ugurbil K, Brown TR, et al. Studies of anaerobic and aerobic glycolysis in Saccharomyces cerevisiae. *Biochemistry.* 1986;25: 203–211.
5. Cohen SM, Rognstad R, Shulman RG, Katz J. A comparison of ^{13}C nuclear magnetic resonance and ^{13}C tracer studies of hepatic metabolism. *J Biol Chem.* 1981;256:3428–3432.
6. Cohen SM, Shulman RG, McLaughlin AC. Effects of ethanol on alanine metabolism in perfused mouse liver studied by ^{13}C NMR. *Proc Natl Acad Sci USA.* 1979;76:4808–4812.
7. Cohen SM. Simultaneous ^{13}C and ^{31}P NMR studies of perfused rat liver. Effects of insulin and glucagon and a ^{13}C NMR assay of free Mg^{2+}. *J Biol Chem.* 1983;258:14291–14308.
8. Bailey IA, Gadian DG, Matthews PM, et al. Studies of metabolism in the isolated, perfused rat heart using ^{13}C NMR. *FEBS Lett.* 1981;123:315–318.
9. Sherry AD, Nunnally RL, Peshock RM. Metabolic studies of pyruvate- and lactate-perfused guinea pig hearts by ^{13}C NMR. *J Biol Chem.* 1985;260: 9272–9279.
10. Lavanchy N, Martin J, Rossi A. Glycogen metabolism: A ^{13}C-NMR study of the isolated perfused rat heart. *FEBS Lett.* 1984;178:34–38.
11. Hoekenga DE, Brainard JR, Hutson JY. Rates of glycolysis and glycogenolysis during ischemia in glucose-insulin-potassium-treated perfused hearts: A ^{13}C, [31]P Nuclear Magnetic Resonance Study. *Circ Res.* 1988;62:1065–1074.
12. Chance EM, Seeholzer SH, Kobayashi K, Williamson JR. Mathematical analysis of isotope labeling in the citric acid cycle with applications to ^{13}C NMR studies in perfused rat hearts. *J Biol Chem.* 1983;258:13785–13794.
13. Neurohr KJ, Barrett EJ, Shulman RG. In vivo carbon-13 nuclear magnetic resonance studies of heart metabolism. *Proc Natl Acad Sci USA.* 1983;80: 1603–1607.
14. London RE. [13]C labeling studies of metabolic regulation. *Prog NMR Spectroscopy.* 1988;20:337–383.
15. Malloy CR, Sherry AD, Jeffrey FMH. Evaluation of carbon flux and substrate selection through alternate pathways involving the citric acid cycle of the heart by ^{13}C NMR spectroscopy. *J Biol Chem.* 1988;263:6964–6971.
16. Malloy CR, Sherry AD, Jeffrey FMH. Analysis of tricarboxylic acid cycle of the heart using ^{13}C isotope isomers. *Am J Physiol.* 1990;259:H987–H995.
17. Katz J, Wals P, Lee WNP. Isotopomer studies of gluconeogenesis and the Krebs cycle with ^{13}C-labeled lactate. *J Biol Chem.* 1993;268:25509–25521.

18. Robitaille PML, Rath DP, Abduljalil AM, et al. Dynamic ^{13}C NMR analysis of oxidative metabolism in the in-vivo canine myocardium. *J Biol Chem.* 1993;268:26296–26301.
19. Robitaille PML, Rath DP, Skinner TE, et al. Transaminase reaction rates, transport activities and TCA cycle analysis by post-steady state ^{13}C NMR. *Magn Reson Med.* 1993;30:262–266.
20. Ackerman JJH, Grove TH, Wong GG, et al. Mapping of metabolites in whole animals by ^{31}P NMR using surface coils. *Nature.* 1980;283:167–170.
21. Pruski JC, Abduljalil AM, Robitaille PM. Improved cardiac gating and ventilation timing in animal experiments. *Magn Reson Med.* 1992;27:329–337.
22. Ugurbil K, Garwood M, Bendall MR. Amplitude and frequency-modulated pulses to achieve 90° plane rotations with inhomogeneous B_1 fields. *J Magn Reson.* 1987;72:177–185.
23. Silver MS, Joseph RI, Hoult DI. Selective spin inversion in nuclear magnetic resonance and coherent optics through an exact solution of the Bloch-Riccati equation. *Phys Rev A.* 1985;31:2753–2755.
24. Skinner TE, Robitaille PML. General solutions for tailored modulation profiles in adiabatic excitation. *J Magn Reson.* 1992;98:14–23.
25. Skinner TE, Robitaille PM. Adiabatic excitation using sin2 amplitude cos2 frequency modulation functions. *J Magn Reson.* 1993;103A:34–39.
26. Neeley JR, Liebermeister H, Battersby EJ, Morgan HE. Effect of pressure development on oxygen consumption by isolated rat heart. *Am J Physiol.* 1967;212:804–814.
27. Mason GF, Rothman DL, Behar KL, Shulman RG. NMR Determination of the TCA cycle rate and the α-ketoglutarate/glutamate exchange rate in rat brain. *J Cereb Blood Flow Metab.* 1992;12:434–447.
28. Weiss RG, Gloth ST, Kalil-Filho R, et al. Indexing tricarboxylic acid cycle flux in intact hearts by carbon-13 nuclear magnetic resonance. *Circ Res.* 1992;70:392–408.
29. Lewandowski ED, Hulbert C. Dynamic changes in ^{13}C NMR spectra of intact hearts under conditions of varied metabolite enrichment. *Magn Reson Med.* 1991;19:186–190.
30. Lewandowski ED. Nuclear magnetic resonance evaluation of metabolic and respiratory support of work load in intact rabbit hearts. *Circ Res.* 1992;70:576–582.
31. Lewandowski ED. Metabolic heterogeneity of carbon substrate utilization in mammalian heart: NMR determinations of mitochondrial versus cytosolic compartmentation. *Biochemistry.* 1992;31:8916.
32. Safer B. The metabolic significance of the malate-aspartate cycle in the heart. *Circ Res.* 1975;37:527–533.
33. LaNoue KF, Schoolwerth AC. Metabolite transport in mitochondria. *Ann Rev Biochem.* 1979;48:871–922.
34. LaNoue KF, Bryla J, Bassett DJP. Energy-driven aspartate efflux from heart and liver mitochondria. *J Biol Chem.* 1974;249:7514–7521.
35. LaNoue KF, Tischler ME. Electrogenic characteristics of the mitochondrial glutamate-aspartate antiporter. *J Biol Chem.* 1974;249:7522–7528.
36. Schoolwerth AC, LaNoue KF, Hoover WJ. Glutamate transport in rat kidney mitochondria. *J Biol Chem.* 1982;258:1735–1739.
37. Safer B, Williamson JR. Mitochondrial-cytosolic interactions in perfused rat heart. *J Biol Chem.* 1973;248:2570–2579.
38. Yu X, Alpert NM, Damico LA, Lewandowski ED. Kinetic analysis of ^{13}C turnover in intact hearts at varied flux rates due to workload and oxidation. *Proc Soc Magn Reson.* 1994;87.

39. Yu X, White LT, Doumen C, et al. Contribution of transaminase flux to dynamic ^{13}C-NMR observation of isotope turnover in intact hearts. Society of Magnetic Resonance, 3rd meeting, Aug 19–25, 1995, Nice, France.
40. Rath DP, Zhang H, Jiang Z, et al. Direct evidence that glutamate pool sizes do not change appreciably with changing workload using post-steady state ^{13}C-NMR Methods. Society of Magnetic Resonance, 2nd meeting, Aug 6–13, 1994, San Francisco, California.
41. Angelos MG, Little CM, Torres CAA, et al. Acetate oxidation in the in-vivo porcine myocardium. American Heart Association Scientific Conference on Current and Future Application of Magnetic Resonance in Cardiovascular Disease, Jan. 15, 1996, San Francisco, California.
42. Rath DP, Zhu H, Tong X, et al. Dynamic analysis of pyruvate oxidation in the in-vivo canine myocardium: PDH activation is insufficient to ensure pyruvate oxidation. Proceedings of the Society of Magnetic Resonance, 2nd meeting, Aug. 6–13, 1994, San Francisco, California.
43. Diem K, Lenter C. eds. Geigy Scientific Tables, Seventh Edition. Geigy Pharmaceuticals, Ardsley, New York, 1975, p. 607.
44. Bing RJ. The metabolism of the heart. *Harvey Lect.* 1955;50:27–70.
45. Taegtmeyer H. Energy metabolism of the heart: From basic concepts to clinical Applications. *Curr Prob Cardiol* 1994;19:57–116.
46. Gordon RS, Cherkes A. Unesterified fatty acid in human blood plasma. II. The transport function of unesterified fatty acid. *J Clin Invest.* 1957;36:810–815.
47. Shipp JC, Opie LH, Challoner DC. Fatty acid and glucose metabolism in the perfused heart. *Nature.* 1961;189:1018–1019.
48. Ballard FB, Danforth WH, Naegle S, Bing RJ. Myocardial metabolism of fatty acids. *J Clin Invest.* 1960;39:717–723.
49. Fournier NC. Uptake and transport of lipid substrates in the heart. *Basic Res Cardiol.* 1987;82:11–18.
50. Stam H, Schroonderwoerd, Hulsmann WC. Synthesis, storage and degradation of myocardial triglycerides. *Basic Res Cardiol.* 1987;82:19–28.
51. Rath DP, Little CM, Zhang H, et al. Sodium pentobarbital versus α-chloralose anaesthesia: Experimental production of substantially different slopes in the transmural CP/ATP ratios within the left ventricle of the canine myocardium. *Circulation.* 1995;91:471–475.

Index